Alphabetical List of Muscles

A

215 Abductor digiti minimi (foot)
159 Abductor digiti minimi (hand)
224 Abductor hallucis
171 Abductor pollicis brevis
166 Abductor pollicis longus
180 Adductor brevis
225 Adductor hallucis
179 Adductor longus
81 Adductor magnus
173 Adductor pollicis
144 Anconeus
53 Arytenoid
Oblique
Transverse
27 Auriculares

B

140 Biceps brachii
192 Biceps femoris
141 Brachialis
143 Brachioradialis
26 Buccinator
120 Bulbospongiosus

C

34 Chondroglossus
116 Coccygeus
139 Coracobrachialis
5 Corrugator supercilii
117 Cremaster
50 Cricothyroid
[Cricothyroideus]

D

133 Deltoid [Deltoideus]
23 Depressor anguli oris
24 Depressor labii inferioris
14 Depressor septi
101 Diaphragm
78 Digastricus [Digastric]

E

149 Extensor carpi radialis brevis
148 Extensor carpi radialis longus
150 Extensor carpi ulnaris
158 Extensor digiti minimi
154 Extensor digitorum
212 Extensor digitorum brevis
211 Extensor digitorum longus
221 Extensor hallucis longus
155 Extensor indicis
168 Extensor pollicis brevis
167 Extensor pollicis longus

F

209 Fibularis brevis
208 Fibularis longus
210 Fibularis tertius
151 Flexor carpi radialis
153 Flexor carpi ulnaris
216 Flexor digiti minimi brevis
(foot)
160 Flexor digiti minimi brevis
(hand)
214 Flexor digitorum brevis
213 Flexor digitorum longus
157 Flexor digitorum profundus
156 Flexor digitorum
superficialis
223 Flexor hallucis brevis
222 Flexor hallucis longus
170 Flexor pollicis brevis
169 Flexor pollicis longus

G

205 Gastrocnemius
190 Gemellus inferior
189 Gemellus superior
32 Genioglossus
77 Geniohyoid [Geniohyoideus]
182 Gluteus maximus
183 Gluteus medius
184 Gluteus minimus
178 Gracilis

H

33 Hyoglossus

I

176 Iliacus
66 Iliocostalis cervicis
90 Iliocostalis lumborum
89 Iliocostalis thoracis
38 Inferior longitudinal
(tongue) [Longitudinalis
inferior]
41 Inferior pharyngeal
constrictor [Constrictor
pharyngis inferior]
84–87 Infrahyoids (see
Sternothyroid,
Thyrohyoid,
Sternohyoid, Omohyoid)
136 Infraspinatus
102 Intercostales externi
103 Intercostales interni
104 Intercostales intimi
219 Interossei, dorsal (foot)
[Interossei dorsales]
164 Interossei, dorsal (hand)
[Interossei dorsales]
165 Interossei, palmar or volar
[Interossei palmares]
220 Interossei, plantar
[Interossei plantares]
69 Interspinales cervicis
98 Interspinales lumborum
97 Interspinales thoracis
70 Intertransversarii cervicis
99 Intertransversarii thoracis
and lumborum
121 Ischiocavernosus

L

52 Lateral cricoarytenoid
[Cricoarytenoideus lateralis]
30 Lateral pterygoid
[Pterygoideus lateralis]
130 Latissimus dorsi
17 Levator anguli oris
115 Levator ani (includes
Puborectalis, Pubococcygeus,
and Iliococcygeus)
15 Levator labii superioris
16 Levator labii superioris
alaeque nasi
3 Levator palpebrae superioris
127 Levator scapulae
46 Levator veli palatini
107 Levatores costarum
60 Longissimus capitis
64 Longissimus cervicis
91 Longissimus thoracis
74 Longus capitis
79 Longus colli
218 Lumbricales (foot)
[Lumbricals]
163 Lumbricales (hand)
[Lumbricals]

M

28 Masseter
31 Medial pterygoid
[Pterygoideus medialis]
21 Mentalis
42 Middle pharyngeal constrictor
[Constrictor pharyngis
medius]
94 Multifidi
48 Musculus uvulae
75 Mylohyoid [Mylohyoideus]

13 Nasalis

54 Oblique arytenoid
[Arytenoideus obliquus]
59 Obliquus capitis inferior
58 Obliquus capitis superior
110 Obliquus externus abdominis
11 Obliquus inferior oculi
111 Obliquus internus
abdominis
10 Obliquus superior oculi
188 Obturator externus
[Obturatorius externus]
187 Obturator internus
[Obturatorius internus]
1 Occipitofrontalis
87 Omohyoid [Omohyoideus]
161 Opponens digiti minimi
172 Opponens pollicis
4 Orbicularis oculi
25 Orbicularis oris

P

36 Palatoglossus
49 Palatopharyngeus
162 Palmaris brevis
152 Palmaris longus
177 Pectineus
131 Pectoralis major
129 Pectoralis minor
186 Piriformis
207 Plantaris
88 Platysma
51 Posterior cricoarytenoid
[Cricoarytenoideus
posterior]
12 Procerus
147 Pronator quadratus
146 Pronator teres
174 Psoas major
175 Psoas minor
114 Pyramidalis

Q

191 Quadratus femoris
100 Quadratus lumborum
217 Quadratus plantae
196–200 Quadriceps femoris
(see Rectus femoris,
Vastus intermedius,
Vastus medialis longus,
Vastus medialis oblique,
Vastus lateralis)

R

113 Rectus abdominis
72 Rectus capitis anterior
73 Rectus capitis lateralis
56 Rectus capitis posterior major
57 Rectus capitis posterior minor
196 Rectus femoris
7 Rectus inferior
9 Rectus lateralis
8 Rectus medialis
6 Rectus superior
125 Rhomboid major
[Rhomboideus major]
126 Rhomboid minor
[Rhomboideus minor]
20 Risorius
71 Rotatores cervicis
96 Rotatores lumborum
95 Rotatores thoracis

45 Salpingopharyngeus
195 Sartorius
80 Scalenus anterior
81 Scalenus medius
65 Semispinalis cervicis
93 Semispinalis thoracis
193 Semitendinosus
128 Serratus anterior
109 Serratus posterior inferior
108 Serratus posterior superior
206 Soleus
123 Sphincter ani externus
122 Sphincter urethrae
63 Spinalis capitis
68 Spinalis cervicis
92 Spinalis thoracis
61 Splenius capitis
67 Splenius cervicis
83 Sternocleidomastoid
[Sternocleidomastoideus]
86 Sternohyoid
[Sternohyoideus]
84 Sternothyroid
[Sternothyroideus]
35 Styloglossus
76 Stylohyoid [Stylohyoideus]
44 Stylopharyngeus
132 Subclavius
105 Subcostales
134 Subscapularis
37 Superior longitudinal
(tongue) [Longitudinalis
superior]
43 Superior pharyngeal
constrictor [Constrictor
pharyngis superior]
145 Supinator
75–78 Suprahyoids (see
Mylohyoid, Stylohyoid,
Geniohyoid, Digastricus)
135 Supraspinatus

T

29 Temporalis
2 Temporoparietalis
185 Tensor fasciae latae
47 Tensor veli palatini
138 Teres major
137 Teres minor
55 Thyroarytenoid
[Thyroarytenoideus]
05 Thyrohyoid
[Thyrohyoideus]
203 Tibialis anterior
204 Tibialis posterior
39 Transverse lingual
[Transversus linguae]
112 Transversus abdominis
22 Transversus menti
119 Transversus perinei
profundus
118 Transversus perinei
superficialis
106 Transversus thoracis
124 Trapezius
142 Triceps brachii

U

48 Uvula (see Musculus uvulae)

V

198 Vastus intermedius
197 Vastus lateralis
199 Vastus medialis longus
200 Vastus medialis oblique
40 Vertical lingual [Verticalis
linguae]

Z

18 Zygomaticus major
19 Zygomaticus minor

DANIELS and WORTHINGHAM'S
Muscle Testing
Techniques of Manual Muscle and Physical Performance Testing

11th EDITION

Dale Avers | PT, DPT, PhD, FAPTA
Professor Emeritus
Department of Physical Therapy Education
College of Health Professions
SUNY Upstate Medical University
Syracuse, New York

Donovan J. Lott, PT, PhD, CSCS
Research Professor
Department of Physical Therapy
University of Florida
Gainesville, Florida

Marybeth Brown | PT, PhD, FAPTA, FACSM
Professor Emeritus
Physical Therapy Program, Biomedical Sciences
University of Missouri
Columbia, Missouri

ELSEVIER

Elsevier
3251 Riverport Lane
St. Louis, Missouri 63043

Notice

Practitioners and researchers must always rely on their own experience and knowledge in evaluating and using any information, methods, compounds or experiments described herein. Because of rapid advances in the medical sciences, in particular, independent verification of diagnoses and drug dosages should be made. To the fullest extent of the law, no responsibility is assumed by Elsevier, authors, editors or contributors for any injury and/or damage to persons or property as a matter of products liability, negligence or otherwise, or from any use or operation of any methods, products, instructions, or ideas contained in the material herein.

Senior Content Strategist: Lauren Willis
Content Development Manager: Lisa Newton
Senior Content Development Specialist: Laura Goodrich
Publishing Services Manager: Deepthi Unni
Senior Project Manager: Kamatchi Madhavan
Design Direction: Maggie Reid

Printed in India

Last digit is the print number: 9 8 7 6 5 4 3 2

Working together
to grow libraries in
developing countries

www.elsevier.com • www.bookaid.org

To those who find human muscle the key to discovering the potentials of movement.

—Dale Avers

To my many instructors, teachers, and mentors (in particular Michael J. Mueller, Jack D. Close, Shirley A. Sahrmann, and Marybeth Brown) who instilled in me a passion and appreciation for human bodily movement. I also dedicate this book to the patients and participants with muscular dystrophy who have taught me so much about muscle and movement.

—Donovan Lott

This book is dedicated to the decades of strong women who made the PT profession a viable entity and to those that have continued to push the scope of practice to new frontiers. My personal thanks also to the strong women who mentored me, particularly Helen J Hislop PT, ScD, Jacquelin Perry PT, MD and Joan Walker PT, PhD. Finally, this book is dedicated to all in our profession who go beyond classroom learning, that continue to question, to learn and figure out new techniques that are important for the ever emerging patient groups that are evolving.

—Marybeth Brown

Helen J. Hislop, PT, PhD, FAPTA—A Tribute

In 2013, the physical therapy profession lost one of the brightest beacons it had ever known. Helen Hislop was an extraordinary woman who changed the course of our profession, in part by implementing heightened standards of academic success and by creating the DPT and PhD degrees during her tenure at the University of Southern California. She also took the editorship of *Physical Therapy*, the professional journal of the American Physical Therapy Association, and transformed it from an anecdotal "how-to" magazine into a scientific journal with genuine credibility in the medical community. The sheer magnitude of her contributions is probably beyond that of any physical therapist in the history of our profession.

One of the most notable achievements in Helen's repertoire was her authorship of four editions of the classic text, *Daniels and Worthingham's Muscle Testing: Techniques of Manual Examination*. First published in 1946, the original Daniels, Williams, and Worthingham book was a how-to manual for testing the patient with poliomyelitis. Although the book was modified to some extent over the next 30 years, the practice of physical therapy changed considerably during that time span, and the earlier muscle testing book did not reflect the expansion of the profession to include the testing of neurological patients, the testing of men and women with orthopedic injuries and joint replacements, and contending with the burgeoning older adult population. Helen became involved in shepherding the book to a more contemporary text beginning with the sixth edition, and when the book was published in 1995, it reflected a sea change. Beautiful anatomical drawings produced under Helen's direction were incorporated, the testing of new patient populations was added, and there was the inclusion of new muscle tests that had evolved from clinical practice that were far more accurate than those described in previous texts, such as the 25× heel rise. Although these changes were the product of Helen's vision, the contributions of her coauthor, Jacqueline Montgomery, MA, PT, were of tremendous importance, as Jackie was a clinician with her finger on the pulse of clinical practice.

In 2010, Helen called to ask if I would become a contributor to the ninth edition, and I agreed. After multiple trips to Helen's home in North Carolina, it became apparent that her declining health was going to preclude completion of the book without a great deal more help. We worked for another year, but with looming deadlines, the need for a move away from "manual" muscle testing, and the inclusion of functional testing, it became necessary to enlist additional help. Dale Avers, PT, DPT, PhD, FAPTA, was asked to be an author, and the ninth edition continued to evolve in response to changing practice.

Even with multiple hospitalizations and further declines in health, Helen continued to be a vital contributor to the ninth edition. At all times, she was "in charge." Her fortitude was extraordinary; once a vision was planted in her brain, there was no dissuading her from the task at hand. She never saw the final completed copy of the ninth edition, but she contributed to each and every one of the enormous changes brought forth in the new book. Even though Helen is gone, her contributions will persist through many more iterations of this text.

Wherever Helen may be, there is no question she is lustily singing Gilbert and Sullivan tunes, engaging those around her in lively and insightful conversation, regaling anyone who will listen with tales of Scottish history, and making people laugh. Hopefully, too, she has caught the "big fish" that eluded her for her entire 84 years.

Rest in peace, dear friend.

— MB

For more than 70 years, *Daniels and Worthingham's Muscle Testing* has been informing students and practitioners about the art and science of manual muscle testing. Over the past seven decades, there have been 10 editions of the text, not including this current edition.

So, why an 11th edition? *Muscle Testing* has evolved into a different entity during its lengthy history. Initially a primer on how to test muscles affected by poliomyelitis, *Daniels and Worthingham's Muscle Testing* book continues to reflect the muscle testing requirements for a far broader scope of practice. Additionally, muscle testing techniques are now appropriate for patients who range in age from young adults to those who have lived 100 or more years (material appropriate for children may be found in other sources). We believe this book is the most up-to-date muscle testing book available, with detailed "how-to" information on hundreds of tests. Importantly, this new edition is continues to be evidence based reflecting our current understanding of anatomy and muscle function, an imperative in our contemporary health care system.

We are enormously grateful to our forebears for the work that went into the creation of this text. We are gratified that Donovan Lott, PT, PhD, CSCS has joined us as an author and future caretaker of this text. Dr. Lott completed his undergraduate degree in Exercise Science at Brigham Young University, his MSPT degree at Washington University School of Medicine, his PhD in Movement Science at Washington University in St. Louis, and a post-doctoral fellowship in muscle physiology at the University of Florida. He is currently a Research Professor at the University of Florida with research interests of skeletal muscle damage, exercise, and the relationship between muscle pathology and functional mobility in people with neuromuscular disease. We are confident Dr. Lott will continue to guide this foundational text to reflect current understandings of muscle function.

We are grateful to reviewers Stephanie Partis, PT, CHT (hand and wrist), Barbara Smith, PT, PhD (respiration), and Meryl Alappattu, PT, DPT, PhD (pelvic floor). We are also grateful to Nasir Williams who posed for several muscle testing techniques in this edition. And finally, we thank the team at Elsevier, including Kamatchi Madhavan and Lauren Willis whose behind-the-scenes work helped bring the book to fruition.

Dale Avers, PT, DPT, PhD, FAPTA
Marybeth Brown, PT, PhD, FAPTA
Donovan Lott, PT, PhD, CSCS

CONTENTS

List of Plates

Plate 1 Flexion and Extension of the Head and Neck, 31
Plate 2 Cardinal Planes of the Scapula, 96
Plate 3 Cross Sections of the Arm Muscles in Chest, 123
Plate 4   Cross Sections of the Arm and Forearm, 172
Plate 5 Motions of the Thumb, 209
Plate 6 Cross Sections of the Thigh, 251
Plate 7 Cross Sections of the Leg, 289

Introduction

Brief History of Muscle Testing, xi
How to Use This Book, xii
Names of the Muscles, xii
Anatomical Authorities, xiii
The Convention of Arrows in the Text, xiii

Chapter 1
Principles of Manual Muscle Testing, 1

Principles, 2
  Grading System, 2
  Overview of Test Procedures, 2
  Criteria for Assigning a Muscle Test Grade, 4
How to Use This Book, 7
  Preparing for the Muscle Test, 7
  Prime Movers, 7
  Exercises, 10
Muscle Testing, 11
  Summary, 12

Chapter 2
Practical Considerations for Manual Muscle Testing, 13

Introduction, 14
The Clinician and the Value of the Muscle Test, 15
Influence of the Patient on the Test, 16
Use of Manual Muscle and Strength Testing in Various Clinical Settings, 17
  Acute Care Facilities, 17
  Acute Rehabilitation Facilities, 17
  Long-Term Care Facilities, 18
  Home Health Setting, 18
  Outpatient Clinics, 18
  Wellness Clinics, 19
  Summary, 19

Limitations of Manual Muscle Testing, 20
  Population Variation, 20
  Objectivity, 20
  Reliability and Validity, 20
  Sensitivity, 20
  Diagnostic Validity, 21
  Ceiling Effect, 21
  Tester Strength, 21
Summary, 22

Chapter 3
Testing the Muscles of the Neck, 25

Testing the Muscles of the Neck, 26
  Introduction, 26
Capital Extension, 27
Cervical Extension, 32
Capital Flexion (Chin Tuck), 36
Cervical Flexion, 40
Flexion to Isolate a Single Sternocleidomastoid, 44
Cervical Rotation, 45

Chapter 4
Testing the Muscles of the Trunk and Pelvic Floor, 47

Trunk Extension, 48
Lumbar Spine, 51
Thoracic Spine 52
Elevation of the Pelvis, 55
Trunk Flexion, 59
Trunk Rotation, 65
Core Tests, 70
  Core Strength, Stability, and Endurance, 70
Quiet Inspiration, 77
  Diaphragm, 79
  Intercostals, 81
Forced Expiration, 82
Pelvic Floor, 85

Chapter 5
Testing the Muscles of the Upper Extremity, 95

Shoulder Girdle Strength Testing, 97
  Introduction, 97
Scapular Abduction (Protraction) and Upward Rotation, 100
Scapular Elevation, 105
Scapular Adduction (Retraction), 108

Scapular Depression and Adduction, 111

Scapular Adduction (Retraction) and Downward Rotation, 114

Latissimus Dorsi, 119

Introduction to Testing the Deltoid, 124

Shoulder Flexion, 125

Shoulder Extension, 129

Shoulder Abduction, 133

Shoulder Horizontal Abduction, 138

Shoulder Horizontal Adduction, 141

Introduction to the Rotator Cuff, 145

Shoulder External Rotation, 146

Shoulder Internal Rotation, 151

Elbow Flexion, 157

Elbow Extension, 162

Forearm Supination, 168

Forearm Pronation, 173

Wrist Flexion, 177

Wrist Extension, 182

Introduction to Muscle Testing of the Hand, 188
   Extrinsic Muscles, 188

Finger PIP and DIP Flexion, 189
   Combined DIP and PIP Tests, 191

PIP Tests, 192

DIP Tests, 194

Finger MCP Extension, 195

Finger MCP Flexion, 198
   Intrinsic Muscles, 198

Finger Abduction, 204

Finger Adduction, 206
   Thumb Muscles, 208

Thumb MCP and IP Flexion, 210

Thumb IP Flexion, 213

Thumb MCP and IP Extension, 214

Thumb Abduction, 218
   Abductor Pollicis Longus, 219
   Abductor Pollicis Brevis, 220

Thumb Adduction, 221

Opposition (Thumb to Little Finger), 225

Grip Strength, 229

Chapter 6
Testing the Muscles of the Lower Extremity, 235

Hip Flexion, 236

Hip Flexion, Abduction, and External Rotation With Knee Flexion, 241

Hip Extension, 244
   Hip Extension Test to Isolate Gluteus
     Maximus, 248

   Hip Extension Tests Modified for Hip Flexion
     Tightness, 250
   Supine Hip Extension Test, 252

Hip External Rotation, 254

Hip Internal Rotation, 258

Hip Abduction and Pelvic Stabilization, 261

Hip Abduction from Flexed Position, 266

Hip Adduction, 268

Knee Flexion, 273
   Hamstring Muscles in Aggregate, 275
   Medial Hamstring Test (Semitendinosus and
     Semimembranosus), 275
   Lateral Hamstring Test (Biceps Femoris), 276

Knee Extension, 278

Ankle Plantar Flexion, 283
   Gastrocnemius and Soleus Combined
     Test, 285

Foot Dorsiflexion and Inversion, 290

Foot Inversion, 293

Foot Eversion With Plantar Flexion, 296

Hallux and Toe Metatarsophalangeal (MP) Flexion, 300
   Hallux MP Flexion, 302
   Toe MP Flexion, 303

Hallux and Toe DIP and PIP Flexion, 304

Hallux and Toe MP and IP Extension, 307

Chapter 7
Alternatives to Manual Muscle Testing, 313

Alternatives to Manual Muscle Testing, 314
   Introduction, 314
   General Testing Considerations, 314
   One-Repetition Maximum Test, 315

Equipment-Based Strength Testing, 317
   Interpretation of Equipment-Based Strength Testing
     Data, 317
   Sitting Unilateral Knee Extension Test, 317
   Power Testing, 326
   Body Weight Testing, 333
   Cyriax Method of Testing
     Contractile Lesions, 334

Chapter 8
Testing Functional Performance, 337

Testing Functional Performance, 338
   Introduction, 338

Chair Stand, 340

Gait Speed, 343

Physical Performance Test and Modified Physical Performance Test, 346

Timed Up and Go, 356

Stair Climb, 359

Floor Rise, 361

Gait, 363

Chapter 9
Handheld Muscle Dynamometry, 369

Handheld Muscle Dynamometry, 370
  Introduction, 370
  Instrumentation, 370
Summary, 373
Shoulder Flexion, 374
Shoulder Extension, 375
Shoulder Abduction, 376
Shoulder External Rotation, 377
Shoulder Internal Rotation, 378
Elbow Flexion, 379
Elbow Extension, 380
Wrist Extension, 381
Hip Flexion, 382
Hip Extension, 383
  Hip Extension Tests Modified for Hip Flexion
    Tightness, 383
Hip Abduction, 384

Hip External Rotation, 385

Hip Internal Rotation, 386

Knee Flexion, 387

Knee Extension, 388

Foot Dorsiflexion and Inversion, 389

Chapter 10
Case Studies, 393

Introduction, 394
Case 1: Shoulder Pain, 394
Case 2: Compromised Gait and Function
         Secondary to Muscle Weakness, 395
Case 3: Fatigue Secondary to Muscle
         Weakness, 397
Case 4: Muscle Weakness Following Nerve
         Injury, 398
Case 5: Muscle Weakness Following Hip
         Surgery, 399
Case 6: Muscle Weakness Following Childbirth, 399

Index, 401

This 11th edition presents manual muscle testing within the context of strength testing. Classic muscle testing is a fundamental skill of every physical therapist and many other health care professionals and is essential to the diagnosis and assessment of movement impairments. However, as manual muscle testing has come under scientific scrutiny, it is obvious that its use to evaluate and assess strength as a component of functional movement patterns and tasks is inadequate. Therefore, in addition to the classic presentation of manual muscle testing, this edition presents alternative methods of strength testing that are valid, objective, and applicable across various settings.

A number of noteworthy changes have been made in the new edition. First and foremost, it is a modern 21st-century text that has been thoroughly researched. Each test presented is backed by evidence, and the utility of each muscle testing approach is presented in context with alternative options. Throughout the text, there are updated testing methods. Origins, insertions, and actions of key muscles for each manual muscle test are now included and precede the description of most test procedures. Additionally, for each specific muscle (e.g., serratus anterior, tibialis anterior), there are exercises that the therapist can use to strengthen weak muscles in patients. Each recommended exercise has been demonstrated, in most instances, to elicit at least 40% of maximum voluntary strength. Thus exercises are sufficiently rigorous to induce genuine strength increases in patients.

Muscle strength is a critical component of functional movement. Assessment must include accurate measurement of the quantity of strength within the context of functional tasks and movement. Especially for the lower extremities, methods that allow the expansion of the findings of manual muscle testing from an impairment to a function level are needed. Quantitative assessment promotes accurate assessment of progress and patient performance within the context of age-based normative values. Although few "hard numbers" of threshold strength levels exist for specific functional movements, we have identified the known muscles that have been correlated with a specific task and, in some cases, have suggested values that may serve as a target for the minimum strength required for a specific functional task.

The manual muscle testing portion of this book, as in previous editions, directs its focus on manual procedures. For the most part, joint motions (e.g., hip flexion), rather than individual muscles (e.g., iliopsoas), are the focus of this text because of the contributions of more than one muscle to a movement. Although prime movers of a movement can be identified, secondary or accessory movers may be equally important and should not be overlooked or underestimated. Rarely is a prime mover the only active muscle, and rarely is it used under isolated control for a given movement. For example, knee extension is the prerogative of the five muscles of the quadriceps femoris, yet none of these five extend the knee in isolation from its synergists. Regardless, definitive

activity of any muscle in a given movement can be precisely detected by electromyography, and such studies, when they exist, are now included as important pieces of evidence in this updated text.

Range of motion in this book is presented only to illustrate the range required to test a movement correctly. A consensus of typical ranges is presented with each test, but the techniques of measurement used are not within the scope of this text.

Brief History of Muscle Testing

Wilhelmine Wright and Robert W. Lovett, MD, Professor of Orthopedic Surgery at Harvard University Medical School, were the originators of the muscle testing system that incorporated the effect of gravity.[1,2] Janet Merrill, PT, Director of Physical Therapeutics at Children's Hospital and the Harvard Infantile Paralysis Commission in Boston, an early colleague of Dr. Lovett, stated that the tests were used first by Wright in Lovett's office gymnasium in 1912.[3] The seminal description of the tests used largely today was written by Wright and published in 1912[1]; this was followed by an article by Lovett and Martin in 1916[4] and by Wright's book in 1928.[5] Miss Wright was a precursor of the physical therapist of today, there being no educational programs in physical therapy in her time, but she headed Lovett's physical therapeutic clinic. Lovett credits her fully in his 1917 book, *Treatment of Infantile Paralysis*,[6] with developing the testing for polio. In Lovett's book, muscles were tested using a resistance-gravity system and graded on a scale of 0 to 6. Another early numerical scale in muscle testing was described by Charles L. Lowman, MD, founder and medical director of Orthopedic Hospital, Los Angeles.[7] Lowman's system (1927) covered the effects of gravity and the full range of movement on all joints and was particularly helpful for assessing extreme weakness. Lowman further described muscle testing procedures in the *Physiotherapy Review* in 1940.[8]

H.S. Stewart, a physician, published a description of muscle testing in 1925 that was very brief and not anatomically or procedurally consistent with what is done today.[9] His descriptions included a resistance-based grading system not substantially different from current use: maximal resistance for a normal muscle, completion of the motion against gravity with no other resistance for a grade of fair, and so forth. At about the time of Lowman's book, Arthur Legg, MD, and Janet Merrill, PT, wrote a valuable small book on poliomyelitis in 1932. This book, which offered a comprehensive system of muscle testing, was used extensively in physical therapy educational programs during the early 1940s; muscles were graded on a scale of 0 to 5, and a plus or minus designation was added to all grades except 1 and 0.[10]

Among the earliest clinicians to organize muscle testing and support such testing with sound and documented kinesiologic procedures in the way they are used today were Henry and Florence Kendall. Their earliest published documents on comprehensive manual muscle testing became available in 1936 and 1938.[11,12] The 1938 monograph on muscle testing was published and distributed to all Army hospitals in the United States by the US Public Health Service. Another early contribution came from Signe Brunnström and Marjorie Dennen in 1931; their syllabus described a system of grading movement, rather than individual muscles, as a modification of Lovett's work with gravity and resistance.[13]

The first comprehensive text on muscle testing was written by Lucille Daniels, MA, PT; Marian Williams, PhD, PT; and Catherine Worthingham, PhD, PT, published in 1946.[14] These three authors prepared a comprehensive handbook on the subject of manual testing procedures that was concise and easy to use. It remains one of the most used texts the world over and is the predecessor for all subsequent editions of *Daniels and Worthingham's Muscle Testing*, including this edition.

The Kendalls (together and then Florence alone after Henry's death in 1979) developed and published work on muscle testing and related subjects for more than six decades[15-17] Their first edition of *Muscles: Testing and Function* appeared in 1949.[15] Earlier, the Kendalls had developed a percentage system ranging from 0 to 100 to express muscle grades as a reflection of normal; they reduced the emphasis on this scale, only to return to it in the latest edition (1993), in which Florence again advocated the 0 to 10 scale.[17] The contributions of the Kendalls should not be considered as limited to grading scales, however. Their integration of muscle function with posture and pain in two separate books[15,16] and then in one other book[17] is a unique and extremely valuable contribution to the clinical science of physical therapy.

Muscle testing procedures used in national field trials that examined the use of gamma-globulin in the prevention of paralytic poliomyelitis were described by Carmella Gonnella, Georgianna Harmon, and Miriam Jacobs, all physical therapists.[18] The later field trials for the Salk vaccine also used muscle testing procedures.[19] The epidemiology teams at the Centers for Disease Control and Prevention were charged with assessing the validity and reliability of the vaccine. Because there was no other method of accurately "measuring" the presence or absence of muscular weakness, manual muscle testing techniques were used.

A group from the D.T. Watson School of Physiatrics near Pittsburgh, which included Jesse Wright, MD, Mary Elizabeth Kolb, PT, and Miriam Jacobs, PT, PhD, devised a test procedure that eventually was used in the field trials.[20] The test was an abridged version of the complete test procedure but did test key muscles in each functional group and body part. It used numerical values that were assigned grades, and each muscle or muscle group also had an arbitrary assigned factor that corresponded (as closely as possible) to the bulk of the tissue. The bulk factor multiplied by the test grade resulted in an "index of involvement" expressed as a ratio.

Before the trials, Kolb and Jacobs were sent to Atlanta to train physicians to conduct the muscle tests, but it was decided that experienced physical therapists would be preferable to maintain the reliability of the test scores.[20] Lucy Blair, then the Poliomyelitis Consultant in the American Physical Therapy Association, was asked by Catherine Worthingham of the National Foundation for Infantile Paralysis to assemble a team of experienced physical therapists to conduct the muscle tests for the field trials. Kolb and Jacobs trained a group of 67 therapists in the use of the abridged muscle test.[20] This work of determining the presence or absence of weakness and paralysis had an enormous impact on the eventual approval of the Salk vaccine. A partial list of participants was appended to the Lilienfeld paper in the *Physical Therapy Review* in 1954.[19]

How to Use This Book

The general principles that govern manual muscle testing are described in Chapter 1. Chapter 2 describes the purposes and limitations of manual muscle testing, placing manual muscle testing in the context of strength testing across settings. Chapters 3 through 7 present traditional and updated techniques for testing motions of skeletal muscle groups in the body region covered by that chapter. Chapter 4 reflects additional changes to practice through the expansion of the trunk muscle strength testing section, particularly trunk endurance, and new updates to the respiratory and pelvic floor sections. Chapter 7 describes methods of strength testing using equipment and instruments, and Chapter 8 is devoted to functional tests, which have become critical for successful documentation. Students should learn manual muscle testing within the context of strength testing to avoid some of the limitations described in Chapter 2. Chapter 9 describes manual testing using a handheld dynamometer and includes normative values where they exist. Chapter 10 provides updated case studies to describe different methods of strength testing in various patient populations and settings.

For instant access to anatomical information without carrying a large anatomy text to a muscle testing session, see the Ready Reference Anatomy section in the eBook *included with print purchase* on Elsevier eBooks+ (eBooks.Health.Elsevier.com). This chapter is a synopsis of muscle anatomy, muscles as part of motions, muscle innervations, and myotomes.

To assist readers, each muscle has been assigned an identification number based on a regional sequence, beginning with the head and face and proceeding through the neck, thorax, abdomen, perineum, upper extremity, and lower extremity. This reference number is retained throughout the text for cross-referencing purposes. Two lists of muscles with their reference numbers are presented, one alphabetical and one by region, to assist readers in finding muscles in the Ready Reference section. These can also be found on the inside front and back covers of the book.

Names of the Muscles

Muscle names have conventions of usage. The most formal usage (and the correct form for many journal manuscripts) is the terminology established by the Federative International Committee on Anatomical Terminology (FCAT) in 1998. However, common usage often neglects these prescribed names in favor of shorter or more readily pronounced names. The authors of this text make no apologies for not keeping strictly to formal usage. Most of the muscles cited follow Terminologia

Anatomica. Others are listed by the names in most common use. The alphabetical list of muscles (see the inside front cover of the book) gives the name used in this text and the correct Terminologia Anatomica term, when it differs, in brackets.

Anatomical Authorities

The authors of this book relied on the American and British versions of *Gray's Anatomy* Neumann's Kinesiology of the Musculoskeletal System as principal references for anatomical and kinesiological information, as well as Sabotta's *Atlas of Human Anatomy*. Because proficiency in muscle testing can only be achieved if the practitioner has a thorough understanding of anatomy, anatomical drawings are presented throughout the book, many in cross-section format, and descriptions of origins and insertions and functions are provided in multiple places, in detail and in abbreviated form.

The Convention of Arrows in the Text

Red arrows in the text denote the direction of movement of a body part, either actively by the patient or passively by the examiner. The length and direction of the arrow indicate the relative excursion of the part.

Black arrows in the text denote resistance by the examiner.

It is important to remind the reader that mastery of muscle testing, whether performed manually or using a strength-testing device, requires substantial practice. The only way to acquire proficiency in clinical evaluation procedures is to practice over and over again. As experience with patients matures over time, the nuances that can never be fully described for the wide variety of patients encountered by the clinician will become as much intuition as science. Muscle testing continues to be among the most fundamental skills of the physical therapist and others who are concerned with abnormalities of human motion. The skill of manual muscle testing is a critical clinical tool that every physical therapist must not only learn but also master. A physical therapist who aspires to be recognized as a master clinician will not achieve that status without acquiring exquisite skills in manual muscle testing and precise assessment of muscle performance.

References

1. Wright WG. Muscle training in the treatment of infantile paralysis. *Boston Med Surg J.* 1912;167:567–574.
2. Lovett RW. Treatment of infantile paralysis. Preliminary report. *JAMA.* 1915;64:2118.
3. Merrill J. *Personal letter to Lucille Daniels dated January 5;* 1945.
4. Lovett RW, Martin EG. Certain aspects of infantile paralysis and a description of a method of muscle testing. *JAMA.* 1916;66:729–733.
5. Wright WG. *Muscle Function.* New York: Paul B. Hoeber; 1928.
6. Lovett RW. *Treatment of Infantile Paralysis.* 2nd ed. Philadelphia: Blakiston's Son & Co.; 1917.
7. Lowman CL. A method of recording muscle tests. *Am J Surg.* 1927;3:586–591.
8. Lowman CL. Muscle strength testing. *Physiotherap Rev.* 1940;20:69–71.
9. Stewart HS. *Physiotherapy: Theory and Clinical Application.* New York: Paul B. Hoeber; 1925.
10. Legg AT, Merrill J. Physical therapy in infantile paralysis. In: Mock, ed. *Principles and Practice of Physical Therapy.* Vol. 2. Hagerstown, MD: W.F. Prior; 1932.
11. Kendall HO. Some interesting observations about the after care of infantile paralysis patients. *J Excep Child.* 1936;3:107.
12. Kendall HO, Kendall FP. *Care during the recovery period of paralytic poliomyelitis. U.S. Public Health Bulletin No. 242.* Washington, D.C.: U.S. Government Printing Office; 1938.
13. Brunnstrom S, Dennen M. *Round table on muscle testing.* New York: Annual Conference of the American Physical Therapy Association, Federation of Crippled and Disabled, Inc. (mimeographed); 1931.
14. Daniels L, Williams M, Worthingham CA. *Muscle Testing: Techniques of Manual Examination.* Philadelphia: W.B. Saunders; 1946.
15. Kendall HO, Kendall FP. *Muscles: Testing and Function.* Baltimore: Williams & Wilkins; 1949.
16. Kendall HO, Kendall FP. *Posture and Pain.* Baltimore: Williams & Wilkins; 1952.
17. Kendall FP, McCreary EK, Provance PG. *Muscles: Testing and Function.* 4th ed. Baltimore: Williams & Wilkins; 1993.
18. Gonella C, Harmon G, Jacobs M. The role of the physical therapist in the gamma globulin poliomyelitis prevention study. *Phys Ther Rev.* 1953;33:337–345.
19. Lilienfeld AM, Jacobs M, Willis M. Study of the reproducibility of muscle testing and certain other aspects of muscle scoring. *Phys Ther Rev.* 1954;34:279–289.
20. Kolb ME. Personal communication, October 1993.

Principles of Manual Muscle Testing

Principles

Grading System

Overview of Test Procedures

Criteria for Assigning a Muscle Test Grade

How to Use this Book

Preparing for the Muscle Test

Prime Movers

Exercises

Muscle Testing

Summary

Functional movement and physical activity require muscle strength. Muscle strength is defined as the ability of the muscle to exert force. Muscle endurance is the ability of the muscle to continue to perform without fatigue. Muscle testing typically measures muscle isometric strength (no limb movement), although a few tests in this book (heel rise and sit to stand) are tests more of muscle endurance but performed isotonically (with limb movement). This chapter will provide an overview of manual muscle testing performed to assess muscle strength for a specific movement.

GRADING SYSTEM

Grades for a manual muscle test are recorded as numeric ordinal scores ranging from zero (0), which represents no discernable muscle activity, to five (5), which represents a maximal or best-possible response, or as great a response as can be evaluated by a manual muscle test. Because this text is based on specific actions (e.g., elbow flexion), a muscle test may be a test of the summed effect of the muscles involved in the action rather than a test of an individual muscle (e.g., biceps brachii). In the case of multiple muscles contributing to a single action, the muscle grade assigned represents the performance of all muscles contributing to that action, with the emphasis on the prime mover.

The numeric 0 to 5 system of grading is the most commonly used muscle strength scoring convention across health care professions. The muscle testing scale is ordinal in that the numbers have no relationship to each other. Each numeric grade (e.g., 4) can be paired with a word grade (e.g., good) that describes the test performance in qualitative, but not quantitative, terms (see following table). Use of these qualitative terms is an outdated convention and is not encouraged because these terms tend to misrepresent the strength of the tested action. For example, knee extension strength that may be 50% less than its absolute or potential strength (certainly not "normal") is still often graded as a 5 because of the amount of force still generated.[1] The knee extension action graded as 4 may generate forces as low as 10% of maximal expected force, a level clearly not appropriately described as "good."[1] Because of the problematic implications of the qualitative grading scale terms, qualitative terms have been removed from this book. The numeric grades are based on several factors that will be addressed later in this chapter.

Numeric Score	Qualitative Score	Definition
5	Normal (N)	Completes full active range of motion against gravity and can hold the test position against maximum resistance
4	Good (G)	Completes full active range of motion against gravity but cannot hold the test position against maximum resistance
3	Fair (F)	Completes full active range of motion against gravity (no resistance)
2	Poor (P)	Moves the body part with gravity minimized
1	Trace activity (T)	Movement is detected visually or with palpation, but no movement occurs
0	Zero (no activity) (0)	No discernable contraction visually or through palpation

OVERVIEW OF TEST PROCEDURES

Break Test

Manual resistance is applied to a limb or other body part only after the clinician has observed the patient's ability to perform range of motion against gravity. The term *resistance* is always used in this book to denote a concentric force provided by the tester that acts in opposition to contracting muscles. Manual resistance should always be applied opposite to the line of pull of the muscle or muscles being tested. The patient is asked to hold the body segment at midrange (for two-joint muscles) or near end range (for one-joint muscles). At this point, the patient is instructed to not allow the clinician to "break" the hold while the clinician applies manual resistance for 2 to 3 seconds, matching the isometric force of the muscle, then continuing to exert force until the maximal effort is overcome, if possible.[2] For example, in the muscle test of elbow flexion for all the elbow flexors, a seated patient is asked to flex the elbow to its end range (Grade 3) and then position the elbow in midrange (for two-joint muscle). The clinician applies resistance just proximal to the wrist, trying to "break" the muscle's hold and thus allow the forearm to move downward into extension. This is called a break test, and it is the procedure most commonly used in manual muscle testing. The break test may be a more relevant measure to represent true strength and therefore is the preferred test and is used in this text. However, there are alternatives to the break test for grading specific muscle actions, and they are described next.

Make Test

An alternative to the break test is the use of manual resistance against the line of pull of the muscle or muscle group being tested (i.e., opposite the direction of the movement) that matches the patient's resistance but does not overcome it. During the muscle contraction, the clinician gradually, over approximately 3 seconds, increases the amount of manual resistance against the muscle's action until the resistance matches the patient's ability to hold the joint in the test position. The make test is considered a submaximal test and therefore is not as reliable as the break test because the patient may be exerting only the amount of effort that matches the clinician. Chapter 2 will elaborate on this issue.

Active Resistance Test

In the active resistance test, manual resistance is applied opposite the line of pull of the muscle being tested throughout the range, starting at the muscle's fully lengthened position. The amount of resistance matches the patient's resistance but allows the joint to move through the full range. This kind of manual muscle test requires considerable skill and experience to perform and is not reliable; thus, its use is not recommended as a testing procedure. However, it may be effective as a therapeutic exercise technique.

Application of Resistance

The principles of manual muscle testing presented here and in all published sources since 1921 follow the basic tenets of muscle length-tension relationships, as well as those of joint mechanics.[2,3,4] For example, in the case of elbow flexion, when the elbow is straight, the biceps are long, but the lever arm is short. As the elbow flexes, leverage increases and becomes maximal at 90°, where the muscles are most efficient and are likely to be strongest. However, as flexion continues, the biceps shorten, and the lever arm again decreases in length and efficiency.

The point in the range where application of resistance is ideal depends on whether the muscle is a two-joint muscle or one-joint muscle. Two-joint muscles are typically tested in midrange where length-tension is more favorable.

Critical to the accuracy of manual muscle testing and scoring is the location of the applied resistance and the consistency of resistance and technique across all patients. The placement of resistance is typically near the distal end of the body segment to which the tested muscle attaches. Because force is a product of the distance from the muscle's origin, the clinician's hand placement even a few inches away from the ideal hand placement can affect the output.[5] However, there are exceptions to this rule. One exception is when resistance cannot be provided effectively without moving to a body segment distal to its attachment. For example, to muscle test shoulder and

hip internal and external rotators, resistance is applied through the hand placed on the distal forearm or lower leg, respectively. Another exception involves patients with a shortened limb segment as in an amputation. The patient with a transfemoral amputation presents a challenge in applying a challenging force to assess the gluteus medius because of the shortened limb. Even if the patient could hold against maximum resistance while abducting the hip, the weight of the lower limb is so reduced and the lever arm for resistance application is so short that a Grade 5 cannot be assumed regardless of the resistance applied. A patient holding against maximum resistance may still struggle with the force demands of walking with a prosthesis. If a variation is used, the clinician should make a note of the placement of resistance to ensure consistency in testing.

The application of manual resistance should never be sudden or uneven (jerky). The clinician should apply resistance with full patient awareness and in a somewhat slow and gradual manner, slightly exceeding the muscle's force as it builds over 2 to 3 seconds to achieve the maximum tolerable intensity. Applying resistance that slightly exceeds the muscle's generated force will likely encourage a maximum effort and an accurate break test.

The clinician should also understand that the weight of the limb plus the influence of gravity is part of the test response. Heavier limbs and longer limb segments put a higher demand on the muscles that move them, such as the leg moving against gravity compared to the hand moving against gravity. When the muscle contracts in a parallel direction to the line of gravity, it is noted as "gravity minimal." It is suggested that the commonly used term "gravity eliminated" be avoided because, of course, gravity eliminated can never occur except in a zero-gravity environment.

Weakened muscles are tested in a plane horizontal to the direction of gravity with the body part supported on a smooth, flat surface in such a way that friction force is minimal (Grades 2, 1, and 0). A powder board may be used to minimize friction. For stronger muscles that can complete a full range of motion in a direction against the pull of gravity (Grade 3), resistance is applied perpendicular to the line of gravity (Grades 4 and 5). Acceptable variations to antigravity and gravity-minimal positions are discussed in individual test sections.

Stabilization

Stabilization of the body or segment is crucial to assigning accurate muscle test grades. Patients for whom stabilization is particularly important include those with weakness in the stabilizing muscles (e.g., scapular stabilizers) when testing the shoulder muscles and those who are particularly strong in the joint action being tested.

Numerous muscles, some seemingly remote from the joint of interest, can contribute as stabilizers to the performance of tested muscle actions. However, manual muscle testing is meant to test the prime mover of the joint action and minimize the input of other muscles.

To give an extreme example, shoulder abduction on the left side should not be dependent on the trunk muscles on the right side. Therefore, a patient with weak trunk muscles and limited sitting balance should be supported and stabilized either through patient positioning or by a stabilizing hand on the right shoulder.

A muscle or muscle group that is particularly strong may also require patient stabilization if the full capacity of a muscle group is to be accurately tested.[6] For example, a tester may not be able to break the knee extension action of a patient who is allowed to rise off of a support surface during the performance of a break test. However, the same patient, properly stabilized by the clinician, an assistant, or a belt during testing, may not be able to hold against maximum clinician resistance, thus causing a "break" in the muscle contraction that indicates the patient has a muscle Grade 4 rather than 5.

Patient Effort

To obtain an accurate grade in manual muscle testing, the patient must be instructed to exert their maximum effort. The clinician should also be prepared to provide strong, if not maximum, resistance to help elicit the patient's maximum effort. Maximum effort should not be confused with maximum output. To achieve maximum effort, the clinician should consider using vocal encouragement, similar to a coach's methods. Without maximum, voluntary effort, an accurate grade cannot be determined. This is true regardless of age or ability.

CRITERIA FOR ASSIGNING A MUSCLE TEST GRADE

The grade given on a manual muscle test comprises both subjective and objective factors. Subjective factors include the clinician's impression of the amount of resistance given during the actual test and the amount of resistance the patient actually holds against during the test. Objective factors include the ability of the patient to complete a full range of motion or to hold the test position once placed there, the ability to move the part against gravity, or an inability to move the part at all. All these factors require clinical judgment, which makes manual muscle testing a skill that requires considerable practice and experience to master. An accurate test grade is important not only to establish the presence of an impairment but also to assess the patient's longitudinal status over time. Clinical reasoning is necessary for the clinician to determine the causes for the lack of ability to complete the full range or hold the position, ascertain which is most applicable, and decide whether manual muscle testing is appropriate.

Consistent with a typical orthopedic or neurological exam, the patient is first asked to perform the active movement of the muscle to be tested independently without clinician or mechanical assistance. This active movement informs the clinician of the patient's willingness and ability to move the body part, of the available range in the related joint(s), and whether there are limitations to full range, such as pain, excess tone, or weakness. Active movement without resistance and through the full range of the action being tested is the equivalent of a Grade 3. Active movement is also called active range of motion and begins every muscle test to help determine the appropriate test position and amount of resistance to apply.

Grade 5 Muscle

A grade of 5 is assigned when a patient can complete full active range of motion (active movement) against gravity (Grade 3) followed by holding the test position against maximum resistance without a break in the muscle's contraction. Grade 5 is a measure of absolute or potential strength, not expected strength. If the clinician can break a patient's hold, a Grade 5 should *not* be assigned. The clinician should recognize that some muscles, such as the quadriceps, will be overestimated because of the absolute strength of the muscle. In fact, it is doubtful that a manual muscle test can discern absolute strength of the quadriceps. Chapters 7 and 8 describe alternate tests to accurately assess absolute strength.

The inherent wide range of "normal" muscle performance (Grade 5) typically leads to a considerable underestimation of a muscle's capability.[7] If the clinician has no experience in examining people who are free of disease or injury, it is unlikely that there will be any realistic or accurate assessment of what is Grade 5 and how much normality can vary. In general, a student learns manual muscle testing by practicing on classmates, but this provides only minimal experience compared with what is needed to master the skill necessary to test a wide variety of patients. It should be recognized, for example, that the average clinician cannot "break" knee extension in a reasonably fit young person, even by doing a handstand on their leg! A clinician may not be aware of the underestimation of the muscle contraction unless quantitative measures of strength are also used, such as in a sit-to-stand test for the quadriceps. Contributing to an underestimation of weakness is the inability of some clinicians (oftentimes female) to apply adequate resistance to elicit the patient's maximum effort.[8]

Grade 4 Muscle

Grade 4 is assigned when the patient can complete full active range of motion (active movement) against gravity but is not able to withstand a break test against the clinician's maximum resistance. Appropriate stabilization is critical to determine the true difference between a Grade 5 and Grade 4 muscle. A Grade 4 muscle "gives" or "yields" to some extent at the end of its test position with maximal or submaximal resistance. When maximal resistance results in a break or give, irrespective of age or disability, the muscle is assigned a Grade 4. However, if pain limits the ability to generate a maximal effort against the force applied by the clinician, evaluation of actual strength may not be realistic or accurate and should be documented as such. For example, in the presence of pain that limited the ability to generate a maximal contraction, documentation might say "Elbow flexion appeared strong but painful" or "Elbow flexion appeared weak and painful." Documentation such as this helps differentiate between a neurological cause of the inability to generate a maximum contraction and other causes such as pain.

Grade 3 Muscle

The Grade 3 muscle test is based on an objective measure of movement throughout the joint's range against gravity. For a Grade 3 to be assigned, the individual muscle or muscle group can complete a full range of motion against the resistance of gravity. This is also called "active range of motion." Even if a tested muscle can move through the full range against gravity and tolerate a small or "mild" amount of resistance, the muscle is assigned a Grade 3.

Direct force measurements have demonstrated that the force level of the Grade 3 muscle is quite low (less than 5% of normal for knee extension) so that a much greater span of functional loss exists between Grades 3 and 5 than between Grades 3 and 1.[9] A Grade 3 may represent a *functional threshold* for some muscle actions tested (e.g., elbow flexion during feeding); however, a Grade 3 may fall far short of the functional requirements of many lower extremity muscles during weight-bearing activities, particularly for such muscle groups as the hip abductors and the ankle plantar flexors. The clinician must be sure that muscles given a Grade 3 are not in the joint "locked" position during the test (e.g., locked elbow when testing elbow extension).

Grade 2 Muscle

Grade 2 is assigned to a muscle or muscle group that can move the body segment when gravity is minimized. This position is typically described as the horizontal plane of motion. Movement in this plane may be eased by use of a powder board or other such friction-minimizing surface.

Grade 1 Muscle

Grade 1 is assigned when the clinician can detect visually or by palpation some contractile activity in one or more of the muscles that participate in the action being tested (provided that the muscle is superficial enough to be palpated). The clinician also may be able to see or feel a tendon pop up or tense as the patient tries to perform the movement. However, there is no movement of the body part as a result of this contractile muscle activity.

Patient positioning is less important in Grade 1 testing because a Grade 1 muscle can be detected in almost any position. When a Grade 1 muscle is suspected, the clinician should passively move the part into the test position and ask the patient to hold the position and then relax; this will enable the clinician to palpate the muscle or tendon, or both, during the patient's attempts to contract the muscle and also during relaxation. Care should be taken to avoid substitution of other muscles.

Grade 0 Muscle

Grade 0 muscle is assigned when the clinician's palpation or visual inspection fail to provide evidence of contraction. This does not mean there is no muscle activation. In fact, electromyography may demonstrate that some activation is present. Thus, the phrase "no discernable contraction" defines a Grade 0 in this text.

Plus (+) and Minus (–) Grades

Use of plus (+) or minus (–) delineations to manual muscle test grades is discouraged. Avoiding the use of plus or minus signs restricts manual muscle test grades to those that are meaningful, defendable, and reliable. The use of pluses and minuses adds a level of subjectivity that lacks reliability, especially for grades of 3 or greater. However, in the case of Grade 2, described earlier, there is a considerable difference between the muscle that can complete full range in a gravity-minimized position (horizontal position) and the one that cannot complete full range but can achieve some joint movement. Therefore, Grade 2– is acceptable when the muscle can complete partial range of motion in the horizontal plane, gravity minimized. The difference between Grade 2 and Grade 1 muscles represents such a broad functional difference that a minus sign may be important in assessing even minor improvements in function. The clinician is encouraged to supplement the grade with descriptive documentation of the quality of movement.

Grade 4 Muscle Revisited

Grade 4 has a huge range of strength ability, spanning from the limb tolerating a small amount of resistance notwithstanding a maximal break test effort. In fact, considerable discussion has occurred about the validity of Grade 4. In one study, comparing manual muscle testing with isokinetic dynamometry, Dvir found that up to 86% of the muscle strength potential is spanned by Grade 4.[10] More recently, Bohannon found that force values for muscles that were graded as "normal" ranged from 80 to 625 Newtons,[7] an astronomical difference, further demonstrating how difficult it is to distinguish a "good" muscle from a "normal" muscle.

Accurate muscle grades are especially challenging to assign to older adults. By the time a person reaches the age of 80 years, approximately 50% of their muscle mass and strength may be lost due to natural decline.[11] Older adults may not be familiar or comfortable in exerting maximum effort, and clinicians may have an ageist bias that assumes older adults do not need the same strength requirements as a younger person, and so, they may grade more generously. Unfortunately, these lower expectations may result in the assignment of a grade of "normal" (5) or worse, "within normal limits" (WNL), even though the individual's strength is half of what it used to be. Functionally, this same 80-year-old assigned "normal" strength may be unable to get out of a chair without pushing on the arms or to ascend stairs without pulling on the railing. Certainly, this person's functional performance is not WNL or within functional limits (WFL). Inaccurate muscle grading based on the patient's age, sex, presumed strength, or because the clinician cannot apply adequate resistance must be avoided.

There are numerous instances in which a Grade 4 muscle cannot meet its functional demands. When the gluteus medius is graded as a 4, a patient will display a positive Trendelenburg sign. This is one of the reasons the test position requires so much effort. When the soleus is graded a 4, the heel rise fails to occur during the latter portion of the stance phase of gait, which reduces gait speed.[12] When the abdominals are Grade 4, there is difficulty stabilizing the pelvis while arising from bed or when sitting up, and this often results in back pain. Calling a muscle "good," rather than Grade 4, simply is not "good" enough. Based on Dvir's and Bohannon's findings, it is these author's opinions that many more Grade 4s should be assigned, rather than Grade 5, especially considering the aging patient population.

As noted previously, there is no other term in muscle testing that is more problematic than the term "good" used to denote numerical Grade 4. Too often, clinical practitioners, including therapists and physicians, construe the term "good" in the literal sense, interpreting "good" to mean the muscle's strength is totally adequate. This assumption, that a Grade 4 is adequate, is quite erroneous considering the enormous span of muscle strength within Grade 4. If used in the qualitative sense, the assumption that a Grade 4/good is adequate may deprive the patient of beneficial rehabilitation.

It is unclear how a grade of "good" became synonymous with achievement of a satisfactory end point of treatment. Certainly, the pressure from third-party payers to discharge patients as soon as possible does not help the clinician to fulfill the minimum goal of reaching "prior level of function." Nonetheless, the opportunity for patients to recover muscle strength to the fullest extent possible is a primary goal of an intervention. If this goal is not met, patients (especially aging individuals) may lose their independence or find themselves incapable of returning to a desired sport or activity because their weak muscles fatigue too quickly. Athletes who have not fully recovered their potential strength before returning to a sport are far more likely to suffer a reinjury, potentially harming themselves further.

In summary, a "good" muscle is not always good. Everything must be done to ensure accuracy in manual muscle test grading and to provide the intervention necessary to fully restore strength and function to "normal." Substituting the numerical system of 5 to 0 for the subjective terms "good" or "normal" in manual muscle testing assessment is a start in the right direction as is being aware of the span of absolute or potential strength of individual muscles. Chapters 7 to 9 will assist with this familiarization.

Available Range of Motion

When muscle shortness ("tightness"), a contracture, or fixed joint limitation (e.g., total knee replacement) limits joint range of motion, the patient performs only within the range available. In this circumstance, the *available range* is the full passive range of motion for that patient at that time, even though it is not "normal." This is the range used to assign a muscle testing grade. For example, the normal knee extension range is 135 degrees to 0 degrees. A patient with a 20-degree knee flexion contracture is tested for knee extension strength in the middle of the ideal range, where the muscle is considered the strongest. If this range (in sitting) can be completed with maximal resistance, the grade assigned would be a 5. If the patient cannot actively complete that range because of a structural issue but can hold against maximum resistance, the grade assigned may still be a 5. However, the clinician should document the patient's muscle grade within the limited range. For example, "knee extension is graded a 5 in the presence of a 20-degree knee flexion contracture" or "the presence of the patient's 20-degree knee flexion contracture did not appreciable affect the patient's ability to exert maximum force, achieving a Grade 5."

Screening Tests

In the interests of time and cost-efficient care, it is often unnecessary to perform a muscle test on each muscle of the body. As the strength of various muscle actions tend to be correlated and internally consistent,[7] a systematic testing of a limited number of muscle actions often will suffice. Three screening indexes warrant mentioning. Each was developed with a specific diagnostic group in mind and allows for the calculation of a total score. The first, the Motricity Index, was developed for patients with stroke and includes three muscle actions of the upper limb (shoulder elevation, elbow flexion, and hand grasp) and three muscle actions of the lower limb (hip flexion, knee extension, and ankle dorsiflexion).[9] The second, the Motor Index Score, was developed for patients with spinal cord injury and includes muscle actions representative of key nerve root levels in the upper and lower limbs (elbow flexion [C5], wrist extension [C6], elbow extension [C7], finger flexion [C8], small finger abduction [T1], hip flexion [L2], knee extension [L3], ankle dorsiflexion [L4], great toe extension [L5], and ankle plantarflexion [S1]).[13] The final test, the Medical Research Council Sum Score, was produced to capture weakness in patients with Guillain-Barré but has since been used with other patients with dispersed weakness. It includes most of the actions included in the Motricity Index (shoulder abduction, elbow flexion, wrist extension, hip flexion, knee extension, and ankle dorsiflexion).[14]

Never should the clinician use phrases such as WNL or WFL for a screening exam. If a nonspecific strength exam is performed (e.g., through observation of tasks), documentation is better served with terms like "patient demonstrated no difficulty performing task," rather than making a judgment about the degree of strength present.

To screen for muscles that need definitive testing, the clinician can use a number of techniques to identify movements that do and do not need testing. Observation of the patient before the examination will provide valuable clues to muscular weakness and performance deficits. For example, the clinician can do the following:

- Observe the patient as they enter the treatment area to detect gross abnormalities of gait or other aspects of mobility.
- Observe the patient doing other everyday activities such as rising from a chair, completing admission or history forms, or removing street clothing.
- Ask the patient to walk on the toes and then on the heels.
- Ask the patient to grip the clinician's hand.
- Perform gross checks of bilateral muscle groups, such as reaching toward the floor, overhead, and behind the back.

If evidence from the previous "quick checks" suggests a deficit in movement, in the interest of time and to optimize the patient's clinic visit, manual muscle testing can quickly be focused to the region observed to be weak.

PREPARING FOR THE MUSCLE TEST

For the test session to be successful, the clinician and the patient must work in harmony. This means that some basic principles and inviolable procedures must be second nature to the clinician.

1. The patient should be as free as possible from discomfort or pain for the duration of each test. It may be necessary to allow some patients to move or be positioned differently between tests.
2. The environment for testing should be quiet and non-distracting. The ambient temperature should be comfortable for the partially disrobed patient.
3. The testing surface must be firm to help stabilize the body part being tested. The ideal is a firm surface, minimally padded or not padded at all. The firm surface will not allow the trunk or limbs to "sink in." Friction of the surface material should be kept to a minimum. When the patient is reasonably mobile, a plinth or table is fine, but its width should not be so narrow that the patient is afraid of falling or sliding off. Sometimes a low mat table is the more practical choice. The height of the table should be adjustable to allow the clinician to use proper leverage and body mechanics.
4. Patient position should be carefully organized so that position changes in a test sequence are minimized. The patient's position must permit adequate stabilization of the part or parts being tested by virtue of body weight or with help provided by the clinician.
5. All materials needed for the test must be at hand. This is particularly important when the patient is anxious for any reason or is too weak to be safely left unattended. Materials needed include the following:
- Manual muscle test documentation forms (Fig. 1.1)
- Pen, pencil, or computer
- Pillows, towels, pads, and wedges for positioning
- Sheets or other draping linen
- Goniometer
- Stopwatch
- Specific equipment for specific functional tests
- Test forms for functional tests
- Interpreter (if needed)
- Assistance for turning, moving, or stabilizing the patient
- Emergency call system (if no assistant is available)
- Reference material

PRIME MOVERS

Within each chapter are tables indicating the muscles involved in the action that is tested (e.g., shoulder flexion). When prime movers have been identified for a particular action, they are in boldface type. For example,

DOCUMENTATION OF MANUAL MUSCLE TESTS

		Date of Examination				Examiner's Initials		

LEFT						RIGHT		
3	2	1				1	2	3
			CERVICAL					
			Capital extension					
			Cervical extension					
			Capital flexion (chin tuck)					
			Cervical flexion					
			Cervical rotation					
			TRUNK					
			Trunk extension combined					
			Lumbar					
			Thoracic					
			Elevation of the pelvis					
			Trunk flexion					
			Trunk rotation					
			Core tests					
			Prone plank					
			Side bridge endurance test					
			Timed partial curl up test					
			Isometric trunk flexor endurance test					
			Front abdominal power test					
			Unilateral supine bridge test					
			Maximal inspiratory pressure					
			Maximal expiratory pressure					
			Cough					
			Pelvic floor					
			UPPER EXTREMITY					
			Scapular abduction and upward rotation (serratus)					
			Scapular elevation					
			Scapular adduction (retraction)					
			Scapular depression and adduction					
			Scapular adduction (retraction) and downward rotation (rhomboids)					
			Latissimus dorsi					
			Shoulder flexion					
			Shoulder extension					
			Shoulder abduction					
			Shoulder horizontal abduction (posterior deltoid)					
			Shoulder horizontal adduction (pectoralis major)					
			Shoulder external rotation					
			Shoulder internal rotation (subscapularis)					
			Elbow flexion (combined)					
			Elbow extension					
			Forearm supination					
			Forearm pronation					
			Wrist flexion combined					
			Flexor carpi radialis					
			Flexor carpi ulnaris					

FIGURE 1.1 Documentation of Manual Muscle Examination.

MANUAL MUSCLE TESTS - Page 2

			Date of Examination	Examiner's Initials			
LEFT						**RIGHT**	
3	2	1		1	2	3	

3	2	1		1	2	3
			Wrist extension combined			
			Extensor carpi radialis longus and brevis			
			Extensor carpi radialis ulnaris			
			Hand			
			Finger proximal phalanges (PIP) and distal phalanges (DIP) flexion			
			Combined			
			Flexor digitorum superficialis (PIP)			
			Flexor digitorum profundus (DIP)			
			Finger MCP extension			
			Extensor digitorum			
			Extensor indicis			
			Extensor digiti minimi			
			Finger MCP flexion			
			Finger abduction			
			Dorsal interossei			
			Abductor digiti minimi			
			Finger adduction (palmar interossei)			
			Thumb MCP and IP flexion			
			Flexor pollicis brevis			
			Flexor pollicis longus			
			Thumb MCP and IP extension (extensor pollicis brevis and longus)			
			Thumb abduction			
			Abductor pollicis longus			
			Abductor pollicis brevis			
			Thumb adduction (adductor pollicis)			
			Opposition			
			Opponens pollicis			
			Opponens digiti minimi			
			Grip strength			
			LOWER EXTREMITY			
			Hip flexion			
			Hip flexion, abduction, and external rotation with knee flexion (sartorius)			
			Hip extension combined			
			Gluteus maximus			
			Supine hip extensor test			
			Hip abduction			
			Hip adduction			
			Hip external rotation			
			Hip internal rotation			
			Knee flexion combined			
			Medial hamstring test (semitendinosus and semimembranosus)			
			Lateral hamstring test (biceps femoris)			

FIGURE 1.1, cont'd

MANUAL MUSCLE TESTS - Page 3

| | Date of Examination | | | Examiner's Initials | | |

LEFT					RIGHT		
3	2	1			1	2	3
			Knee extension				
			Ankle plantar flexion combined				
			Soleus				
			Foot dorsiflexion and inversion				
			Foot inversion				
			Foot eversion with plantar flexion				
			Hallux and toe MP flexion				
			Hallus MP flexion				
			Toe MP flexion				
			Hallux and toe DIP and PIP flexion				
			Hallux and toe MP and IP extension				

Comments:

Diagnosis _____ Onset _____ Age _____ Birth date _____

Patient Name _____

last   first   middle   ID number

FIGURE 1.1, cont'd

the prime mover of shoulder flexion is the anterior deltoid muscle, and therefore this muscle is bolded. In other instances, there is no distinct prime mover and, thus, no bolding. The movement of back extension, for example, involves a dozen muscles, none of which is a prime mover, and therefore there are no muscle names bolded. Our intent in highlighting the prime movers is to help the student more readily understand which muscles are critical for many important movements and to have a better understanding of which muscles to strengthen when weakness is present.

EXERCISES

Specific exercises have been included in the text where there is electromyographic evidence of isometric maximal voluntary contraction (MVC). Clinically, motions that evoke higher electromyographic activities (%MVC) have been interpreted to be more challenging to a muscle.[15] The following scale is used when interpreting %MVC:

MVIC	Percentages
Low	0%–20%
Moderate	21%–40%
High	41%–60%
Very high	>60%

An MVC of greater than 40% is considered necessary for strengthening.[16,17]

We have included exercises that are known to elicit >40% MVC in the suggested exercise. These exercises should be considered challenging and used when the rehabilitation has progressed. The clinician should also be aware of the different types of contractions applied in muscle testing and exercise (see Box 1.1).

BOX 1.1 Types of Contractions

Concentric contraction refers to the shortening of a muscle as it contracts, as in the flexion portion of a biceps curl or extension of the elbow when lifting an object overhead. Concentric activity is generally the primary motion of the muscle.

Eccentric contraction refers to the lowering phase of a movement, when the muscle lengthens, as in lowering the weight to the chest during the bench press or lowering oneself into a chair. Eccentric muscle activity is seen in many mobility-related functional tasks such as stepping down a curb or in gait.

Isometric contraction refers to the creation of muscle tension without joint movement. Isometric contractions are often used when the limb is immobilized, such as postsurgery. Isometric contractions are used with handheld dynamometry, discussed in Chapter 9.

The inherent limitations in evaluating muscle strength necessary for functional movement and sporting activity requires alternate forms of muscle testing. Chapter 7 describes alternatives to manual muscle testing, including the one-repetition maximum test, equipment-based strength testing, power testing, and body weight testing. Reference scores for some tests are provided. Chapter 8 describes the testing of functional performance with selected tests that are directed related to muscle strength. Finally, Chapter 9 describes the use of handheld muscle dynamometer in assessing strength, a method that can be more objective in that instead of an ordinal scale to grade a muscle's strength, an objective number in kilograms of force is derived.

SUMMARY

From the foregoing discussion, it should be clear that manual muscle testing is an exacting clinical skill. Practice, practice, and more practice on a variety of patient types create the experience essential to building the skill to an acceptable level of clinical proficiency, to say nothing of clinical mastery. Accurate muscle testing is one piece of the clinical puzzle. Since this text is not a kinesiology text, this text should be supplemented with a greater study of combined muscle and joint actions to supply additional pieces of the clinical puzzle.

REFERENCES

1. Bohannon RW. Measuring knee extensor muscle strength. *Am J Phys Med Rehabil.* 2001;80:13–18.
2. Holt KL, Raper DP, Boettcher CE, Waddington GS, Drew MK. Hand-held dynamometry strength measures for internal and external rotation demonstrate superior reliability, lower minimal detectable change and higher correlation to isokinetic dynamometry than externally-fixed dynamometry of the shoulder. *Phys Ther Sport.* 2016;21:75–81.
3. Soderberg GL. *Kinesiology: Application to Pathological Motion.* Baltimore: Williams & Wilkins; 1997.
4. Neumann DA. *Kinesiology of the Musculoskeletal System: Foundations for Rehabilitation.* St. Louis: Elsevier; 2017.
5. Bohannon RW. Considerations and practical options for measuring muscle strength. A narrative review. *Biomed Res Int.* 2019:8194537.
6. Magnusson SP, Geismar RA, Gleim G, et al. The effect of stabilization on isokinetic knee extension and flexion torque production. *J Athlet Train.* 1993;28:221–225.
7. Bohannon RW, Corrigan D. A broad range of forces is encompassed by the maximum manual muscle test grade of five. *Percept Mot Skills.* 2000;90:747–750.
8. Mulroy SJ, Lassen KD, Chambers SH, et al. The ability of male and female clinicians to effectively test knee extension strength using manual muscle testing. *J Orthop Sports Phys Ther.* 1997;26:192–199.
9. Demeurisse G, Demol O, Roboye E. Motor evaluation in hemiplegia. *Eur Neurol.* 1980;19:382–389.
10. Dvir Z. Grade 4 in manual muscle testing: the problem with submaximal strength assessment. *Clin Rehabil.* 1997;11:36–41.
11. Piering AW, Janowski AP, Moore MT, et al. Electromyographic analysis of four popular abdominal exercises. *J Athl Train.* 1993;28:120–126.
12. Perry J. *Gait Analysis: Normal and Pathological Function.* 2nd ed. Thorofare, NJ: Slack, Inc.; 2010.
13. Lazar RB, Yarkony GM, Ortolano D, et al. Prediction of functional outcome by motor capability after spinal cord injury. *Arch Phys Med Rehabil.* 1989;70:819–822.
14. Hough CL, Lieu BK, Caldwell ES. Manual muscle strength testing of critically ill patients: feasibility and interobserver agreement. *Crit Care.* 2011;15(1):R43.
15. Smith J, Padgett DJ, Kaufman KR, et al. Rhomboid muscle electromyography activity during 3 different manual muscle tests. *Arch Phys Med Rehabil.* 2004;85(6):987–992.
16. Ayotte NW, Stetts DM, Keenan G, et al. Electromyographical analysis of selected lower extremity muscles during 5 unilateral weight-bearing exercises. *J Orthop Sports Phys Ther.* 2007;37:48–55.
17. Escamilla RF, Lewis C, Bell D, et al. Core muscle activation during Swiss ball and traditional abdominal exercises. *J Orthop Sports Phys Ther.* 2010;40:265–276.

CHAPTER 2

Practical Considerations for Manual Muscle Testing

Introduction

The Clinician and the Value of the Muscle Test

Influence of the Patient on the Test

Use of Manual Muscle and Strength Testing in Various Clinical Settings

    Acute Care Facilities

    Acute Rehabilitation Facilities

    Long-Term Care Facilities

Home Health Setting

Outpatient Clinics

Wellness Clinics

Summary

Limitations of Manual Muscle Testing

    Population Variation

    Objectivity

    Reliability and Validity

    Sensitivity

    Diagnostic Validity

    Ceiling Effect

    Tester Strength

Summary

INTRODUCTION

Manual muscle testing (MMT) is well recognized as the most common strength-testing technique in rehabilitation, neurology, and orthopedics, having first appeared during the poliomyelitis epidemic in New England before World War I. A brief history of MMT is described elsewhere in this text. MMT has the advantage of being well established and efficient, requires no equipment, is relatively easy to learn, and can be utilized anywhere. MMT serves unique purposes that can vary according to the setting in which it is practiced. Although MMT is an essential and foundational skill in a clinician's examination techniques, it also has its limitations. Appreciating these limitations and learning how to compensate for them helps to make MMT as relevant nowadays as it was when first conceptualized.

The knowledge and skill of the clinician determine the accuracy and defensibility of a manual muscle test. Specific elements include:

- Knowledge of the location and anatomical features of the muscles in a test. In addition to knowing the muscle attachments, the clinician should be able to visualize the location of the tendon and its muscle in relationship to other tendons and muscles and other structures in the same area (e.g., the tendon of the extensor carpi radialis longus lies on the radial side of the tendon of the extensor carpi radialis brevis at the wrist).
- Knowledge of the direction of muscle fibers and their alignment in each muscle.
- Knowledge of the function of the participating muscles (e.g., synergist, prime mover, agonist, and antagonist).
- Consistent use of a standardized method for each test procedure.
- Consistent use of proper positioning and stabilization techniques for each test procedure. Stabilization of the proximal segment of the joint being tested is achieved in several ways. These include patient position (via body weight), the use of a firm surface for testing, patient muscle activation, manual fixation by the clinician, or external fixation such as with a belt.
- Ability to identify patterns of substitution in a given test and how they can be detected based on a knowledge of which other muscles can be substituted for the one(s) being tested.
- Ability to detect contractile activity during both contraction and relaxation, especially in the minimally active muscle.
- Sensitivity to differences in contour and the bulk of the muscles being tested in contrast to the contralateral side or expectations based on such things as body size, occupation, activity level, sex, or age.
- Awareness of any deviation from reference values for range of motion and the presence of any joint laxity or deformity.
- Understanding that the muscle belly must not be grasped at any time during a manual muscle test except specifically to assess muscle mass.
- Ability to identify muscles with the same innervation that will ensure a comprehensive muscle evaluation and accurate interpretation of test results (because the weakness of one muscle in a myotome should require examination of all muscles within that myotome).
- Relating the diagnosis to the sequence and extent of the test (e.g., the patient with C7 complete tetraplegia will require definitive muscle testing of the upper extremity but only confirmatory tests in the trunk and lower extremities).

- Ability to modify test procedures when necessary while understanding the influence of the modification on the result and thus not compromising the accuracy of the test result.
- Knowledge of fatigue on the test results, especially muscles tested late in a long testing session, and a sensitivity to fatigue in certain diagnostic conditions such as myasthenia gravis or multiple sclerosis.
- Understanding of the effect of sensory and perceptual loss on movement. The clinician also may inadvertently *influence* the test results and should be especially alert when testing in the following situations:
  - The patient with open wounds or other conditions requiring gloves, which may blunt palpation skills.
  - The patient who must be evaluated under difficult conditions, such as in an intensive care unit with multiple tubes and monitors or immediately after surgery; the patient in traction; the patient for whom turning is contraindicated; the patient on a ventilator; and the patient in shackles or restraints.
  - The patient with limited understanding of the test, such as in the presence of delirium or dementia.
  - The patient who cannot assume test positions, such as the prone position.
- Documentation of any deviations from the established test position.
- Avoidance of the temptation to use shortcuts or "tricks of the trade" before mastering the basic procedures, lest such shortcuts become an inexact personal standard. One such pitfall is not using the established test position (e.g., patient sitting in a chair) but still using the standard grading system. Another common pitfall is assigning a lower muscle grade when the patient could not successfully perform a test at a higher grade but without actually testing in the position required for the lower grade.

For example, when testing trunk flexion, a patient just partially clears the scapula from the surface, with the hands resting lightly on the side of the head (the position for the Grade 5 test), thus not earning a Grade 5. The temptation may exist to assign a Grade 4 to the result because the patient could not achieve a Grade 5, but this may "overrate" the true strength of trunk flexion unless the patient is actually tested with the arms across the chest to confirm Grade 4.

The skilled and conscientious clinician never ignores a patient's comments and must be a good listener, not just to the patient's questions but also to the meaning of the words the patient uses. This quality is an essential element of good communication and is the primary means of encouraging understanding and respect between clinician and patient. The patient is the best guide to a successful muscle test.

Early Kendall Examination

Accuracy in giving examinations depends primarily on the clinician's knowledge of the isolated and combined actions of muscles in individuals with normal muscles, as well as in those with weak or paralyzed muscles.

The fact that muscles act in combination permits substitution of a strong muscle for a weaker one. For accurate muscle examinations, no substitutions should be permitted; that is, the movement described as a test movement should be done without shifting the body or turning the part to allow other muscles to perform the movement for the weak or paralyzed group. The only way to recognize substitution is to know normal function and realize the ease with which a normal muscle performs the exact test movement.

Kendall, H. O. & Kendall, F. P. From *Care During the Recovery Period in Paralytic Poliomyelitis.* Public Health Bulletin No. 242. Washington, DC: U.S. Government Printing Office; 1939: 26.

The intrusion of a living, breathing, feeling person into the testing situation may distort scoring for the unwary clinician. The following circumstances should be recognized:
- There may be variation in the assessment of the true effort expended by a patient in a given test (reflecting the patient's desire to do well or to seem more impaired than is actually the case).
- The patient's willingness to endure discomfort or pain may vary (e.g., the stoic, the complainer, the high competitor).
- The patient's ability to understand the test requirements may be limited in some cases because of cognitive impairments, comprehension, and language challenges.

- The motor skills required for the test may be beyond those possessed by some patients, making it impossible for them to perform as requested.
- Lassitude and depression may cause the patient to be indifferent to the test and the clinician.
- Cultural, social, and gender issues may be associated with palpation and exposure of a body part for testing.
- Muscle mass and available force differences between muscles can cause considerable differences in results and grading (e.g., the gluteus medius versus a finger extensor). There is huge variability in maximum torque between such muscles, and the clinician must use care not to assign a grade that is inconsistent with muscle size and potential force output.

MMT is used in many different types of health care settings. In this section, we will discuss some of the more common applications of MMT in various clinical and therapeutic settings, with emphasis on the specific challenges often seen in each. The student should be aware that the examples provided here are not limited to these settings only.

ACUTE CARE FACILITIES

Patients seen in acute care facilities can be either acutely ill or recovering from a recent surgical procedure. Often, patients in acute care are older adults of varying physical abilities. The MMT is often used to assess the patient's mobility status to inform a treatment and discharge plan. A manual muscle exam performed as part of a general assessment may provide information concerning the amount of assistance the patient requires and whether the patient will need an assistive device. Assessing the patient's strength to help ensure safe transfers from bed to chair, to a standing position, or on and off the toilet is an essential part of the acute care patient management process. A strength assessment may also inform the clinician of the patient's ability to follow directions and/or to verbalize concerns such as following a stroke or in the presence of delirium or other cognitive loss.[1,2]

Strength assessment may also indicate the presence of pain. The identification of painful muscles before asking a patient to do an activity such as transfers will save time in the long run (and from a potentially adverse situation). Strength assessment can take several forms, such as a manual muscle test, a 10-repetition maximum (RM) such as in a seated shoulder dip, or a chair rise test.

A muscle exam for the postoperative patient informs the clinician of the integrity of the patient's nervous system. The clinician may be the first person requiring the patient to move voluntarily after surgery and thus may be the first one to observe the patient's ability to contract a muscle on command. Although nerve damage as a result of surgery is rare, clearly, the consequences of assuming an attitude of "all is well" and finding out during a transfer that the patient cannot control part of an extremity would have undesirable consequences. A muscle exam in this scenario might take the form of isometric contractions, especially in the presence of contraindications to joint movement or suspected postsurgical pain (e.g., in a newly repaired fractured hip). If testing is done in a manner that differs from the established procedures, documentation should describe how the test was performed. For example, isometric testing of the hip flexors following a posterior approach hip arthroplasty could be documented as "contraction of hip flexors elicited with leg extended due to precautions."

Key movements that should be assessed for viability and the presence of strength necessary to perform transfers or gait include elbow extension, hand grip, shoulder depression, knee extension, hip abduction, hip extension, ankle plantarflexion, and ankle dorsiflexion. Functional tests that might be useful in assessing the patient include gait speed, chair stand, timed transfer, and the timed up-and-go test (see Chapter 8).

Special considerations for the acute care setting may include the patient's rapid fluctuations in response to medications, illness, or pain. Reassessment may be necessary when any changes in strength are documented along with the clinician's insights into why the changes are occurring. Clearly, strength gains are not possible in the short time a typical patient is in acute care but, rather, should be attributed to increased confidence in moving, less pain, better understanding of the movement to be performed, motor learning, and so forth.

ACUTE REHABILITATION FACILITIES

Strength assessment in the acute rehabilitation setting may be performed as a baseline assessment to determine progress over time and to identify key impairments that affect the patient's mobility-related and other functional goals. Knowledge of community-based reference scores for mobility such as chair stands, distance walked, stair climbing speed, floor transfer ability, and gait speed will inform the clinician's clinical decision-making. (See Chapter 8 for a more complete description of these tests.) A standard manual muscle test and/or a 10-RM strength assessment are other methods used to assess relevant strength abilities.

As in the acute care setting, assessment of strength for mobility tasks is critical in the acute rehabilitation setting. Recognition of the importance of key muscle groups in specific mobility tasks such as the plantar flexors in gait speed is key to informed clinical decision-making.

Special considerations for the acute rehabilitation setting often include rapid change over a short period. Positive changes may be attributed to increased comfort and less pain, less apprehension, neuroplasticity, and a change in medications. Negative changes may be attributed to, for example, a decline in medical status, pain, or depression. Muscle fatigue resulting from an extended inpatient stay, poor fitness, and excessive sedentary behavior or general body fatigue related to frailty or post–acute care implications may affect the perception of strength. The patient may not be able to assume a proper test position because of postsurgical restrictions or a lack of range of motion, requiring the clinician to do a strength screen rather than a strength test. Although a screen may be appropriate, the screen cannot serve as an accurate baseline because of the lack of standardization. Functional testing may be more informative and accurate in these situations. The clinician should take special care to document any deviations from the standardized manual muscle test.

LONG-TERM CARE FACILITIES

Strength testing and assessment approaches used in long-term care settings are similar to those used in acute rehabilitation. Strength assessment can serve as a baseline to identify key impairments that impact a patient's fall risk, mobility, and other functional goals as well as to determine the patient's progress over time. Strength screening can be part of a required annual assessment for long-term residents. Strength in the form of a chair stand test or grip strength is a key component of the diagnosis of frailty and therefore can inform prognosis.[3]

Frailty is a common geriatric syndrome, characterized by decreased reserve and increased vulnerability to adverse outcomes, including falls, hospitalization, institutionalization, and death.[4] The majority of residents in long-term care are considered frail.[5] A profound loss of strength is a significant cause of frailty and serves as a diagnostic criterion. Box 2.1 lists the diagnostic criteria for frailty. Based on these criteria, strength assessment and functional testing are essential in the examination and intervention of nursing home residents.[4]

Although a natural consequence of aging is a gradual loss of strength and power, it should not be assumed that older adults are functionally weaker than younger adults.[6-8] Because MMT has a ceiling effect with regard to functional mobility and activities of daily living tasks (ADLs), the clinician should not lower their expectations or overestimate strength in frail older adults. *Criteria for grading remain the same for people of all ages and conditions.* Because the ceiling effect of a manual muscle test can be so profound, especially in regard to function, functional testing may be a better option for strength testing and assessment in the long-term care setting.[9] Community criterion reference values exist that guide the long-term care clinician in establishing appropriate goals and expectations (see Box 2.2). Older adults might be better served with strength training options such as a leg press or latissimus pulldown rather than the cuff weights or a recumbent bicycle or cross-trainer that are commonly used in long-term care settings. The student is referred to Chapter 7 for alternative strength measurement options.

HOME HEALTH SETTING

Assessment of home health patients' strength and function for the purpose of comparison with community-based reference data and for identification of impairments related to function are the primary purposes of MMT and alternative strength-testing methods in the home health setting. Returning a patient to community-based mobility may prevent frailty and increase the patient's quality of life. Lower extremity strength is a primary component of these goals. Box 2.2 lists community

BOX 2.1 Diagnostic Criteria for Frailty

Diagnostic criteria for frailty include the presence of three or more of the following[4,10]:
1. Unintentional weight loss (>10 lb in past year)
2. General feeling of exhaustion on 3 or more days/week (self-report)
3. Weakness (grip strength in lowest 20%; <23 lb for women; <32 lb for men)
4. Slow walking speed (lowest 20%; ≤0.8 m/s)
5. Low levels of physical activity (in kcal/week, lowest 20%; 270 kcal/week for women; 383 kcal/week for men; equivalent to sitting quietly and/or lying down for the vast majority of the day)

The presence of one or two of these characteristics indicates prefrailty.

BOX 2.2 Community Mobility Requirements

To be considered mobile, an individual should be able to:
Walk 300 m minimum per errand[12]
Perform multiple errands during one trip outside the home[13]
Carry a package weighing 7.5 lb[13]
Change direction while walking[14]
Step onto and off of a curb without support
Achieve a gait speed of >0.8 m/s
Make postural transitions including stooping, lifting, reaching, and reorientation of head, independent of change in direction[13]
Climb stairs
Navigate slopes and uneven surfaces[13]
Step over objects

mobility requirements that can be used as outcome goals for home health patients and serve to guide strength testing. The authors recommend that functional goals drive the strength assessment. In addition, for a homebound patient to receive home health services, the Centers for Medicare and Medicaid Services require patients to demonstrate "considerable and taxing effort in leaving the home," a criterion that has strength implications.[11] A weaker individual will expend more effort and energy doing the same task than a stronger individual.

OUTPATIENT CLINICS

Strength testing and assessment in outpatient clinics provide essential information, such as the (1) origin of the patient's pain, (2) quality of the contraction, (3) symmetry between sides and between the primary mover (agonist) and opposing muscles (antagonist), and (4) weakness within a kinetic chain (body segments linked by a series of joints).[15] This information aids in making a differential diagnosis. It can also provide a baseline assessment for changes over time. Challenges of MMT in the outpatient setting can include the presence of pain that prohibits a full, voluntary contraction and limitations of range of motion, such as with retraction and upward rotation of the scapula at the shoulder. Although a weak and painful or strong and painful contraction can be diagnostic, it can preclude the assessment of quantitative strength.[16] The ceiling effect of MMT often prevents an accurate assessment of strength quantity. Therefore, we recommend that quantitative strength be assessed through a 1-RM or 10-RM strength assessment when pain permits (see Chapter 7) or assessed with a muscle dynamometer (Chapter 9). It is useful to assess the noninvolved side to ascertain asymmetry.

Careful differentiation is required to use strength assessment and testing for diagnostic (as opposed to quantification) purposes. For example, the Cyriax method (see Chapter 7) maintains the joint in a neutral, relaxed position while assessing the muscle's contraction in various directions while keeping noncontractile (e.g., connective tissues) elements on slack. This method can reveal the presence of a contractile lesion if pain is produced during a contraction.[16] Alternatively, if the contraction is not painful while the joint is in a neutral position, an inert lesion, such as a bone spur or capsular inflammation, may be implicated. Of course, documentation of the method used is critical to the accurate measurement of progress.

The presence of pain, joint restriction, or muscle tightness may prevent the patient from assuming the correct testing position for accurate assessment of muscle testing. Although this text advocates testing the muscle in standardized positions, pain or other factors may not allow the standardized position to be used. The student should be aware that substitution patterns are more difficult to discern if an alternate position is used; thus, specific muscle strength quantification may not be possible. However, the clinician can document asymmetric differences, points in the range where pain exists or does not

exist, and the nature of the pain that may aid the clinician in making an accurate diagnosis.

Another challenge for clinicians in outpatient settings is the variety of patients seen on a given day. For example, a clinician may see a college or professional athlete in the same afternoon as a frail older adult. Careful discernment of appropriate strength testing is critical to avoid overestimation or underestimation of strength limitations. Using alternative muscle strength assessments as described in Chapters 7 to 9 may be useful to avoid biases.

WELLNESS CLINICS

Muscle screening provides feedback to participants regarding their abilities relative to age-matched reference samples that may impact functional abilities such as gait speed and chair stands. Although individual MMT is not routinely done as part of a wellness screening, functional movements such as floor transfers, 30-second sit-to-stands, or hand grip tests are useful to ascertain individual fitness levels and risk of disability. The information gleaned from a wellness assessment may indicate the need for an individualized assessment of strength to maintain age-based expectations of function.[17,18]

SUMMARY

MMT has utility in all clinical settings. However, it is incumbent on the clinician to judiciously use MMT when and if appropriate and to choose alternative forms of testing (e.g., functional and instrumented tests) when the information obtained from MMT is inadequate or inappropriate.

Even though muscle testing has tremendous value, there are situations in which it is not particularly informative, nor even accurate. Some of the clinical scenarios in which muscle testing is not optimal have already been discussed (e.g., in the presence of pain), but more detail will be presented in the next section.

As alluded to in Chapter 2, MMT has significant limitations. When MMT was first developed, the majority of patients seen by clinicians had polio with profound and variable muscle weakness. The current patient population has changed enormously, and clinicians now see hundreds of patient types who range in age from infancy to 100-plus years and with a variety of orthopedic, cardiovascular, and neurological conditions. As a result, the muscle testing system designed to pick up profound weakness in patients with polio is now used on healthy, fit individuals and individuals with a variety of medical and functional concerns. Muscle testing has changed simultaneously to more accurately reflect the needs of clients, and MMT is only one approach among many. Each form of testing has its advantages and disadvantages, as will be noted in this chapter and elsewhere in this book. The major limitations of traditional MMT are discussed in the following section.

POPULATION VARIATION

Many articles that report MMT results are based on studies of normal adults or specific subpopulations such as athletes, sedentary individuals, and older adults. Children and adolescents occupy a separate category. In addition, results of muscle testing values are reported for individuals with a wide variety of pathologies, including Parkinson disease, cerebral palsy, and muscular dystrophy. Because of this wide variation, it is necessary to utilize a variety of testing procedures. While some testers believe that the assigned grade should be modified based on age or ability, the authors strongly disagree and discourage this practice. Rather, MMT interpretation requires knowledge of the strength requirements of the task.

OBJECTIVITY

MMT, as originally described, suffers from a lack of objectivity, where objectivity is defined as a test not dependent primarily on the judgment of the clinician.[19,20] As discussed in Chapter 1, the ordinal scale of 5 to 0 used to assign muscle strength grades is not objective, and the use of qualitative terms such as "good" and "fair" further reduces its objectivity. However, it does provide useful information in a clinical assessment. Although clinical judgment is inherently a subjective assessment and cannot be discounted, the examination aspect of the patient encounter should primarily consist of objective measures.

RELIABILITY AND VALIDITY

Reliability in MMT varies considerably according to the muscle tested, the strength of the muscle, the experience of the clinician, the age of the patient, and the particular condition being tested. For example, in a study of 102 boys ages 5 to 15 years with Duchenne muscular dystrophy, intrarater reliability ranged from 0.65 to 0.93, with the proximal muscles having the higher reliability values.[21] The muscles with gravity minimized also had higher reliability values. In another study of physical therapists comparing MMT to handheld muscle dynamometry (HHD) in 11 patients, reliability was high and differentiated between grades at all levels.[22] In muscles with grades less than 3, reliability declined.[23-26] Yahyaei-Rad examined the reliability of MMT in a small study of 11 patients with neuropathy or myopathy. The author found MMT to have fair interexaminer reliability (0.62 to 0.82), with the measurement of proximal muscles having better reliability than that of distal muscles and Grade 2 being assessed with the most reliability (>0.86). Reliability also decreased for the muscles of the lower extremity.[26,27]

Because MMT as originally described is subjective, the historical and conventional acceptability for reliability is that, among clinicians and in successive tests with the same clinician, the results should be within one-half of a grade (or within a plus or minus of the base grade).[30] Others maintain that within the same grade is acceptable, pluses and minuses notwithstanding.[29] However, even if this historical convention is used, clinicians are unreliable in differentiating between the grades of 4 and 5.[9,25]

Clearly, the reliability of MMT is of concern, and yet MMT remains an important screening and diagnostic tool. Clinicians, especially novices, must be cautious about their test procedures and make vigorous attempts to standardize their methods. Reliability is increased by adhering to the same procedure for each test (one or several clinicians), providing clear instructions to the subject, having a quiet and comfortable environment for the test, and being conscious of age or gender biases. To further enhance the reliability of the manual muscle test, the following steps should be taken[29,30]:

- Ensure proper positioning to optimize the prime mover
- Ensure adequate stabilization of regional anatomy
- Observe the way the patient or subject assumes and maintains the test position
- Use consistent timing, pressure, and position
- Avoid preconceived impressions regarding the test outcome
- Use nonpainful contact and provide for a nonpainful execution of the test

SENSITIVITY

MMT also lacks sensitivity to change. Years ago, Beasley reported that patients with various neurological disorders who had Grade 4 knee extension forces were approximately 43% of Grade 5, rather than the traditionally defined 75% of Grade 5.[24] In the same study, the Grade 3 group generated force that was only 9%

of Grade 5, rather than traditionally assumed 50% of Grade 5.[24] Similarly, inadequate sensitivity was reported for detecting muscle force deficits when comparing compromised muscles to those that are Grade 5.[25] Clinicians have not shown the ability to accurately discern small or even moderate strength gains, thus making overgrading common.

DIAGNOSTIC VALIDITY

MMT is useful in the assessment of weakness of muscles directly involved with pain, injury, and neuromusculoskeletal disorders.[30] The Cyriax[16] method of discerning between contractile and noncontractile tissue is an example of muscle testing on the painful limb (see Chapter 7). In a study to detect differences between sides using MMT, the test accuracy had a sensitivity ranging from 62.9% to 72.3%, increasing with more pronounced strength differences.[30]

CEILING EFFECT

MMT has wide variability in the range of forces reported for a given grade, especially in the upper range of the scale. For example, in a subset of four studies, men with an MMT Grade 5 for knee extension and also concurrently tested with HHD demonstrated values ranging from 85.4 to 650.0 Newtons.[9] In addition, all settings with a variety of patient types were represented in the four studies. Grade 5 represented 86% of the range of measurable forces (Grades 3 to 5), and yet, knee extension forces of more than 800 Newtons are not unusual for young men.[30] Thus, MMT suffers from a profound ceiling effect. Many patients may be classified as having Grade 5 strength while exhibiting strength deficits only appreciated through more objective means such as functional testing. This ceiling effect may also mask changes in strength that have functional and prognostic consequences. Thus, it is not recommended that a change in a MMT grade be used as a goal or an objective measure of progress greater than the grade of 3 because of the issues described earlier. Rather, alternative forms of strength testing should be used (see Chapters 7 to 9).

Another concern about the applicability of MMT is its lack of accuracy in identifying impairments related to function, secondary to the curvilinear relationship of strength and function. The curvilinear relationship suggests that strength gains are not apparent when greater than a relative threshold. The relative threshold for some lower-level functional tasks (e.g. feeding oneself or walking unsupported) requires relatively low strength (compared to absolute strength potential). This threshold can easily be exceeded by the strength gain. Alternatively, traditional MMT may not reflect the amount of strength needed to perform strenuous functional tasks such as getting up from the floor or throwing a baseball because they exceed what a clinician can manually resist. When a basic manual muscle test screen reveals test grades that are greater than Grade 3, and in particular, where there are side-to-side differences, the clinician should rely on instrumented or functional testing to further clarify deficiencies and to differentiate between Grades 4 and 5 (see Chapters 7 to 9).

HHD may address some of the aspects of reliability. Because HHD records a number, it does not require the clinician to execute a judgment about a grade. However, other issues of MMT still hold true for HHD, such as tester strength, discussed later. HHD is further discussed in Chapter 9.

TESTER STRENGTH

A break test in MMT requires the clinician to exert a greater force than the patient in any given muscle. When testing a very strong individual, such as a weightlifter or football player, a greater amount of force on the part of the clinician may not be possible. Differences have been recorded in MMT forces between female and male clinicians, leading to an underestimation of the patient's quadriceps strength.[31] Mulroy and colleagues also found that female therapists overgraded the strength of the quadriceps in 14 of 19 patients, in part because of the patient's strength being greater than the clinician's.[31] Male clinicians assigned too high a grade in 2 of 19 patients.[31] A possible contributor to this discrepancy may be that women traditionally have 35% less upper body strength than men.[25]

SUMMARY

MMT appears to be both reliable and valid in the presence of profound weakness, such as that seen in neuromuscular diseases. However, when used in individuals with near-normal (Grade 5) levels of strength, it is recommended that MMT be used as a screening tool that informs alternative forms of strength testing such as those described in Chapters 7 to 9.

1. Bittner EA, Martyn JA, George E, et al. Measurement of muscle strength in the intensive care unit. *Crit Care Med.* 2009;37:S321–S330.

2. Andrews AW, Bohannon RW. Short-term recovery of limb muscle strength after acute stroke. *Arch Phys Med Rehabil.* 2003;84:125–130.

3. Vermeulen J, Neyens JC, van Rossum E, et al. Predicting ADL disability in community-dwelling elderly people using physical frailty indicators: a systematic review. *BMC Geriatr.* 2011;11:33.

4. Fried LP, Tangen CM, Walston J, et al. Frailty in older adults: evidence for a phenotype. *J Gerontol A Biol Sci Med Sci.* 2001;56A:M146–M156.

5. Fried TR, Mor V. Frailty and hospitalization of long-term stay nursing home residents. *J Am Geriatr Soc.* 1997;45:265–269.

6. Bortz WM. A conceptual framework of frailty: a review. *J Gerontol.* 2002;57A:M283–M288.

7. Visser M, Kritchevsky SB, Goodpaster B, et al. Leg muscle mass and composition in relation to lower extremity performance in men and women aged 70-79: the health, aging and body composition study. *J Am Geriatr Soc.* 2002;50:897–904.

8. Schwartz RS. Sarcopenia and physical performance in old age: introduction. *Muscle Nerve Suppl.* 1997;5:S10–S12.

9. Bohannon RW, Corrigan D. A broad range of forces is encompassed by the maximum manual muscle test grade of five. Percept Mot.

10. Xue QL, Bandeen-Roche K, Varadhan R, et al. Initial manifestations of frailty criteria and the development of frailty phenotype in the women's health and aging study II. *J Gerontol A Biol Sci Med Sci.* 2008;63:984–990.

11. U.S. Department of Health and Human Services. *Centers for Medicare & Medicaid Services, Home Health Services. Chapter 7: Medicare Benefit Policy Manual;* 2022:24–25. http://www.cms.gov/Regulations-and-Guidance/Guidance/Manuals/downloads/bp102c07.pdf. Accessed February 10, 2023.

12. Chang M, Cohen-Mansfield J, Ferrucci L, et al. Incidence of loss of ability to walk 400 meters in a functionally limited older population. *J Am Geriatr Soc.* 2004;52:2094–2098.

13. Shumway-Cook A, Patla AE, Stewart A, et al. Environmental demands associated with community mobility in older adults with and without mobility disabilities. *Phys Ther.* 2002;82:670–681.

14. Perry J, Garrett M, Gronley JK, et al. Classification of walking handicap in the stroke population. *Stroke.* 1995;26:982–989.

15. Maffiuletti NA. Assessment of hip and knee muscle function in orthopaedic practice and research. *J Bone Joint Surg Am.* 2010;92:220–229.

16. Cyriax JH. *Textbook of Orthopaedic Medicine: Diagnosis of Soft Tissue Lesions.* Vol. 1. 8th ed. London: Bailliere Tindall; 1982:14–21.

17. Rikli R, Jones J. Development and validation of a functional fitness test for community-residing older adults. *J Aging Phys Act.* 1999;7:129–161.

18. Rikli R, Jones J. Functional fitness normative scores for community-residing older adults, ages 60-94. *J Aging Phys Act.* 1999;7:162–181.

19. Knepler C, Bohannon RW. Subjectivity of forces associated with manual muscle test scores of 3+, 4-, and 4. *Percept Mot Skills.* 1998;87:1123–1128.

20. Bohannon RW. Objective measures. *Phys Ther.* 1989;69:590–593.

21. Florence JM, Pandya S, King WM, et al. Intrarater reliability of manual muscle test (medical research council scale) grades in Duchenne's muscular dystrophy. *Phys Ther.* 1992;72:115–122; discussion 122–126.

22. Wadsworth CT, Krishnan R, Sear M, et al. Intrarater reliability of manual muscle testing and hand-held dynametric muscle testing. *Phys Ther.* 1987;67:1342–1347.

23. Frese F, Brown M, Norton BJ. Clinical reliability of manual muscle testing: middle trapezius and gluteus medius muscles. *Phys Ther.* 1987;67:1072–1076.

24. Beasley WC. Quantitative muscle testing: principles and application to research and clinical services. *Arch Phys Med Rehabil.* 1961;42:398–425.

25. Wintz M. Variations in current manual muscle testing. *Phys Ther Rev.* 1959;39:466–475.

26. Cuthbert SCJ, Goodheart GJ. On the reliability and validity of manual muscle testing: a literature review. *Chiropr Osteopat.* 2007;15:4.

27. Yahyaei-Rad M. Inter-examiner reliability of the manual muscle strength testing. *J Basic Appl Sci Res.* 2012;2(12):13134–13138.

28. Lamb R. Manual muscle testing. In: Rothstein JM, ed. *Measurement in Physical Therapy.* New York: Churchill-Livingstone; 1985:47–55.

29. Palmer ML, Epler ME. *Fundamentals of Musculoskeletal Assessment Techniques.* 2nd ed. Philadelphia: Lippincott Williams & Wilkins; 1998.

30. Bohannon RW. Manual muscle testing: does it meet the standards of an adequate screening test? *Clin Rehabil.* 2005;19:662–667.

31. Mulroy SJ, Lassen KD, Chambers SH, et al. The ability of male and female clinicians to effectively test knee extension strength using manual muscle testing. *J Orthop Sports Phys Ther.* 1997;26:192–199.

CHAPTER

Testing the Muscles
of the Neck

Testing the Muscles of
the Neck

Capital Extension

Cervical Extension

Capital Flexion (Chin
Tuck)

Cervical Flexion

Flexion to Isolate a Single
Sternocleidomastoid

Cervical Rotation

INTRODUCTION

The neck musculature contributes approximately 80% of the mechanical stability of the cervical spine.[1] Thus, measurement of cervical muscle strength is important and relevant in many conditions. Trauma-related conditions such as whiplash or concussion, disease/disorder-related conditions such as rheumatoid arthritis, neuromuscular diseases such as Guillain-Barré syndrome, and posture-ergonomic–related conditions make cervical muscle testing especially relevant.[2] A grade of 3 out of 5, the strength equivalent to moving against gravity, is sufficient for many functional activities but may not be sufficient to resist trauma such as concussion or a whiplash movement.[2] Because individuals with neck pain have reduced maximal isometric neck strength and endurance capacity, individuals with cervical pain should be manually muscle tested.[3] Appropriate screening should be done before manual muscle testing of the cervical spine is performed if trauma or pathology is the source of the pain.

Isometric measurement is the most common and reliable method of assessing cervical muscle strength and will be the only procedure discussed here. Because studies have shown the deep cervical flexors are inhibited more often in the presence of neck pain,[4] differentiation between the deep cervical flexors (longus capitis and colli), which are responsible for the chin tuck movement and provide support of cervical lordosis and cervical joints,[5] and superficial cervical flexors (sternocleidomastoid and others), responsible for cervical flexion, is important.

Reliability of muscle testing of the cervical spine is affected by the lack of a fixed axis. This is particularly true with regard to the location of the thoracic support in prone extension. Reliability is also affected by the lack of bilaterality for comparison purposes and the lack of reference values.

Cervical flexion muscle strength is influenced by the position of the neck and maintenance of the normal lordosis. Cervical muscle strength is also affected by the position of the head over the thorax. In this text, we recommend resistance be placed at the mandible, below the chin.[2]

Assessments for cervical flexion musculature should include neck flexor muscle endurance tests.[6] For testing the endurance of the short neck flexors, a recent meta-analysis demonstrated moderate interrater reliability (intercorrelation coefficient [ICC] = 0.76) and good intrarater reliability (ICC = 0.86).[7] Another systematic review recommended lifting the head with a slight chin tuck (page 42) as the most reliable (ICC > 0.85).[3] Individuals with neck pain–related disorders have significantly less cervical strength and endurance.[3] Dvir and Prushansky found women's cervical spine strength to be approximately 40% that of men.[2]

As noted in Chapter 1, when obvious prime movers exist for a particular movement, they are bolded in the tables. However, in this chapter, there are no identifiable prime movers for capital extension, cervical extension, or capital flexion. It is the simultaneous contraction of a number of capital and cervical muscles that produces each of these three movements. Figures and tables are included in the chapter outlining the attachments, innervations, and functions for the muscles of capital extension (Figs. 3.1, 3.2 and Table 3.1), cervical extension (Figs. 3.6, 3.7 and Table 3.2), capital flexion (Figs. 3.12, 3.13 and Table 3.3), and cervical flexion (Figs. 3.19, 3.20 and Table 3.4).

POSTERIOR

FIGURE 3.1

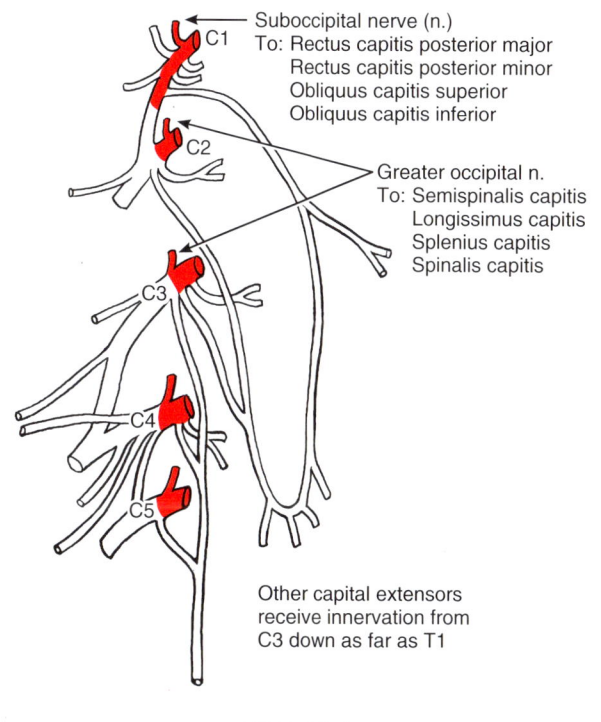

Suboccipital nerve (n.)
To: Rectus capitis posterior major
Rectus capitis posterior minor
Obliquus capitis superior
Obliquus capitis inferior

Greater occipital n.
To: Semispinalis capitis
Longissimus capitis
Splenius capitis
Spinalis capitis

Other capital extensors
receive innervation from
C3 down as far as T1

FIGURE 3.2

Range of Motion

0°–25°

Table 3.1 CAPITAL EXTENSION

I.D.	Muscle	Origin	Insertion	Function
56	Rectus capitis posterior major	Axis (spinous process)	Occiput (inferior nuchal line laterally)	Capital extension Rotation of head to same side Lateral bending of head to same side
57	Rectus capitis posterior minor	Atlas (tubercle of posterior arch)	Occiput (inferior nuchal line medially)	Capital extension
60	Longissimus capitis	T1-T5 vertebrae (transverse processes) C4-C7 vertebrae (articular processes)	Temporal bone (mastoid process, posterior surface)	Capital extension Lateral bending and rotation of head to same side
58	Obliquus capitis superior	Atlas (transverse process)	Occiput (between superior and inferior nuchal lines)	Capital extension of head on atlas (muscle on both sides) Lateral bending to same side (muscle on that side)
59	Obliquus capitis inferior	Axis (lamina and spinous process)	Atlas (transverse process, inferior-posterior surface)	Capital extension of head on atlas (muscle on both sides) Lateral bending to same side (muscle on that side)
61	Splenius capitis	Ligamentum nuchae C7-T4 vertebrae (spinous processes)	Temporal bone (mastoid process) Occiput (below superior nuchal line)	Capital extension Rotation of head to same side (debated) Lateral bending of head to same side
62	Semispinalis capitis (distinct medial part often named Spinalis capitis)	C7-T6 vertebrae (transverse processes) C4-C6 vertebrae (articular processes)	Occiput (between superior and inferior nuchal lines)	Capital extension (muscles on both sides) Rotation of head to opposite side (debated) Lateral bending of head to same side
63	Spinalis capitis	Medial part of Semispinalis capitis, usually blended inseparably	Occiput (between superior and inferior nuchal lines)	Capital extension

Grade 5 and Grade 4

Position of Patient: Prone with head off end of table. Arms at sides.

Instructions to Clinician: Stand at side of patient next to the head. Ask patient to tilt the head up and look at the wall. If sufficient range is present, use one hand to provide resistance over the occiput (Fig. 3.3). Place the other hand beneath the overhanging head for support should it give way with resistance. Resistance is applied directly opposite to the movement of the tilt of the head. Care should be made to test the head tilt and not push the neck into flexion.

Test: Patient extends head by tilting chin upward. (Cervical spine is not extended.)

Instructions to Patient: "Look at the wall. Hold it. Don't let me push your head down."

Grading

Grade 5: Patient completes available range of motion without substituting cervical extension. Tolerates maximum resistance. (This is a strong muscle group.)

Grade 4: Patient completes available range of motion without substituting cervical extension. Tolerates strong to moderate resistance.

Grade 3

Position of Patient: Prone with head off end of table, with head supported by clinician. Arms at sides.

Instructions to Clinician: Stand at side of patient's head. One hand should remain under the head to support it should the muscles fail to hold position (Fig. 3.4).

Instructions to Patient: "Look at the wall."

Test: Patient completes available range without resistance.

FIGURE 3.4

FIGURE 3.3

Grade 2, Grade 1, and Grade 0

Position of Patient: Supine with head on table. Arms at sides. Note: The gravity-minimized position (side lying) is not recommended for any tests of the neck for Grades 2 and below because test artifacts are created by the clinician in attempting to support the head without aiding the motion.

Instructions to Clinician: Stand at end of table, facing patient. Support head with two hands under the occiput. Place fingers just at the base of the occiput, lateral to the vertebral column to attempt to palpate the capital extensors (Fig. 3.5). Head may be slightly lifted off table to reduce friction.

Test: Patient attempts to look back toward clinician without lifting head from the table.

Instructions to Patient: "Tilt your chin up" OR "Look back at me. Don't lift your head."

Grading

Grade 2: Patient completes limited range of motion.

Grade 1 and Grade 0: Palpation of the capital extensors at the base of the occiput just lateral to the spine may be difficult; the splenius capitis lies most lateral, and the recti lie just next to the spinous process.

Clinical Relevance

Clinicians are reminded that the head is a heavy object suspended on thin support (neck). Whenever testing with patient's head off the table, care should be used for the patient's safety and comfort, especially in the presence of suspected or known neck or trunk weakness or pain. Always place a hand under the head to be ready to support it should the muscles give way.

FIGURE 3.5

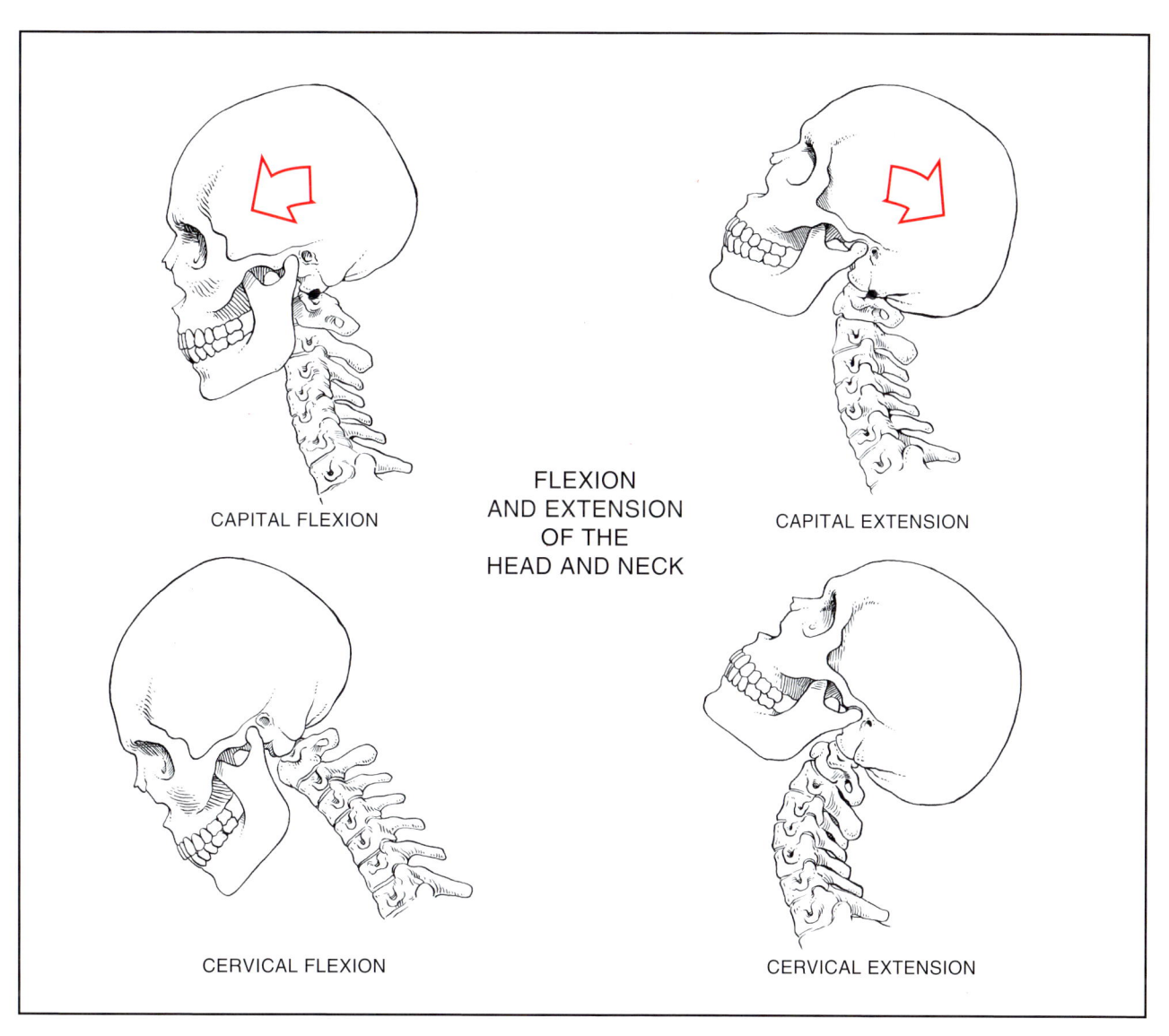

CAPITAL FLEXION

FLEXION
AND EXTENSION
OF THE
HEAD AND NECK

CAPITAL EXTENSION

CERVICAL FLEXION

CERVICAL EXTENSION

PLATE I

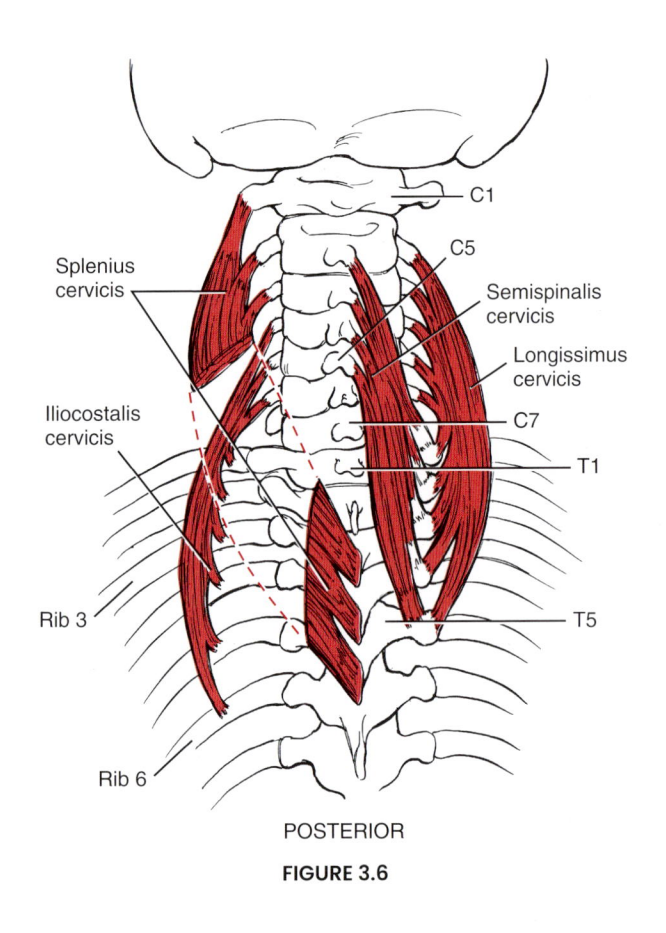

Splenius cervicis

Iliocostalis cervicis

Rib 3

Rib 6

C1

C5

Semispinalis cervicis

Longissimus cervicis

C7

T1

T5

POSTERIOR

FIGURE 3.6

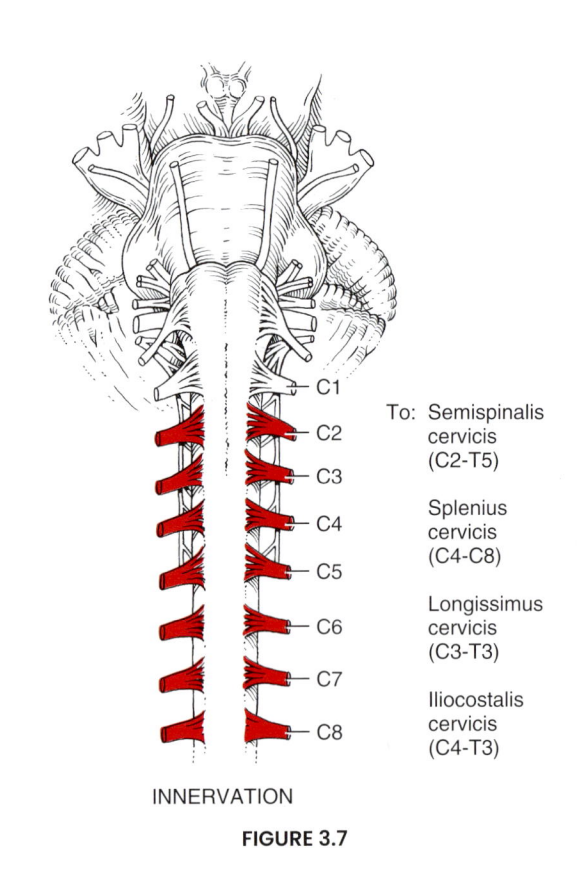

C1

C2

C3

C4

C5

C6

C7

C8

To: Semispinalis cervicis (C2-T5)

Splenius cervicis (C4-C8)

Longissimus cervicis (C3-T3)

Iliocostalis cervicis (C4-T3)

INNERVATION

FIGURE 3.7

Range of Motion
0° to <30°

Table 3.2 **CERVICAL EXTENSION**

I.D.	Muscle	Origin	Insertion	Function
64	Longissimus cervicis	T1-T5 vertebrae (transverse processes) variable	C2-C6 vertebrae (transverse processes)	Extension of the cervical spine (both muscles) Lateral bending of cervical spine to same side (one muscle)
65	Semispinalis cervicis	T1-T5 vertebrae (transverse processes)	Axis (C2)-C5 vertebrae (spinous processes)	Extension of the cervical spine (both muscles) Rotation of cervical spine to opposite side (one muscle) Lateral bending to same side
66	Iliocostalis cervicis	Ribs 3–6 (angles)	C4-C6 vertebrae (transverse processes, posterior tubercles)	Extension of the cervical spine (both muscles) Lateral bending to same side (one muscle) Depression of ribs (accessory)
67	Splenius cervicis (may be absent or variable)	T3-T6 vertebrae (spinous processes)	C1-C3 vertebrae (transverse processes)	Extension of the cervical spine (both muscles) Rotation of cervical spine to same side (one muscle) Lateral bending to same side (one muscle) Synergistic with opposite sternocleidomastoid
124	Trapezius (upper)	Occiput (protuberance and superior nuchal line, middle one-third) C7 (spinous process) Ligamentum nuchae T1-T12 vertebrae occasionally	Clavicle (posterior border of lateral one-third)	Elevation of scapula and shoulder ("shrugging") (with levator scapulae) Rotation of head to opposite side (one) Capital extension (both) Cervical extension (both)
68	Spinalis cervicis (often absent)	C7 and often C6 vertebrae (spinous processes) Ligamentum nuchae T1-T2 vertebrae occasionally	Axis (spinous process) C2-C3 vertebrae (spinous processes)	Extension of the cervical spine

Others

69	Interspinales cervicis			
70	Intertransversarii cervicis			
71	Rotatores cervicis			
94	Multifidi			
127	Levator scapulae			

Cervical extensor muscles are limited to those that act only on the cervical spine with motion centered in the lower cervical spine.

Grade 5 and Grade 4

Position of Patient: Prone with head off end of table. Arms at sides.

Instructions to Clinician: Stand next to patient's head. Ask patient to lift head while looking at the floor. If sufficient range is present, place hand applying resistance over parieto-occipital area (Fig. 3.8). Place other hand below the chin, ready to support the head should it suddenly give way during resistance.

Test: Patient extends neck without tilting chin.

Instructions to Patient: "Push up on my hand but keep looking at the floor. Hold it. Don't let me push your head down."

Grading

Grade 5: Patient holds test position against strong resistance. Clinician must use clinical caution because these muscles are not strong, and their maximum effort will not tolerate much resistance.

Grade 4: Patient holds test position against moderate resistance.

Grade 3:

Position of Patient: Prone with head off end of table. Arms at sides.

Instructions to Clinician: Stand next to patient's head with one hand supporting (or ready to support) the forehead (Fig. 3.9).

Test: Patient extends neck without looking up or tilting chin.

Instructions to Patient: "Lift your forehead from my hand, and keep looking at the floor."

Grading

Grade 3: Patient holds test position but without resistance.

FIGURE 3.9

FIGURE 3.8

Alternate Test for Grade 3: This test should be used if there is known or suspected trunk extensor weakness. The clinician should always have an assistant participate to provide protective guarding under the patient's forehead. This test is identical to the preceding Grade 3 test except that stabilization is provided by the clinician to the upper back by the forearm placed over the upper back with the hand cupped over the shoulder (Fig. 3.10).

FIGURE 3.10

Grade 2, Grade 1, and Grade 0

Position of Patient: Supine with head fully supported by table. Arms at sides.

Instructions to Clinician: Stand at the patient's head, facing the patient. Place both hands under the patient's head. Fingers should be distal to the occiput at the level of the cervical vertebrae for palpation (Fig. 3.11). Ask patient to push head into clinician's hands without any tilt.

Test: Patient attempts to extend neck into table without tilt.

Instructions to Patient: "Try to push your head down into my hands."

Grading

Grade 2: Patient moves through small range of neck extension by pushing into clinician's hands.

Grade 1: Contractile activity palpated in cervical extensors.

Grade 0: No discernable palpable muscle activity.

Clinical Relevance

Patients with a loss of cervical lordosis may have weak cervical extensors. Weak cervical extensors may be a risk factor for cervical kyphosis and dropped head syndrome.[8]

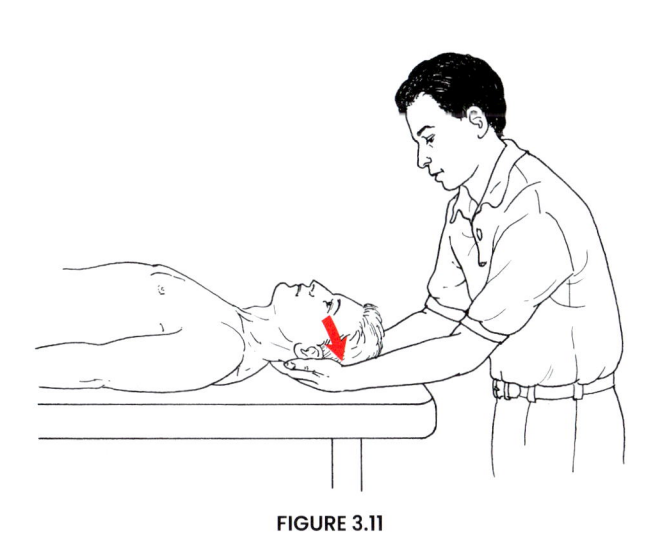

FIGURE 3.11

CAPITAL FLEXION (CHIN TUCK)

(Deep cervical flexors)

ANTERIOR

FIGURE 3.12

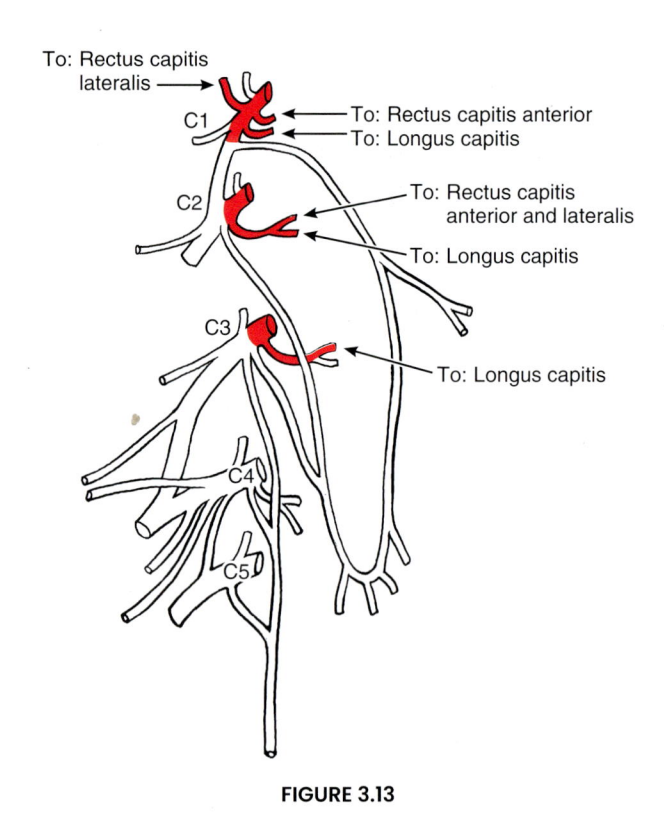

FIGURE 3.13

Range of Motion
0°–10°–15°

Table 3.3 CAPITAL FLEXION (CHIN TUCK)

I.D.	Muscle	Origin	Insertion	Function
72	Rectus capitis anterior	Atlas (C1) transverse process and lateral mass	Occiput (basilar part, inferior surface)	Capital flexion Stabilization of atlanto-occipital joint
73	Rectus capitis lateralis	Atlas (transverse process)	Occiput (jugular process)	Lateral bending of head to same side (obliquity of muscle) Assists head rotation Stabilizes atlanto-occipital joint (assists) Capital flexion
74	Longus capitis	C3-C6 vertebrae (transverse processes, anterior tubercles)	Occiput (basilar part, inferior surface)	Capital flexion Rotation of head to same side (muscle of one side)
Others				
Suprahyoids				
75	Mylohyoid			
76	Stylohyoid			
77	Geniohyoid			
78	Digastric			

(Deep cervical flexors)

The deep cervical flexors (longus capitis, rectus capitis, and colli) achieve capital flexion (nodding), called the chin tuck movement. The longus capitis and longus colli provide an active element of vertical stability to the cervical spine.[9] The weight of the head makes up one-seventh of body weight. Forward head posture (FHP) is the structural forward positioning of the head away from the center line of the body. In FHP, upper cervical vertebrae are extended and lower cervical vertebrae are flexed, increasing the force required to support the head by up to 3.6 times more than normal aligned posture.[10] In FHP, there is increased extension in the upper cervical joints and at the atlanto-occipital joint, causing the face to be directed upward (Fig. 3.14). FHP results in lengthening of the lower cervical flexors (sternocleidomastoid, scalenes, and upper cervical [capital] extensors) and results in weakness of the lower cervical extensors and upper capital flexors. FHP is commonly accompanied by thoracic kyphosis.

Starting Position of Patient: In all capital and cervical tests, the patient is supine with head supported on table and arms at sides (Fig. 3.15). The clinician should be aware of and avoid the tendency of the patient to use thoracic extensors to retract the head and cervical spine when exerting a maximal effort during testing of capital flexion.

FIGURE 3.14

FIGURE 3.15

CAPITAL FLEXION (CHIN TUCK)

(Deep cervical flexors)

Grade 5 and Grade 4

Position of Patient: Supine with head on table. Arms at sides.

Instructions to Clinician: Stand at head of table, facing patient. Ask patient to tuck chin. If sufficient range is present, place cupped hands under the mandible to give resistance against chin tuck, in an upward direction (Fig. 3.16).

Test: Patient tucks chin into neck without raising head from table. No motion should occur at the cervical spine. This is the motion of nodding.

Instructions to Patient: "Tuck your chin and keep your eyes straight ahead. Don't lift your head from the table. Hold it. Don't let me lift up your chin."

Grading

Grade 5: Patient holds test position against maximum resistance. These are very strong muscles.

Grade 4: Patient holds test position against moderate resistance.

Grade 3:

Position of Patient: Supine with head supported on table. Arms at sides.

Instructions to Clinician: Stand at head of table, facing patient.

Test: Patient tucks chin without lifting head from table (Fig. 3.17).

Instructions to Patient: "Tuck your chin into your neck. Do not raise your head from the table."

FIGURE 3.17

FIGURE 3.16

Grading

Grade 3: Patient completes available range of motion without resistance.

Grade 2, Grade 1, and Grade 0

Position of Patient: Supine with head supported on table. Arms at sides.

Instructions to Clinician: Stand at head of table, facing patient. Ask patient to tuck chin.

Test: Patient attempts to tuck chin (Fig. 3.18).

Instructions to Patient: "Try to tuck your chin into your neck."

Grading

Grade 2: Patient completes partial range of motion.

Grade 1: Contractile activity may be palpated in capital flexor muscles, but it is difficult, and only minimal pressure should be used.

Grade 0: No discernable contractile activity.

FIGURE 3.18

Clinical Relevance

- Palpation of small and deep muscles of capital flexion may be a difficult task unless the patient has severe atrophy. It is NOT recommended that much pressure be put on the neck when palpating. Remember that the ascending arterial supply (carotids) to the brain runs quite superficially in this region.
- In patients with lower motor neuron lesions that do not affect cranial nerves, capital flexion is seldom lost. This can possibly be attributed to the suprahyoid muscles, which are innervated by cranial nerves. The suprahyoid muscles also play an important role in speech, tongue movement, and swallowing[9] (all of which can be assessed to identify recruitment and activity of these muscles).
- When capital flexion is impaired or absent, there usually is serious impairment of the cranial nerves, and other central nervous system (CNS) signs are present that may require further evaluation by the clinician.

- Endurance of the neck flexors can be assessed by a cervical flexion test where the patient is in hook-lying position and asked to lift their head and neck 1 inch above the table while maintaining a maximal chin tuck position.[11] The time is recorded for how long the patient can maintain this position. Endurance of the deep cervical flexors decreases approximately one-third with neck pain (40 seconds compared with 23 seconds).[11]
- Forward head posture (FHP) is common in individuals who sit for long periods viewing a screen or who use bifocals (see Fig. 3.14).
- Capital flexors may be weak in the presence of FHP.
- For those patients with a thoracic kyphosis that is severe enough to prevent the head from lying flat or even reaching the table in a supine position, use pillows to support the cervical area so the head is in line with the trunk before testing.

ANTERIOR

FIGURE 3.19

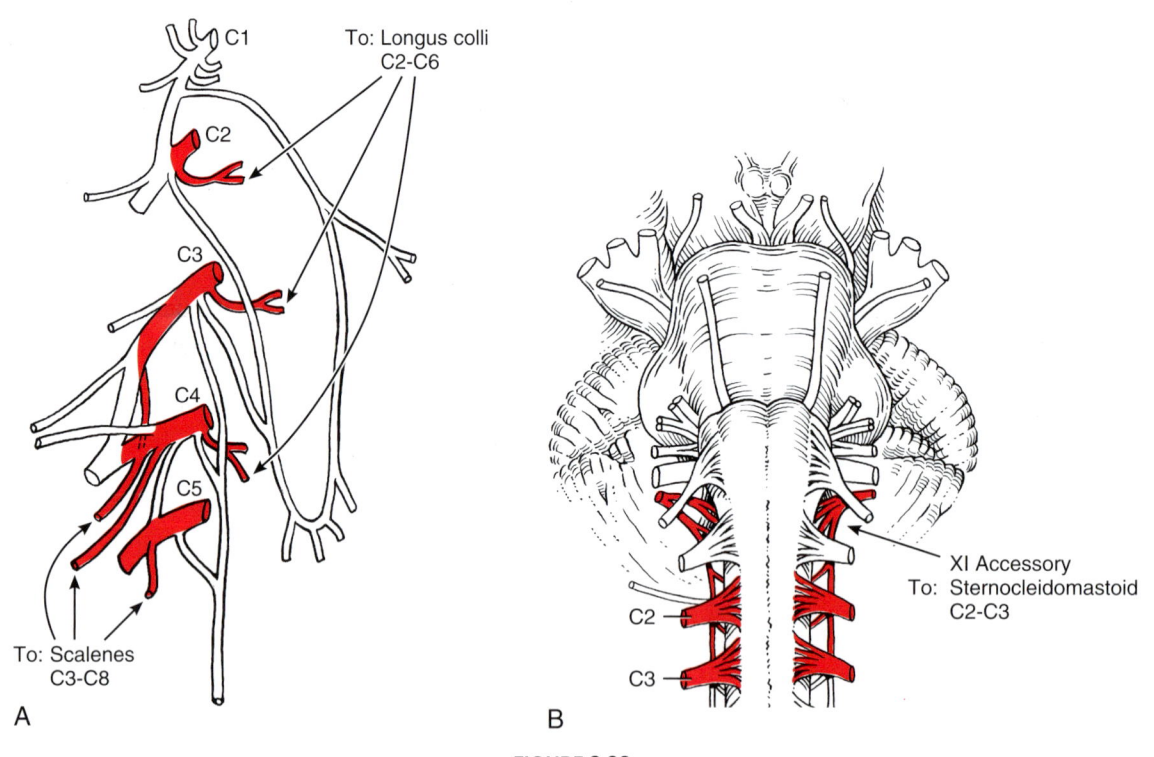

A

To: Scalenes
C3-C8

To: Longus colli
C2-C6

B

XI Accessory
To: Sternocleidomastoid
C2-C3

FIGURE 3.20

Range of Motion
0°–35°–45°

Table 3.4 **CERVICAL FLEXION**

I.D.	Muscle	Origin	Insertion	Function
83	Sternocleidomastoid			Bilateral action: Flexion of cervical of cervical spine Unilateral action Lateral bending of cervical spine to same side Rotation of head to opposite side Capital extension (posterior fibers) Raises sternum in forced inspiration
	Sternal head	Sternum (Manubrium, upper anterior aspect)	Two heads blend in middle of neck; occiput (lateral half of superior nuchal line)	
	Clavicular head	Clavicle (medial one-third superior and anterior surfaces)	Temporal bone (mastoid process)	
79	Longus colli			Cervical flexion (weak) Cervical rotation to opposite side (inferior oblique head) Lateral bending (superior and inferior oblique heads) (debatable)
	Superior oblique head	C3-C5 vertebrae (transverse processes)	Atlas (anterior arch, tubercle)	
	Vertical intermediate head	T1-T3 and C5-C7 vertebrae (anterolateral bodies)	C2-C4 vertebrae (anterior bodies)	
	Inferior oblique head	T1-T3 vertebrae (anterior bodies)	C5-C6 vertebrae (transverse processes, anterior tubercles)	
80	Scalenus anterior	C3-C6 vertebrae (transverse processes, anterior tubercles)	First rib (scalene tubercle)	Flexion of cervical spine (both muscles) Elevation of 1st rib in inspiration Rotation of cervical spine to same side Lateral bending of neck to same side

Others

81	Scalenus medius			
82	Scalenus posterior			

Infrahyoids

84	Sternothyroid			
85	Thyrohyoid			
86	Sternohyoid			
87	Omohyoid			

Chin tuck position should be gently maintained when testing the cervical flexors, avoiding an extended cervical position.

Grade 5 and Grade 4

Position of Patient: Supine, with knees bent and feet on the table (hook lying), arms at sides.[3]

Instructions to Clinician: Stand next to patient's head. Ask patient to lift head from table while keeping chin tucked in with eyes towards ceiling. If sufficient range is present, place hand for resistance on patient's chin. Only use two fingers (Fig. 3.21). Other hand may be placed on chest, but stabilization is needed only when the trunk is weak.

Test: Patient lifts head straight up from the table while tucking their chin. This is a weak muscle group.

Instructions to Patient: "Lift your head from the table; keep your chin tucked in while looking at the ceiling. Do not lift your shoulders off the table. Hold it. Don't let me push your head down."

Grading

Grade 5 and Grade 4: Patient is able to hold test position against moderate to mild two-finger resistance.

Grade 3

No resistance is used (Fig. 3.22).

FIGURE 3.21

FIGURE 3.22

Grade 2, Grade 1, and Grade 0

Position of Patient: Supine with head supported on table. Arms at sides.

Instructions to Clinician: Stand at head of table, facing patient. Index fingers of each hand are placed over the sternocleidomastoid muscles to palpate them during test (Fig. 3.23).

Test: Patient rolls head from side to side, keeping head supported on table.

Instructions to Patient: "Roll your head to the left and then to the right."

Grading

Grade 2: Patient completes partial range of motion. The right sternocleidomastoid produces the roll to the left side and vice versa.

Grade 1: No motion occurs, but contractile activity in one or both muscles can be detected.

Grade 0: No motion and no discernable contractile activity detected.

FIGURE 3.23

Substitution

The platysma may attempt to substitute for weak or absent sternocleidomastoid muscles during cervical or combined flexion. When this occurs, the corners of the mouth pull down; a grimacing expression or "what do I do now?" expression is seen. Superficial muscle activity will be apparent over the anterior surface of the neck, with skin wrinkling.

Grade 5, Grade 4, and Grade 3

Position of Patient: Supine with head supported on table and turned to the left (to test right sternocleidomastoid).

Instructions to Clinician: Stand at head of table, facing patient. Ask patient to raise head from table while keeping head turned. If sufficient range is present, place hand applying resistance on the temporal area above the ear for resistance (Fig. 3.24).

Test: Patient raises head from table.

Instructions to Patient: "Lift up your head, keeping your head turned."

Grading

Grade 5: Patient holds test position and tolerates strong resistance. This is usually a very strong muscle group.

Grade 4: Patient holds test position and tolerates moderate resistance.

Grade 3: Patient completes available range of motion without resistance (Fig. 3.25).

Grade 2, Grade 1, and Grade 0

Position of Patient: Supine with head supported on table.

Instructions to Clinician: Stand at head of table, facing patient. Place index finger of each hand alongside the head and neck to palpate the sternocleidomastoid (see Fig. 3.23).

Test: Patient attempts to roll head from side to side.

Instructions to Patient: "Roll your head to the right and then to the left."

Grading

Grade 2: Patient completes partial range of motion.

Grade 1: Palpable contractile activity in the sternocleidomastoid but no movement.

Grade 0: No discernable contractile activity.

FIGURE 3.25

FIGURE 3.24

Fifty percent of the total neck rotation occurs between C1 and C2 before any rotation is noted throughout the remainder of the cervical spine.[12]

Grade 5, Grade 4, and Grade 3

Position of Patient: Supine with cervical spine in neutral (flexion and extension). Head supported on table with face turned as far to one side as possible. Sitting is an alternative position for all tests.

Instructions to Clinician: Stand at head of table, facing patient. Ask patient to turn head. If sufficient range exists, place hand for resistance over the side of patient's head above the ear (Grades 5 and 4 only).

Test: Patient rotates head to neutral against maximum resistance. This is a strong muscle group. Repeat for rotators on the opposite side. Alternatively, have patient rotate from left side of face on table to right side of face on table.

Instructions to Patient: "Turn your head and face the ceiling. Hold it. Don't let me turn your head back."

Grading

Grade 5: Patient holds test position with maximum resistance.

Grade 4: Patient holds test position with moderate resistance.

Grade 3: Patient rotates head through full available range of motion to both right and left without resistance.

Grade 2, Grade 1, and Grade 0

Position of Patient: Sitting. Trunk and head may be supported against a high-back chair. Head posture neutral.

Instructions to Clinician: Stand directly in front of patient.

Test: Patient tries to rotate head from side to side, keeping the neck in neutral (chin neither down nor up).

Instructions to Patient: "Turn your head as far to the left as you can. Keep your chin level." Repeat for turn to right.

Grading

Grade 2: Patient completes partial range of motion.

Grade 1: Contractile activity in sternocleidomastoid or posterior muscles visible or evident by palpation. No movement.

Grade 0: No discernable palpable contractile activity.

Participating Muscles in Cervical Rotation (With ID Numbers)

56.	Rectus capitis posterior major	74.	Longus capitis
59.	Obliquus capitis inferior	79.	Longus colli (Inferior oblique)
60.	Longissimus capitis	80.	Scalenus anterior
61.	Splenius capitis	81.	Scalenus medius
62.	Semispinalis capitis	82.	Scalenus posterior
65.	Semispinalis cervicis	83.	Sternocleidomastoid
67.	Splenius cervicis	124.	Trapezius
71.	Rotatores cervicis	127.	Levator scapulae

Supplemental Video Resources

Visit Elsevier eBooks+ (eBooks.Health.Elsevier.com) to access supplemental videos about the following tests:
- Capital Extension
- Cervical Extension
- Capital Flexion
- Cervical Flexion
- Combined Flexion to Isolate a Single Sternocleidomastoid
- Cervical Rotation

REFERENCES

1. Panjabi MM, Cholewicki J, Nibu K, et al. Critical load of the human cervical spine: an in vitro experimental study. *Clin Biomech (Bristol, Avon)*. 1998;13(1):11–17.

2. Dvir Z, Prushansky T. Cervical muscles strength testing: methods and clinical implications. *J Manip Physiol Ther*. 2008;31(7):518–524.

3. de Koning CH, van den Heuvel SP, Staal JB, et al. Clinimetric evaluation of methods to measure muscle functioning in patients with non-specific neck pain: a systematic review. *BMC Musculoskelet Disord*. 2008;19(9):142.

4. Jull GA, O'Leary SP, Falla DL. Clinical assessment of the deep cervical flexor muscles: the craniocervical flexion test. *J Manip Physiol Ther*. 2008;31(7):525–533.

5. Falla D, Jull G, Dall'Alba P, et al. An electromyographic analysis of the deep cervical flexor muscles in performance of craniocervical flexion. *Phys Ther*. 2003;83(10):899–906.

6. Blanpied PR, Gross AR, Elliott JM, et al. Neck pain: revision 2017. *J Orthop Sports Phys Ther*. 2017;47(7):A1–A83. https://doi.org/10.2519/jospt.2017.0302. PMID: 28666405.

7. Selistre LFA, Melo CS, Noronha MA. Reliability and validity of clinical tests for measuring strength or endurance of cervical muscles: a systematic review and meta-analysis. *Arch Phys Med Rehabil*. 2021;102(6):1210–1227. https://doi.org/10.1016/j.apmr.2020.11.018. Epub 2020 Dec 28. PMID: 33383030.

8. Alpayci M, Şenköy E, Delen V, et al. Decreased neck muscle strength in patients with the loss of cervical lordosis. *Clin Biomech (Bristol, Avon)*. 2016;33:98–102.

9. Neumann DA. *Kinesiology of the Musculoskeletal System: Foundations for Rehabilitation*. St. Louis, MO: Elsevier; 2017. ISBN: 978-0-323-28753-1.

10. Park SY, Yoo WG. Effects of the sustained computer work on upper cervical flexion motion. *J Phys Ther Sci*. 2014;26:441–442.

11. Harris KD, Heer DM, Roy TC, et al. Reliability of a measurement of neck flexor muscle endurance. *Phys Ther*. 2005;85:1349–1355.

12. Schäfer AGM, Schöttker-Königer T, Hall TM, et al. Upper cervical range of rotation during the flexion-rotation test is age dependent: an observational study. *Ther Adv Musculoskelet Dis*. 2020;12:1–9. https://www.ncbi.nlm.nih.gov/pmc/articles/PMC7607754/.

4

Testing the Muscles of the Trunk and Pelvic Floor

Trunk Extension

Lumbar Spine

Thoracic Spine

Elevation of the Pelvis

Trunk Flexion

Trunk Rotation

Core Tests

Core Strength, Stability, and Endurance

Quiet Inspiration

Diaphragm

Intercostals

Forced Expiration

Pelvic Floor

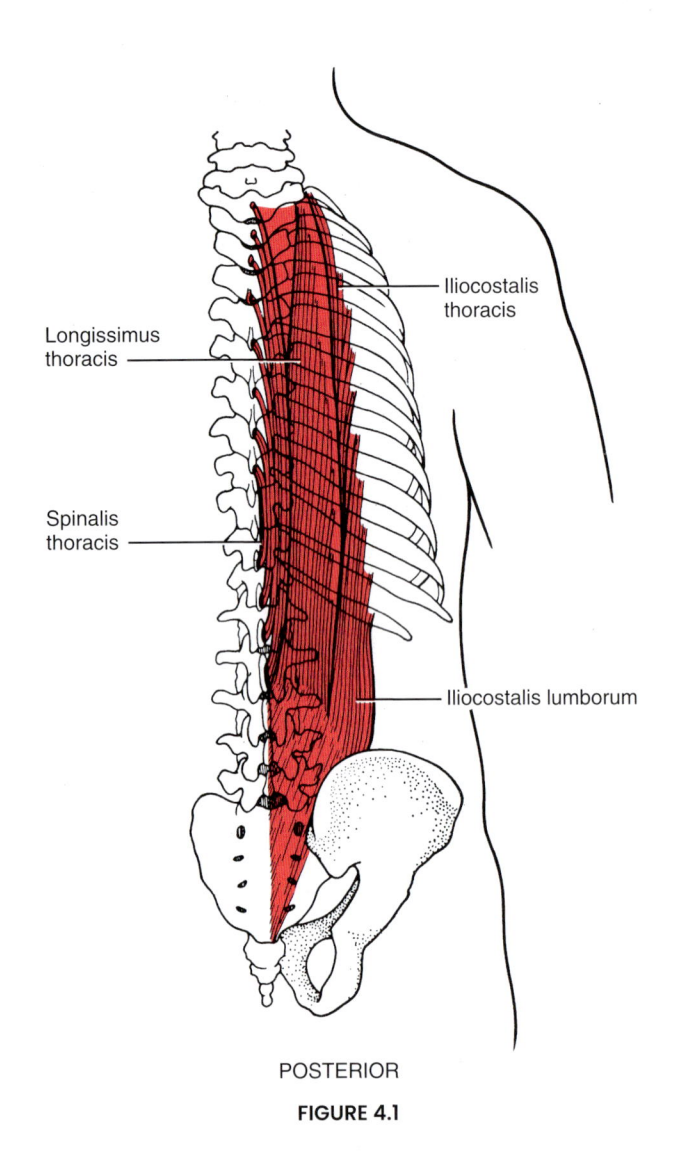

Iliocostalis
thoracis

Longissimus
thoracis

Spinalis
thoracis

Iliocostalis lumborum

POSTERIOR

FIGURE 4.1

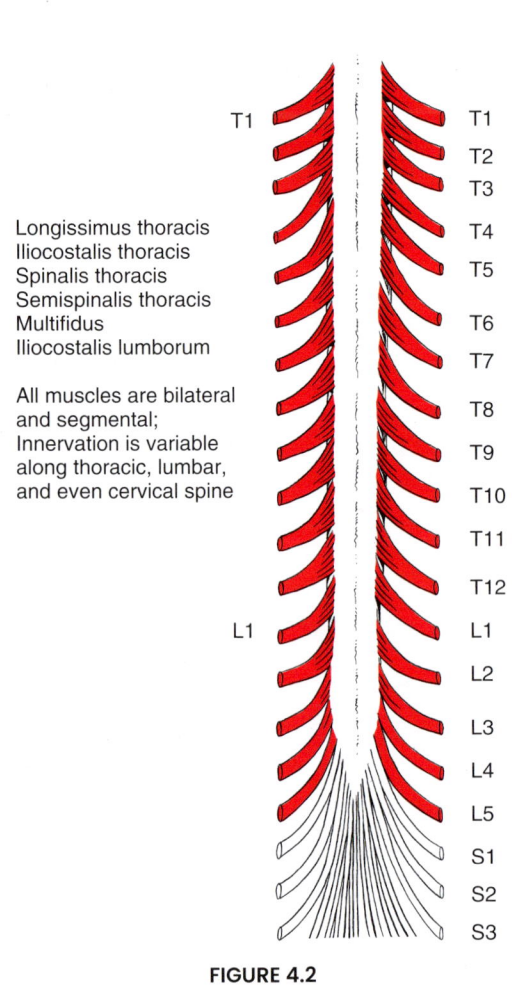

Longissimus thoracis
Iliocostalis thoracis
Spinalis thoracis
Semispinalis thoracis
Multifidus
Iliocostalis lumborum

All muscles are bilateral
and segmental;
Innervation is variable
along thoracic, lumbar,
and even cervical spine

FIGURE 4.2

Range of Motion	
Thoracic spine: 0°–10°	
Lumbar spine: 0°–25°	

Table 4.1 TRUNK EXTENSION

I.D.	Muscle	Origin	Insertion	Function
89	Iliocostalis thoracis	Ribs 12 up to 7 (angles)	Ribs 6 up to 1 (angles) C7 vertebra (transverse processes)	Extension of the spine Lateral bending of spine to same side (muscles on one side) Depression of ribs
90	Iliocostalis lumborum	Tendon of erector spinae (anterior surface) Thoracolumbar fascia Sacrum (posterior surface)	Ribs 6–12 (angles)	Extension of spine Lateral bending of spine (muscles on one side) Depression of ribs (lumborum) Elevation of pelvis
91	Longissimus thoracis	Tendon of erector spinae Thoracolumbar fascia L1-L5 vertebrae (transverse processes)	T1-T12 vertebrae (transverse processes) Ribs 2–12 (between angles and tubercles)	Extension of the spine Lateral bending of spine to same side (muscles on one side) Depression of ribs
92	Spinalis thoracis (often indistinct)	Common tendon of erector spinae T11-L2 vertebrae (spinous processes)	T1-T4 vertebrae (or to T8, spinous processes) Blends with semispinalis thoracis	Extension of spine
93	Semispinalis thoracis	T6-T10 vertebrae (transverse processes)	C6-T4 vertebrae (spinous processes)	Extension of thoracic spine
94	Multifidi	Sacrum (posterior) Erector spinae (aponeurosis) Ilium (PSIS) and crest Sacroiliac ligaments L1-L5 vertebrae (mamillary processes) T1-T12 vertebrae (transverse processes) C4-C7 vertebrae (articular processes)	Spinous processes of higher vertebra (may span 2–4 vertebrae before inserting)	Extension of spine Lateral bending of spine (muscle on one side) Rotation to opposite side
95, 96	Rotatores thoracis and lumborum (11 pairs)	Thoracic and lumbar vertebrae (transverse processes; variable in lumbar area)	Next highest vertebra (lower border of lamina)	Extension of thoracic spine Rotation to opposite side
97, 98	Interspinales thoracis and lumborum	Thoracis: (3 pairs) between spinous processes of contiguous vertebrae (T1 T2, T2-T3, T11-T12) Lumborum: (4 pairs) lie between the 5 lumbar vertebrae; run between spinous processes	See origin	Extension of spine
99	Intertransversarii thoracis and lumborum	Thoracis: (3 pairs) between transverse processes of contiguous vertebrae T10-T12 and L1 Lumborum: medial muscles; accessory process of superior vertebra to mamillary process of vertebra below Lateral muscles: fill space between transverse processes of adjacent vertebrae	See origin	Extension of spine (muscles on both sides) Lateral bending to same side (muscles on one side) Rotation to opposite side

Continued

Table 4.1 TRUNK EXTENSION—cont'd

I.D.	Muscle	Origin	Insertion	Function
100	Quadratus lumborum	Ilium (crest and inner lip) Iliolumbar ligament	12th rib (lower border) L1-L4 vertebrae (transverse processes) T12 vertebra (body)	Elevation of pelvis (weak in contrast to lateral abdominals) Extension of lumbar spine (muscles on both sides) Inspiration (via stabilization of lower attachments of diaphragm) Fixation of lower portions of diaphragm for prolonged vocalization, which needs sustained expiration. Lateral bending of lumbar spine to same side (pelvis fixed) Fixation and depression of 12th rib
Other				
182	Gluteus maximus (provides stable base for trunk extension by stabilizing pelvis)			

PSIS, Posterior superior iliac spine.

The importance of spinal extensors' muscle strength and endurance cannot be understated, as they are implicated in back pain, posture, poor bone mass, gait, and balance (Figs. 4.1 and 4.2). For example, in older women with severely flexed posture (>8 cm from occiput to the wall), spinal extensors and abdominal muscles were found to be weaker than in those with mildly flexed posture.[1] Exaggerated postures, such as extreme lumbar lordosis and pelvic tilt, produce greater muscle activity than more optimal postures, and this has implications for clinicians.[2] Muscle function in the neutral zone is important for stabilization of the lumbar spine.[3,4] Stabilization occurs through global and local stabilizers. Global stabilizers include the rectus abdominis and external oblique muscles. These muscles generate a large amount of muscle torque across multiple segments and thus control movement. Local stabilizers are the deeper muscles, having their origin or insertion directly or indirectly on the lumbar vertebrae.

Transversus abdominis (TA) and lumbar multifidus are examples of local stabilizers. This active system of global and local muscles provides lumbar stabilization.[5,6] Trunk flexors and extensors form the core, discussed later in this chapter.

Trunk extensor muscles are tonic or endurance-type muscles, whereas trunk flexors are phasic or shorter acting. Therefore, the maximum force generated per unit of muscle mass should be expected to be different (less for the extensors). Trunk extensor endurance has a role in upright posture and back pain, and therefore, it may be informative to test the patient's hold time via isometric contractions. Trunk extensors also control trunk flexion eccentrically.

Although there is no "gold standard" for the testing of spinal and abdominal muscles, this chapter includes methods from the best evidence as well as time-honored traditional methods.

Grade 5 and Grade 4

Position of Patient: Prone with fingertips lightly touching the side of the head and shoulders in external rotation. The weight of the head and arms essentially substitutes for manual resistance by the clinician.

Instructions to Clinician: Stand at side of patient to stabilize the lower extremities just above the ankles (Fig. 4.3). Ask patient to raise the head, shoulders, and chest off the table. Observe quality of motion and ability to hold the test position.

Alternate Instructions to Clinician: If the patient has hip extension weakness, stabilize the lower extremities by leaning firmly over the patient's body, placing both arms across the pelvis. Note that it is very difficult to stabilize the pelvis adequately in the presence of significant hip weakness (Fig. 4.4).

Test: Patient extends the lumbar spine until the entire trunk is raised from the table (clears umbilicus).

Instructions to Patient: "Raise your head, shoulders, and chest off the table. Come up as high as you can."

Grading

Grade 5 and Grade 4: Clinician distinguishes between Grade 5 and Grade 4 muscles by observing the response (see Figs. 4.3 and 4.4). The Grade 5 muscle holds the test position like a lock; the Grade 4 muscle yields slightly because of an elastic quality at the end point. The patient with Grade 5 back extensor muscles can quickly come to the end position and hold that position without evidence of significant effort. The patient with Grade 4 back extensors can come to the end position but may waver and/or display some signs of increased effort.

FIGURE 4.3

FIGURE 4.4

Grade 5 and Grade 4

Position of Patient: Prone with head and upper trunk extending off the table from about the nipple line (Fig. 4.5). Hands should be lightly touching the side of the head, with shoulders and elbows retracted (back).

Instructions to Clinician: Stand at side of patient to stabilize the lower limbs at the ankle. Ask patient to raise the head, shoulders, and chest to table level. (Note that this position does not require the same degree of stabilization as the lumbar extension tests.)

Test: Patient extends thoracic spine to the horizontal. This will be a small movement, and care should be made not to extend farther than horizontal because further movement will cause lumbar extension.

Instructions to Patient: "Raise your head, shoulders, and chest to table level."

Grading

Grade 5: Patient raises the upper trunk quickly from its forward flexed position to the horizontal with ease and no sign of exertion (Fig. 4.6).

Grade 4: Patient raises the trunk to the horizontal level but does so with obvious effort.

FIGURE 4.5

Grade 3

Note: Grades 3, 2, 1, and 0 tests involve the lumbar and thoracic spine.

Position of Patient: Prone with arms at sides.

Instructions to Clinician: Stand at side of table. Stabilize lower extremities just above the ankles.

Test: Patient extends spine, raising body from the table so that the umbilicus clears the table (Fig. 4.7).

Instructions to Patient: "Raise your head, arms, and chest from the table as high as you can."

Grading

Grade 3: Patient completes the range of motion.

FIGURE 4.6

FIGURE 4.7

Grade 2, Grade 1, and Grade 0:

These tests are identical to the Grade 3 test except that the clinician must palpate the lumbar and thoracic spine extensor muscle masses adjacent to both sides of the spine. The individual muscles cannot be isolated (Figs. 4.8 and 4.9).

Grading

Grade 2: Patient completes partial range of motion.

Grade 1: Contractile activity is detectable but no movement.

Grade 0: No discernable contractile activity.

FIGURE 4.8

FIGURE 4.9

Clinical Relevance

- When spinal extensors are strong and hip extensors are weak, the patient can hyperextend the low back (increased lordosis) but will be unable to raise the trunk without very strong stabilization of the pelvis by the clinician.
- If neck extensors are weak, the clinician may need to support the head as the patient raises the trunk.
- When spinal extensors are weak and hip extensors are strong, the patient will be unable to raise the upper trunk from the table. Instead, the pelvis will tilt posteriorly while the lumbar spine moves into flexion (low back flattens).
- If hip extensor muscles are Grade 4 or better, it may be helpful to use belts to anchor hips to the table, especially if the patient is much larger or stronger than the testing clinician.
- If the patient is unable to provide stabilization through the weight of the legs and pelvis (such as in paraplegia or amputee), the test should be done on a mat table. Position the subject with both legs and pelvis off the mat. This allows the pelvis and limbs to contribute to stabilization, and the clinician holding the lower trunk has a chance to provide the necessary support. (If a mat table is not available, an assistant will be required, and the lower body may rest on a chair.)

Sørensen Lumbar Spine Extension Test

The Biering-Sørensen test or Sørensen test is a measure of isometric endurance capacity of back extensors and perhaps hip extensor muscles.[7,8] The modified Sørensen test is a similar test with patient arms at the side of the trunk, rather than across the chest, as in the original Biering-Sørensen test.

Position of Patient: Prone with trunk flexed off the end of the table at a level between the anterior superior iliac spine (ASIS) and umbilicus. Until the test begins, the patient may stretch arms over a chair (in front of table) to provide support for the trunk (not shown).

Instructions to Clinician: Lean over patient to firmly stabilize the lower limbs and pelvis at the ankles. Ask patient to fold arms across the chest and then raise head, chest, and trunk so the trunk is straight. Use a stopwatch to time the effort, starting it at the "begin" command and stopping it when the patient shows obvious signs of fatigue and begins to falter.[9]

Test: Patient lifts the trunk to the horizontal and maintains test position as long as possible (Fig. 4.10).

Instructions to Patient: "When I say 'begin,' lift your head, chest, and trunk from the table and hold the position as long as you can. I will be timing you."

FIGURE 4.10

Clinical Relevance

- The Sørensen test elicits no greater than 40% to 52% of the maximal voluntary contractile force.[8]
- Back extensor strength declines approximately 40% to 50% from the 3rd to 8th decades of life, markedly reducing endurance time (Table 4.2).[10-12]
- The Sørensen test has been validated as a differential diagnostic test for low back pain.[7,13]
- With a cutoff score of 28 seconds for men and 29 seconds for women, the Sørensen test had a sensitivity of 92.3% and specificity of 76.0% to predict low back pain in men and 84.3% sensitivity and 84.6% specificity for women.[14]

Table 4.2 AGE-BASED NORMS FOR MODIFIED SØRENSEN TEST

Age	Mean Hold Time in Seconds (SD)[a] Males	Mean Hold Time in Seconds (SD) Females
19–29	140[12]	130[90]
30–39	130[12]	120
35–39	97 (43)[90]	93 (55)[90]
40–44	101 (57)[90]	80 (55)[90]
40–49	120[12]	90[90]
45–49	99 (58)[90]	102 (64)[90]
50–54	89 (55)[90]	69 (60)[90]
50–59	90[12]	75[12]
60+	80[12]	90[12]

[a]Numbers in parentheses refer to standard deviation (SD). The standard deviation is only available for some age groups.
[12]Data from 561 healthy, nonsmoking subjects in Nigeria without low back pain.
[90]Data from 508 subjects with and without back pain that comprised equal groups of blue- and white-collar male and female subjects.

Suggested Strength Exercise for Thoracic Spine

Note: no studies obtaining electromyography (EMG) maximum voluntary isometric contraction (MVIC) results were found in the literature. The exercises listed later are recommended after a synthesis of the literature by Heneghan and colleagues.[15]
- Deadlift (creating stiffness in thoracic spine)
- Partner backward fall with arms overhead (creating stiffness in thoracic spine)
- Side pull prowler
- Partner push (creating stiffness in thoracic spine)
- Battle ropes (power)
- Side medicine ball throws (power)

Suggested Strength Exercises for Lumbar Spine[16]

Isolation of lumbar extensors requires adequate restraint of the pelvis to limit involvement of the hip extensors.
- Roman Chair
- Deadlifts
- Squats
- Extension-based resistance machines

Quadratus
lumborum

POSTERIOR

FIGURE 4.11

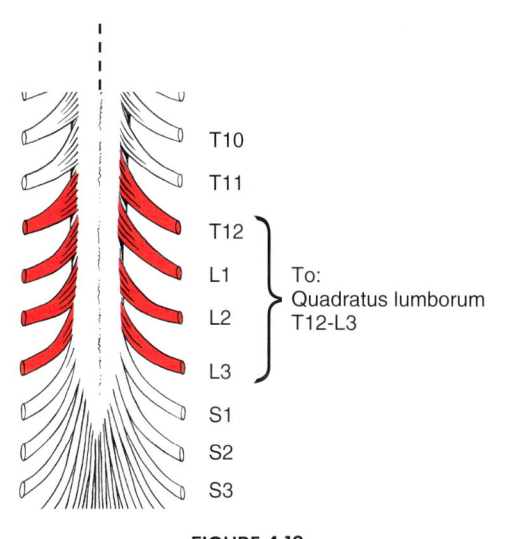

T10

T11

T12

L1

L2

L3

S1

S2

S3

To:
Quadratus lumborum
T12-L3

FIGURE 4.12

Range of Motion

Approximates pelvis to lower ribs;
range not precise.

Table 4.3 **ELEVATION OF THE PELVIS**

I.D.	Muscle	Origin	Insertion	Function
110	Obliquus externus abdominis	Ribs 5–12 (interdigitating on external and inferior surfaces)	Iliac crest (outer border) Aponeurosis from 9th costal cartilage to ASIS; both sides meet at midline to form linea alba Pubic symphysis (upper border)	Flexion of trunk (bilateral muscles) Tilts pelvis posteriorly Elevates pelvis (unilateral) Rotation of trunk to opposite side (unilateral) Lateral bending of trunk (unilateral) Support and compression of abdominal viscera, counteracting effect of gravity on abdominal contents Assists defecation, micturition, emesis, and parturition (i.e., expulsion of contents of abdominal viscera and air from lungs) Important accessory muscle of forced expiration (during expiration it forces the viscera upward to elevate the diaphragm)
111	Obliquus internus abdominis	Iliac crest (anterior two-thirds of intermediate line) Thoracolumbar fascia Inguinal ligament (lateral two-thirds of upper aspect)	Ribs 9–12 (inferior border and cartilages by digitations that appear continuous with internal intercostals) Ribs 7–9 (cartilages) Aponeurosis to linea alba	Flexion of spine (bilateral) Lateral bending of spine (unilateral) Rotation of trunk to same side (unilateral) Increases abdominal pressure to assist in defecation and other expulsive actions Forces viscera upward during expiration to elevate diaphragm Elevation of pelvis
100	Quadratus lumborum	Ilium (crest and inner lip) Iliolumbar ligament	Rib 12 (lower border) L1-L4 vertebrae (transverse processes, apex) T12 vertebra (body; occasionally)	Elevation of pelvis (weak in contrast to lateral abdominals) Extension of lumbar spine (muscles on both sides) Inspiration (via stabilization of lower attachments of diaphragm) Fixation of lower portions of diaphragm for prolonged vocalization, which needs sustained expiration. Lateral bending of lumbar spine to same side (pelvis fixed) Fixation and depression of 12th rib
Others				
130	Latissimus dorsi (if arms are fixed)			
90	Iliocostalis lumborum			

ASIS, Anterior superior iliac spine.

Pelvic elevation is a critical component of gait because it allows the swing leg to clear the floor. The lateral abdominals, in conjunction with the quadratus (Figs. 4.11 and 4.12), produce very strong pelvic elevation, and the clinician should not be able to break a Grade 5 muscle. The hip hike test described later was originally believed to isolate the quadratus lumborum, but a later study revealed the dominance of the abdominals. Even though hip hiking incorporates both abdominals and quadratus,[17] it is still the best differentiation between quadratus and abdominals that we have.

Grade 5 and Grade 4

Position of Patient: Supine or prone. The patient grasps edges of the table, or belts may be used to secure the patient's torso to the table in the presence of upper extremity weakness to provide stabilization during resistance (not illustrated).

Instructions to Clinician: Stand at foot of table, facing patient. Ask patient to hike pelvis. If sufficient range is present, grasp test limb with both hands, using a lumbrical grip just above the ankle, and pull caudally with a smooth, even pull (Fig. 4.13) to provide resistance. Resistance is given as in traction. The Grades 5 and 4 muscles tolerate a very large amount of resistance.

Test: Patient hikes the pelvis on one side, thereby approximating the iliac crest to the inferior margin of the rib cage.

Instructions to Patient: "Hike your pelvis to bring it up to your ribs. Hold it. Don't let me pull your leg down."

Grading

Grade 5: Patient holds test position, and limb does not move with maximal resistance.

Grade 4: Patient holds test position against very strong resistance. Testing this movement requires more than a bit of clinical judgment.

Grade 3 and Grade 2

Position of Patient: Supine or prone. Hip in extension; lumbar spine neutral or extended.

Instructions to Clinician: Stand at foot of table, facing patient. Use one hand to support the leg just above the ankle; keep the other hand under the knee so the limb is slightly off the table to decrease friction (Fig. 4.14).

Test: Patient hikes the pelvis on the test side to bring the rim of the pelvis closer to the inferior ribs.

Instruction to Patient: "Bring your pelvis up to your ribs."

Grading

Grade 3: Patient completes available range of motion.

Grade 2: Patient completes partial range of motion.

FIGURE 4.13

FIGURE 4.14

Grade 1 and Grade 0:

These grades should be avoided to ensure clinical accuracy. The quadratus lumborum lies deep to the paraspinal muscle mass and can rarely be palpated. In people who have extensive truncal atrophy, paraspinal muscle activity may be palpated, and possibly, but not necessarily convincingly, the quadratus lumborum can be palpated.

Substitution

The patient may attempt to substitute with trunk lateral flexion, primarily using the abdominal muscles. Spinal extensors may be used without the quadratus lumborum. In neither case can manual testing detect an inactive quadratus lumborum.

Clinical Relevance

It should be noted that the quadratus lumborum may have functions other than hip hiking, such as maintaining upright posture and enhancing stability of the lumbar spine,[18] although these functions have been less well studied. Quadratus lumborum strength has also implicated in low back pain without consensus.[19]

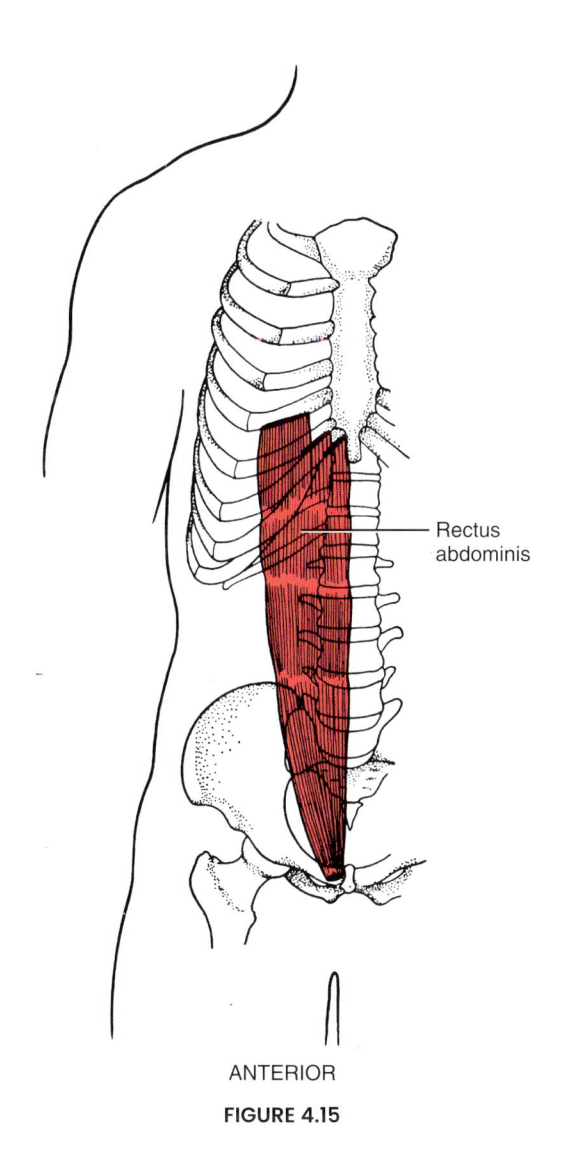

Rectus abdominis

ANTERIOR

FIGURE 4.15

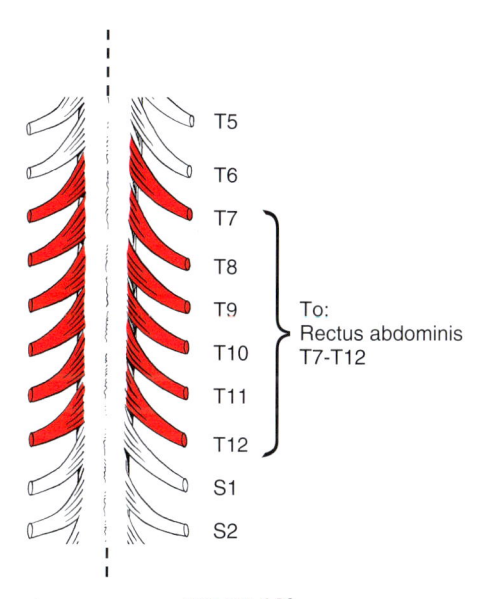

T5
T6
T7
T8
T9
T10
T11
T12
S1
S2

To:
Rectus abdominis
T7–T12

FIGURE 4.16

Range of Motion

0°–80°

Table 4.4 TRUNK FLEXION

I.D.	Muscle	Origin	Insertion	Function
113	Rectus abdominis (paired muscle)	Pubis Lateral fibers (tubercle on crest and pecten pubis) Medial fibers (ligamentous covering of symphysis attaches to contralateral muscle)	Ribs 5–7 (costal cartilages) Sternum (xiphoid ligaments)	Flexion of the spine (draws symphysis pubis and sternum toward each other) Posterior tilt of pelvis
110	Obliquus externus abdominis	Ribs 5–12 (interdigitating on external and inferior surfaces)	Iliac crest (outer border) Aponeurosis from 9th costal cartilage to ASIS; both sides meet at midline to form linea alba	Flexion of the trunk Tilts pelvis posteriorly Elevates pelvis (unilateral) Rotation of trunk to opposite side (unilateral) Accessory muscle of forced expiration
111	Obliquus internus abdominis	Iliac crest (anterior two-thirds of intermediate line) Thoracolumbar fascia Inguinal ligament (lateral two-thirds of upper aspect)	Ribs 9–12 (inferior border and cartilages by digitations that appear continuous with internal intercostals) Ribs 7–9 (cartilages) Aponeurosis to linea alba	Flexion of spine Lateral bending of the spine (unilateral) Rotation of trunk to same side (unilateral) Elevation of pelvis
Others				
174	Psoas major			
175	Psoas minor			

ASIS, Anterior superior iliac spine.

Trunk flexion has multiple elements that include cervical, thoracic, and lumbar motion (Figs. 4.15 and 4.16 and Table 4.4). Measurement is difficult at best and may be done in a variety of ways with considerable variability in results. Compensatory substitution of the neck flexors should be minimized by asking the patient to maintain a neutral neck position with the chin pointed to the ceiling to avoid neck flexion. Legs should be straight to avoid hip flexor activation.[20]

Grade 5

Position of Patient: Supine, with legs straight and fingertips lightly touching the back of the head (Fig. 4.17).

Instructions to Clinician: Stand at side of table at level of patient's chest to ascertain whether scapulae clear table during test (Fig. 4.18). Ask patient to lift head, shoulders, and back off table, keeping the chin pointed to the ceiling. Observe motion for quality and effort. For a patient with no other muscle weakness, the clinician does not need to touch the patient. However, if the patient has weak hip flexors, the clinician should stabilize the pelvis by leaning across the patient on the forearms (see Fig. 4.18).

Test: Patient flexes trunk through range of motion, lifting the trunk until scapulae clear table. The neck should not flex.

Instructions to Patient: "Keep your chin pointed toward the ceiling and lift your head, shoulders, and back off the table."

Grading

Grade 5: Patient raises trunk until inferior angles of scapulae are off the table. (Weight of the arms serves as resistance.)

FIGURE 4.17

FIGURE 4.18

Grade 4

Position of Patient: Supine with arms crossed over chest (Fig. 4.19).

Test: Other than the patient's arm position, all other aspects of the test are the same as for Grade 5.

Grading

Grade 4: Patient raises trunk until scapulae are off the table. Resistance of arms is reduced in the cross-chest position.

Grade 3

Position of Patient: Supine with arms outstretched in full extension above plane of body (Fig. 4.20).

Test: Except for the patient's arm position, all other aspects of the test are the same as for Grade 5. Patient lifts trunk until inferior angles of scapulae are off the table. Position of the outstretched arms "neutralizes" resistance by bringing the weight of the arms closer to the center of gravity.

Instructions to Patient: "Keep your chin pointed to the ceiling as you raise your head, shoulders, and arms off the table."

Grading

Grade 3: Patient lifts trunk until inferior angles of scapulae are off the table.

FIGURE 4.19

FIGURE 4.20

Grade 2, Grade 1, and Grade 0

Testing trunk flexion is rather clear cut for Grades 5, 4, and 3. When testing Grade 2 and below, the results may be ambiguous, but observation and palpation are critical for defendable results. To determine Grades 2 to 0, the patient will be asked, in sequence, to raise the head, do an assisted forward lean, and cough.

Position of Patient: Supine with arms at sides. Knees flexed.

Instructions to Clinician: Stand at side of table. Place the hand used for palpation at the midline of the thorax over the linea alba, and use the four fingers of both hands to palpate the rectus abdominis (Fig. 4.21).

Note: The clinician tests for Grades 2, 1, and 0 in a variety of ways to make certain that muscle contractile activity that may be present is not missed.

Grading

Sequence 1: Head raise (Fig. 4.22): Ask the patient to lift the head from the table. If the scapulae do not clear the table, the Grade is 2. If the patient cannot lift the head, proceed to Sequence 2.

FIGURE 4.21

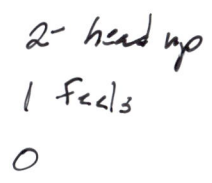

2- head up
1 feels
0

FIGURE 4.22

Sequence 2: Assisted forward lean (Fig. 4.23): The clinician cradles the upper trunk and head off the table and asks the patient to lean forward. If there is depression of the rib cage, the grade is 2. If there is no depression of the rib cage but visible or palpable contraction occurs, the grade assigned should be 1. If there is no activity, the grade is 0; proceed to Sequence 3.

Sequence 3: Cough (Fig. 4.24): Ask the patient to cough. If the patient can cough to any degree and depression of the rib cage occurs, the grade is 2. (If the patient coughs, regardless of its effectiveness, the abdominal muscles are automatically brought into play.) If the patient cannot cough but there is palpable rectus abdominis activity, the grade is 1. Lack of any discernable activity is Grade 0.

FIGURE 4.23

FIGURE 4.24

Clinical Relevance

- In all tests, observe any deviations of the umbilicus. If there is a difference in the segments of the rectus abdominis in response to muscle testing, the umbilicus will deviate toward the stronger part (i.e., cranially if the upper parts are stronger, caudally if the lower parts are stronger, and laterally if one or more segments of *one* rectus is paralyzed).
- It is also important to look for diastasis recti abdominis (separation of abdominal muscles at the linea alba) that can occur in women after childbirth. Women with diastasis recti abdominis at 1 year postpartum had less trunk muscle rotation strength and scored lower on the sit-up test than women without this abdominal deviation.[21]
- If the extensor muscles of the lumbar spine are weak, contraction of the abdominal muscles can cause posterior tilt of the pelvis. If this situation exists, tension of the hip flexor muscles would be useful to stabilize the pelvis; therefore, the clinician should position the patient in hip and knee flexion.
- The thoracic flexion muscle test should be done absolutely correctly—that is, with the neck in neutral to avoid undue strain on the neck and in the presence of known or suspected osteoporosis. Care should be taken in the presence of osteoporosis because repeated trunk flexion can be related to increased risk of compression fractures of the spine. To avoid thoracic flexion, instruct the patient to keep the chin pointed to the ceiling and the elbows flat.
- To avoid cervical strain, have the patient avoid clasping the head with the hands. The hands should not carry any of the head's weight.
- Abdominal-strengthening exercises are performed with spine flexion and without hip flexion to reduce the role of hip flexors and undue disc compression.[20]
- Leg support during a pelvic tilt and fixed feet during spine and hip flexion exercises may decrease the intensity of rectus abdominis activity. Having the feet on the floor or fixed activates the hip flexors.[20]
- In summary, to ensure the patient's spine safety, remember these important guidelines.[20]
  a. Avoid active hip flexion or fixed feet.
  b. Do not allow the patient to pull the head up with the hands behind the head.

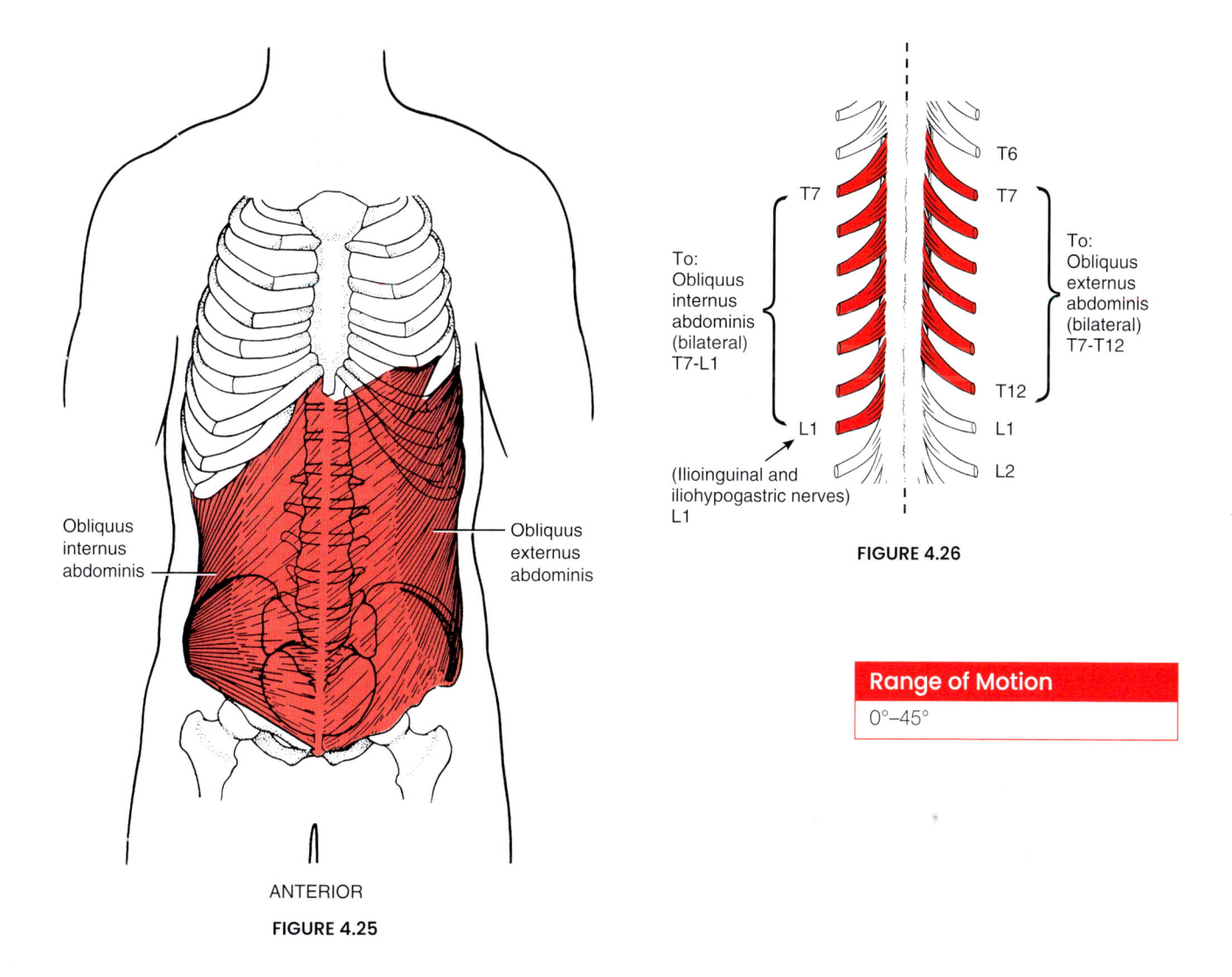

To:
Obliquus
internus
abdominis
(bilateral)
T7-L1

To:
Obliquus
externus
abdominis
(bilateral)
T7-T12

(Ilioinguinal and
iliohypogastric nerves)
L1

FIGURE 4.26

Obliquus
internus
abdominis

Obliquus
externus
abdominis

ANTERIOR

FIGURE 4.25

Range of Motion

0°–45°

Table 4.5 TRUNK ROTATION

I.D.	Muscle	Origin	Insertion	Function
110	Obliquus externus abdominis	Ribs 5–12 (interdigitating on external and inferior surfaces)	Iliac crest (outer border) Aponeurosis from 9th costal cartilage to ASIS; both sides meet at midline to form linea alba Pubic symphysis (upper border)	Flexion of trunk (bilateral muscles) Tilts pelvis posteriorly Elevates pelvis (unilateral) Rotation of trunk to opposite side (unilateral) Lateral bending of trunk (unilateral)
111	Obliquus internus abdominis	Iliac crest (anterior two-thirds of intermediate line) Thoracolumbar fascia Inguinal ligament (lateral two-thirds of upper aspect)	Ribs 9–12 (inferior border and cartilages by digitations that appear continuous with internal intercostals) Ribs 7–9 (cartilages) Aponeurosis to linea alba	Flexion of spine (bilateral) Lateral bending of spine (unilateral) Rotation of trunk to same side (unilateral) Elevation of pelvis
Other				
	Deep back muscles (1 side)			

NOTE: Use caution with trunk rotation in patients with known or suspected osteoporosis.
ASIS, Anterior superior iliac spine.

Trunk rotation is a combined and essential movement of most functional activities. Although the obliques are the primary movers, trunk rotation also involves small oblique extensors and flexors (Figs. 4.25 and 4.26 and Table 4.5).

Grade 5

Position of Patient: Supine with fingertips to the side of the head.

Instructions to Clinician: Stand at the patient's waist level. Ask the patient to lift head and shoulders, moving elbow to opposite hip. Repeat for other side. Observe for adequate range and quality of movement and effort.

Test: With chin pointed to the ceiling, the patient flexes trunk and rotates to one side. This movement is then repeated on the opposite side so that the muscles on both sides can be examined.

Right elbow to left knee tests the right external oblique and the left internal oblique. Left elbow to right knee tests the left external oblique and the right internal oblique (Fig. 4.27). When the patient rotates to one side, the internal oblique muscle is palpated on the side toward the turn; the external oblique muscle is palpated on the side away from the direction of turning (Fig. 4.28).

Substitution

If the pectoralis major is inappropriately active to provide compensatory movement in this test of trunk rotation at any grade, the shoulder will shrug or be raised from the table with limited rotation of the trunk.

Instructions to Patient: "With your chin pointed to the ceiling, lift your head and shoulders from the table, taking your right elbow toward your left knee. Then, with your chin pointed to the ceiling, lift your head and shoulders from the table, taking your left elbow toward your right knee."

Grading

Grade 5: The scapula corresponding to the side of the external oblique function must clear the table for a Grade 5.

FIGURE 4.27

FIGURE 4.28

Grade 4

Position of Patient: Supine with arms crossed over chest.

Test: Other than patient's arm position, all other aspects of the test are the same as for Grade 5. The test is done first to one side (Fig. 4.29) and then to the other.

FIGURE 4.29

FIGURE 4.30

Grade 3

Position of Patient: Supine with arms outstretched above plane of body.

Test: Other than patient's arm position, all other aspects of the test are the same as for Grade 5. The test is done first to the left (Fig. 4.30) and then to the right (Fig. 4.31).

Grading

Grade 3: Patient raises the scapula off the table. The clinician may use one hand to check for scapular clearance (Fig. 4.32).

FIGURE 4.31

Grade 2

Position of Patient: Supine with arms outstretched above plane of body.

Instructions to Clinician: Stand at level of patient's waist. Palpate the external oblique first on one side and then on the other, with one hand placed on the lateral part of the anterior abdominal wall distal to the rib cage (see Fig. 4.32). Continue to palpate the muscle distally in the direction of its fibers until reaching the ASIS.

At the same time, palpate the internal oblique muscle on the opposite side of the trunk. The internal oblique muscle lies under the external oblique, and its fibers run in the opposite diagonal direction.

Clinicians may remember this palpation procedure better if they think of positioning their two hands as if both hands were to be in the pants pockets or grasping the abdomen in pain. (The external obliques run from out to in; the internal obliques run from in to out.)

Instructions to Patient: "Keep your chin pointed to the ceiling while you lift your head, reach toward your right knee." (Repeat to left side for the opposite muscle.)

Test: Patient attempts to raise body and turn toward the right. Repeat toward left side.

Grading

Grade 2: Patient is unable to clear the inferior angle of the scapula from the table on the side of the external oblique being tested. However, the clinician must be able to observe depression of the rib cage during the test activity.

FIGURE 4.32

Grade 1 and Grade 0

Position of Patient: Supine with arms at sides. Hips flexed with feet flat on table.

Instructions to Clinician: Support patient's head as patient attempts to turn to one side (Fig. 4.33). (Turn to the other side in a subsequent test.) Under normal conditions, the abdominal muscles stabilize the trunk when the head is lifted. In patients with abdominal weakness, the supported head permits the patient to recruit abdominal muscle activity without having to overcome the entire weight of the head.

One hand palpates the internal oblique on the side toward which the patient turns (not illustrated) and the external oblique on the side away from the direction of turning (see Fig. 4.33). The clinician assists the patient to raise the head and shoulders slightly and turn to one side. This procedure is used when abdominal muscle weakness is profound.

Instructions to Patient: "Try to lift up and turn to your right." (Repeat for turn to the left.)

Test: Patient attempts to flex trunk and turn to either side.

Grading

Grade 1: The clinician can see or palpate muscular contraction.

Grade 0: No discernable muscle contraction from the obliquus internus or externus muscles.

FIGURE 4.33

Suggested Strength Exercises for Abdominals[22]
• Abdominal slide (prone with hand roller)   • Torso Track   • Ab roller (oblique)   • Crunch (straight and oblique)

CORE STRENGTH, STABILITY, AND ENDURANCE

Core strength, endurance, and stability are important components of nearly every gross motor activity and, as such, deserve to be understood from the perspective of testing. Risk for injury is impacted by delays in core muscle activation, decreased muscle recruitment, muscle fatigue, neuromuscular imbalance, impaired proprioception, and delayed reflex responses.[23] The purpose of the core musculature is to provide trunk stability (stiffness) through intra-abdominal pressure and compression of the spinal segments and to allow movement in all directions and to transfer power to the appendicular skeleton.[24,25] Trunk stiffness is necessary to create anticipatory postural adjustments such as adjusting the center of gravity to affect balance and upper and lower extremity joint forces during upright tasks.[26,27] Cocontraction on the anterior and posterior aspect of the trunk increases intra-abdominal pressure and generates greater trunk stiffness.[24]

Muscular endurance is defined as the ability to sustain a given level of force production over time,[25] and core stability is defined as the ability to use muscular strength and endurance to control the spine over the pelvis and leg when performing functional and athletic activities.[28,29] Core stability requires coordination in addition to core strength and endurance.[30] No one muscle contributes more than 30% to the overall stability of the lumbar spine in a variety of loading conditions.[31] Therefore there is no one single most important stabilizing muscle.[32] The core muscles (Fig. 4.34) are composed of a mixture of fast and slow twitch muscle fibers, although slow twitch fibers dominate the lumbar paravertebral muscles.[33] The back extensors have more capillaries than nonpostural muscles, such as triceps brachii. The deep stabilizing muscles are also made up of slow twitch fibers. Due to this muscle composition, endurance testing may be more appropriate than pure strength testing for these core muscles.[34] In addition, endurance of the core musculature may be more important to function than pure strength.[34]

Although slow twitch muscles may be better suited to endurance-type testing, the combined core muscles are made up of both slow and fast twitch muscles, and thus, there is no one endurance test for the core.[35] These muscles respond to changes in posture, external loading, and spinal intersegmental movement. The global superficial muscles, long muscles capable of generating large movements and torque, are made up of fast twitch fibers. Cocontraction of the internal oblique and TA increases intra-abdominal pressure and stiffness of the spinal segments, resulting in increased spinal stability.[36] It takes

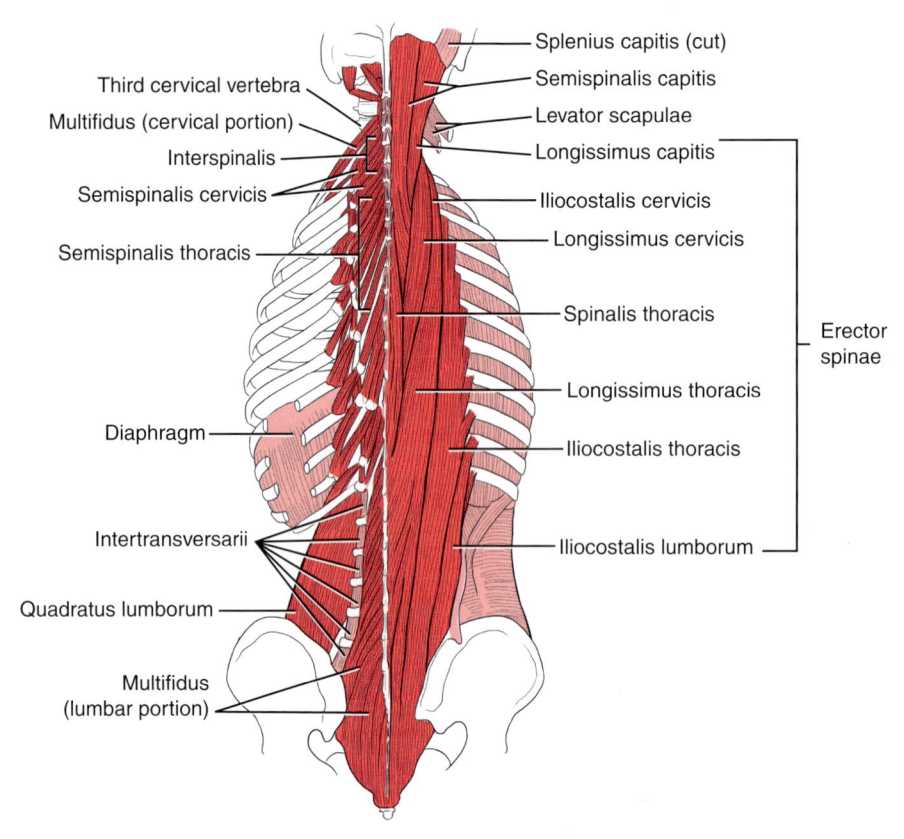

FIGURE 4.34

only 5% to 10% of maximal abdominal and multifidi contraction to stiffen the spine.

Some of the muscles that make up the core are not amenable to individual muscle testing and therefore are tested as *part* of the core. Others form individual and specific functions and can be tested individually (Fig. 4.35). However, when testing the core, all of these muscles are active (Table 4.6).

Rectus abdominis

Transverse abdominis
obliques

Erector spinae
Quadratus lumborum

Gluteals

FIGURE 4.35

Table 4.6 MUSCLES COMPRISING THE CORE[24]

Sagittal Plane	Contribution	Frontal Plane	Contribution
Rectus Abdominis	Active in trunk flexion and in combination with the hamstrings; rotates the pelvis posteriorly	Gluteus medius	Primary lateral stabilizer of tho hip
Transversus abdominis	With assistance from the multifidus, increase spinal stiffness and raise intra-abdominal pressure	Gluteus minimus	Primary lateral stabilizer of the hip
Erector spinae		Quadratus lumborum	Stiffens the spine and may be active in all upright activities
Multifidus		Adductor magnus	All of the medial muscles maintain static alignment in the frontal plane
Gluteus maximus	Transfers forces from the LE to the trunk	Adductor longus	
Hamstrings		Adductor brevis	
		Pectineus	

LE, Lower extremity.

Prone Plank Test (Prone Bridge Test)

The prone plank (bridge) test activates core musculature, specifically the rectus abdominus and internal and external obliques,[37] and assesses abdominal muscle fatigue.[38] The test is reliable.[25,37,39] Correct form consists of maintaining the spine in a neutral position while maintaining scapular adduction and a posterior pelvic tilt.[40] An anterior pelvic tilt reduces electromyography (EMG) activation, so particular attention should be paid to avoid this posturing during this test.[40] The prone plank (bridge) test is correlated with physical fitness; that is, longer test times are related to higher self-reported physical fitness.[39]

Purpose: The plank is a superb challenge to the abdominals and muscles of the shoulder girdle, particularly the pectoralis major and minor, serratus anterior, anterior deltoid, supraspinatus, and infraspinatus.

Position of Patient: Prone on floor or mat.

Instructions to Clinician: From prone, ask patient to lift body weight onto toes and forearms. Elbows should be under the shoulders, with scapulae adducted and hips level with spine like a "plank" (Fig. 4.36). Assess patient's ability to assume a plank position. If successful, explain test to patient.

Time the effort.

Instructions to Patient: "Raise yourself onto your forearms and toes. Keep your body completely straight. Suck your belly button into your spine" (see Fig. 4.36).

Scoring

A full plank position should be held for 120 seconds to be considered a Grade 5 test. Hold times of less than 90 seconds are Grade 4. Ability to assume the test position but unable to hold is a Grade 3. The alternate form (described later) is scored a Grade 2. Table 4.7 contains reference scores for 471 college students and varsity athletes (mean age, 20 years). Table 4.8 contains reference scores for individuals ages 20 to 75.

FIGURE 4.36

Table 4.8 MEAN TIMES OF PRONE PLANK (BRIDGE) TEST IN SAMPLE OF 120 INDIVIDUALS (60 OF WHOM WERE >60)[39]

Group	Age (Mean)	Prone Test Time (Seconds)
Women, 20–35	24.0 (3.5)	152.3 (59.9)
Women, 60–79	66.9 (4.6)	124.7 (78.8)
Men, 20–35	25.4 (4.2)	176.7 (70.5)
Men, 60–79	68.4 (5.2)	127.4 (66.2)
All	46.2 (22.0)	145.3 (71.5)

Table 4.7 PERCENTILE SCORES BY SEX AND SPORTS STATUS, WITH MEAN AGE OF 20 YEARS[25]

Percentile	TIME TO FATIGUE IN THE PLANK TEST (SECONDS)			
	Male (n = 194)	Female (n = 275)	Nonvarsity (n = 109)	Varsity (n = 361)
90th	201	142	151	200
80th	157	108	123	178
70th	137	95	106	149
60th	122	84	94	123
50th	110	72	83	104
40th	97	63	71	92
30th	89	58	62	82
20th	79	48	53	66
10th	62	35	37	59

Alternate Form of Prone Plank Testing

For a patient not able to do a full plank, ask the patient to flex knees and hips and lift the body onto forearms and knees. Elbows should be in line below shoulders. The patient must keep the buttocks in line with the spine, forming a straight line from neck to buttocks while on knees. Time the effort. This alternate form should be scored as a Grade 2. Hint: Make sure pelvis and buttocks are not hiked but in line with the spine. The body must come forward onto forearms to do this Grade 2 test properly.

Clinical Relevance

- Average hold times of 111.8 seconds (SD 9.4) were recorded for individuals who participated in resistance exercise, while scores of 81 seconds (SD 7.7) were recorded for sedentary individuals in a sample of 60 individuals.[37]
- Mean scores for >600 Brazilian navy cadets (18 to 25 years old) demonstrated hold times of 57.5 seconds (SD 7.6) for males and 52.8 seconds (SD 11.4) for females.[41]
- Primary reasons for termination of the test included (in order) shaking, back pain, upper limb pain, unspecified fatigue, abdominal fatigue, upper limb fatigue.[39]

Side Bridge Endurance Test

Purpose: Strength test for core. Quadratus lumborum oblique and transverse muscles are elicited without generating large compression forces on the lumbar spine.[42,43]

Position of Patient: Side-lying with legs extended, resting on lower forearm with elbow flexed to 90°. Upper arm is crossed over chest (Fig. 4.37).

Instructions to Clinician: Stand or sit in front of patient. Ask patient to lift hips off table, keeping the body in a straight line with the contracted core. Time the effort, observing for quality and quantity of effort. Give patient feedback regarding posture; hips and trunk should be level throughout the test (see Fig. 4.37).

Test: Patient lifts hips off the table, holding the elevated position in a straight line with body on a flexed elbow. This position is maintained until the patient loses form, fatigues, or complains of pain. The clinician times the effort.

Instructions to Patient: "When I say 'go!' lift your hips off the table, keeping them in a straight line with your body for as long as you can. I will be timing you."

Scoring: Record the best time of two trials.

FIGURE 4.37

Clinical Relevance

- Mean scores for 31 men and 44 women of good health with a mean age of 23 years:[44] Men: 95 (±32) seconds. Women: 75 (±32) seconds.
- Mean scores for 40 students between the ages of 18 and 25 in Saudi Arabi were 41.6 (30.08) for right side bridge and 38 seconds (26.93) for left side bridge. All subjects were right hand dominant.[45]
- Mean scores for >600 Brazilian Navy cadets (18 to 25 years old) on dominant side demonstrated hold times of 50.8 seconds (13.4) for males and 39.2 seconds (18.5) for females.[41]
- Despite the high reliability of the side bridge test, significant changes in hold times must be observed to confidently assess a true change in strength. One group reported a minimal detectable change (MDC) for the side bridge of 14.02 to 15.13 seconds in asymptomatic individuals ($n = 33$).[46] Other means to help inform clinical decision making for this test include the patient's rating of perceived exertion (RPE).[34]
- Mean hold times ranged from 20 to 203 seconds (mean, 104.8 seconds) for the right side bridge test and from 19 to 251 seconds (mean, 103.0 seconds) for the left side bridge test.[34]
- Exercisers held the side bridge test nearly double the time nonexercisers did (64.9 vs. 31.8 seconds).[47]
- The side bridge test was found to be limited by deltoid muscle and shoulder fatigue.[48]

Timed Partial Curl Up Test[49]

The timed partial curl up test is a standard in the fitness industry and is included here, even though it uses the hook lying position and thus encourages hip flexor activation.

Purpose: Strength test for abdominals.

Position of Patient: Supine in hook lying position on a mat with arms at sides, palms facing down, and the middle fingers touching a piece of tape affixed to the surface parallel to the hand. A second piece of tape is affixed 12 cm (4.7 in) farther than the initial tape for those younger than 45 years and 8 cm (3.1 in) farther for those 45 years and older (Fig. 4.38).

Instructions to Clinician: Stand to the side of patient. Ask patient to perform a slow, controlled sit-up in time, lifting head and scapulae off the mat, while the middle finger reaches to the second tape. If successful, use a metronome set to 40 beats/min to time repetitions. Ask patient to curl up as many times as possible, keeping time with the metronome. The low back should be flattened before curl up.

Test: The individual does as many curl ups as possible without pausing, to a maximum of 75.

Scoring: Refer to The American College of Sports Medicine (ACSM) Norms for partial curl up (Table 4.9).

FIGURE 4.38

Table 4.9 ACSM NORMS FOR PARTIAL CURL UP

Age	20–29		30–39		40–49		50–59		60–69	
Sex	Male	Female	Male	Female	Male	Female	Male	Female	Male	Female
90th percentile	75	70	75	55	75	55	74	48	53	50
80	56	45	69	43	75	42	60	30	33	30
70	41	37	46	34	67	33	45	23	26	24
60	31	32	36	28	51	28	35	16	19	19
50	27	27	31	21	39	25	27	9	16	13
40	24	21	26	15	31	20	23	2	9	9
30	20	17	19	12	26	14	19	0	6	3
20	13	12	13	0	21	5	13	0	0	0
10	4	5	0	0	13	0	0	0	0	0

ACSM, The American College of Sports Medicine.
Data from Pescatello, L.S., Ross, A., Riebe, D., et al. (2014). ACSM's guidelines for exercise testing and prescription (9th ed). Wolters Kluwer/Lippincott Williams & Wilkins.

Isometric Trunk Flexor Endurance Test[24]

Purpose: Measure isometric core endurance.

Position of Patient: Sitting on table with wedge supporting the back at angle of 60° to the table. Hips and knees flexed to 90°, with feet stabilized with a strap. Arms are folded across the chest (Fig. 4.39).

Instructions to Clinician: Ask patient to hold test position when the wedge is pulled back 10 cm. Time effort as soon as wedge is pulled back. Terminate test when the patient can no longer maintain the 60° angle independently.

Scoring: Ages 18 to 55 years (mean, 30 years), mean hold time = 178 seconds.[47]

Exercisers held the test three times as long as nonexercisers (186 seconds vs. 68.25 seconds).[47]

Males and females with mean age of 26.4 (3.2) performed the test in a mean of 304.73 seconds (207.32) with a range of 73.8 to 982.0 seconds.[50]

Front Abdominal Power Test

Purpose: Assess the power component of core stability prestability and poststability training.

Position of Patient: Supine on a mat with arms at sides, feet shoulder width apart, and knees bent to 90° (Fig. 4.40A).

Instructions to Clinician: Place a 2-kg medicine ball into the patient's hands. Then, ask patient to lift arms overhead and explosively project the medicine ball forward, keeping the arms straight. Feet and buttocks should remain on the floor throughout the test. (Note: Feet may be secured manually or with a strap [not shown].) Measure the distance the ball was projected from the tips of the feet to the point where the ball landed. Patient should be sitting upright after the ball is thrown (Fig. 4.40B).

Scoring: We recorded 1.5 to 2 m in a group of 20-year-old men and women (standard error of the mean, 24 cm).[51,52]

FIGURE 4.39

FIGURE 4.40

Unilateral Supine Bridge Test[53]

Purpose: The unilateral supine bridge test assesses lumbopelvic neuromuscular control. This test was found to be correlated with lab-based biomechanical measures of isolated core stability.

Position of Patient: Supine with arms across chest with knees in hook lying.

Instructions to Clinician: Stand to side of patient. Ask patient to lift both hips into a double-leg bridge. When neutral spine and pelvis positions are achieved, ask patient to extend one knee so leg is straight and thighs are parallel to one another (Fig. 4.41). Ask patient to hold position as long as possible, timing the effort. The test is terminated when patient is no longer able to hold a neutral pelvic position, as noted by a 10° change in transverse or sagittal plane alignment. Perform two trials, and average results.

Scoring:
- A sample of 20 healthy male volunteers (mean age, 25.7 years) held the test position for an average of 23.0 seconds (16.5) with a range of 3.1 to 59.5 seconds.[53]
- A sample of 30 sedentary individuals (mean age, 22.4 years [2]) held the test position 79 (9.2) seconds. while 30 resistance-trained individuals (mean age, 22 years [2]) held the test position 100.7 (8.1) seconds.[37]

FIGURE 4.41

Suggested Strength Exercises for Core Strengthening

- The side bridge, lateral step up, lunge, and quadruped with arm and leg lift have been found to be effective exercises for increasing overall core strength. These exercises have electromyography (EMG) amplitude greater than 45% maximum voluntary isometric contraction. Forty-five percent to 50% of one repetition maximum correlates with an increase in strength.[54]
- Longissimus thoracis and lumbar multifidus are most active during bridging, side bridging, unilateral bridging, and quadruped opposite arm/lower extremity lift.[54]
- External oblique and rectus abdominis are most active during prone bridging and side bridging.[54]
- Side bridging was optimal for lower abdominal muscle activation.[54] However, the side bridge exercise may not be well tolerated in patients with low back pain, and it may be best used as an advanced technique when patients have proper physical conditioning and adequate technique.[55] Exercises to reduce low back pain in patients should focus on strengthening, endurance, and trunk coordination.[56]
- Superman exercise produced greatest activation of back stabilizers.[54]
- Transversus abdominis (TA) activity by fine wire EMG was greatest during the prone plank, with contralateral arm and leg lift with maximum voluntary contractions recorded as 50% or less, indicating that the TA activation may be best achieved through low-load exercises focusing on motor learning and control.[57]
- Rectus abdominis activity was found to be highest in a curl up exercise on an unstable surface, such as a BOSU ball, with maximum voluntary contraction (MVC) of approximately 50%.[57]

DIAPHRAGM

FIGURE 4.42

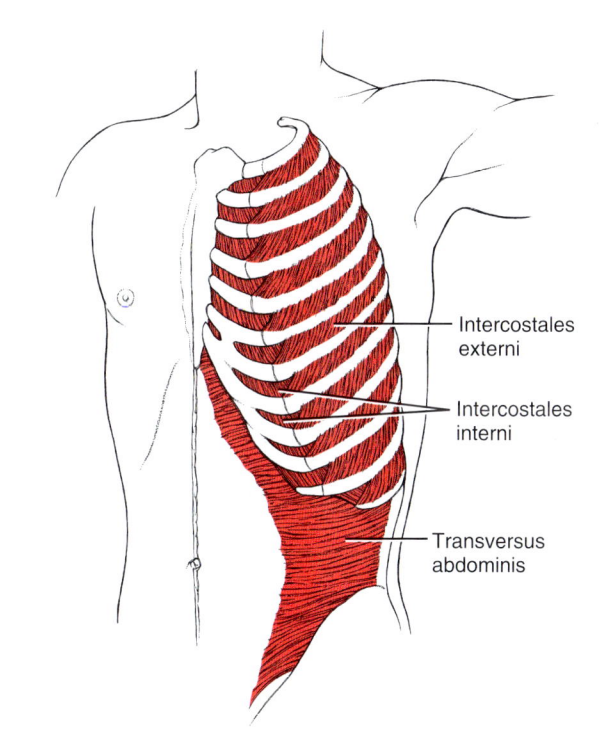

Intercostales externi

Intercostales interni

Transversus abdominis

FIGURE 4.43

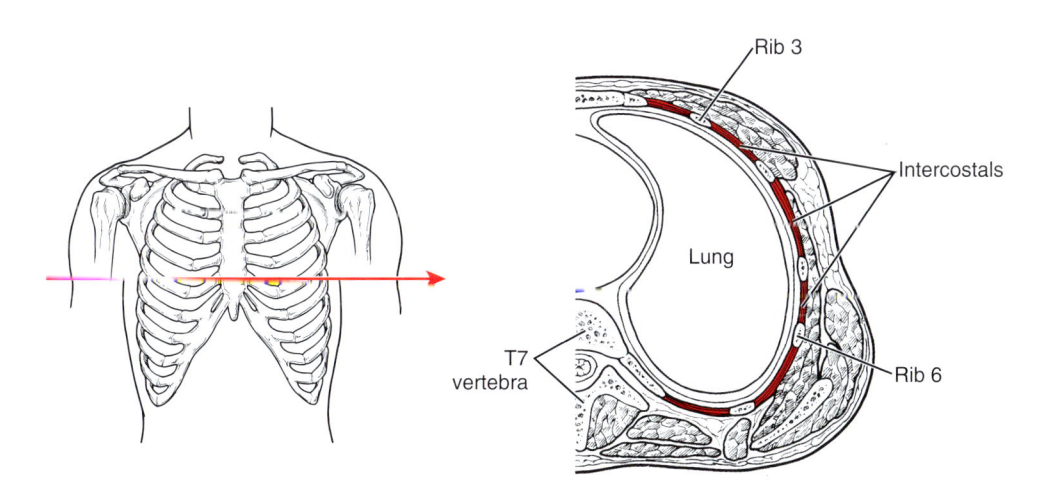

Rib 3

Intercostals

Lung

T7 vertebra

Rib 6

FIGURE 4.44

FIGURE 4.45

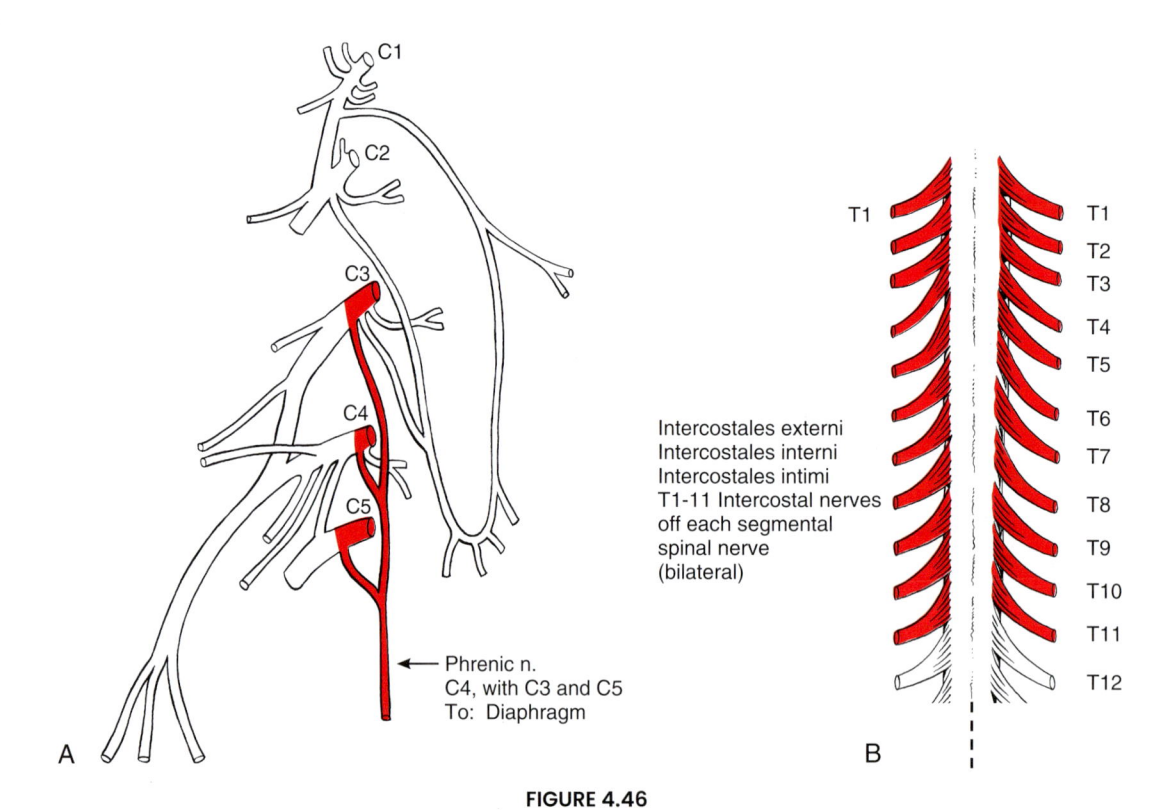

Intercostales externi
Intercostales interni
Intercostales intimi
T1-11 Intercostal nerves
off each segmental
spinal nerve
(bilateral)

Phrenic n.
C4, with C3 and C5
To: Diaphragm

FIGURE 4.46

Range of Motion

Normal chest expansion in forced inspiration varies from 2.0 to 5 cm at the level of the xiphoid dependent on lifestyle (smoker vs. nonsmoker) and nationality, and it declines with age.[58,59]

DIAPHRAGM

The diaphragm (Fig. 4.42) is innervated by the efferent fibers of the left and right phrenic nerves. Breathing at rest is an automatic activity controlled by bulbospinal neurons, leading to diaphragm contractions every 3 to 5 seconds and resulting in inspiratory efforts. In addition to the automatic control of breathing, the diaphragm can also be controlled volitionally via the corticospinal pathway to allow deeper breathing or related activities such as sniffing.[60] Contraction of the diaphragm causes the diaphragm to descend, increasing volume and decreasing pressure within the thoracic cavity. This pressure change creates a pressure gradient that results in movement of air into the airways. As the diaphragm descends, abdominal viscera are compressed, and intra-abdominal pressure increases. Once the viscera cannot be displaced further, additional contraction of the fibers of the diaphragm causes the lower ribs to move in a cephalad and lateral direction, producing a so-called bucket-handle motion.

While the diaphragm generates the majority of resting tidal volume, other synergistic inspiratory muscles are also active while breathing at rest. The scalene muscles, as assessed via needle EMG examination, are active with every inspiratory effort and should be considered a primary muscle of inspiration. Parasternal and upper external intercostal inspiratory EMG activity is also typical during resting breathing.[61] In contrast to inspiration, resting expiration is typically passive. Accessory inspiratory and expiratory muscles can be recruited during periods of increased motor drive, voluntary behaviors, or nonrespiratory movements such as trunk rotation.[62]

If a patient is noted to have significant diaphragm weakness as detected by clinical observation and/or testing, a referral to a physician is recommended. Significant weakness of the diaphragm can contribute to sleep dysfunction, may indicate an underlying neuromuscular condition, and can lead to eventual hypoventilation.

Preliminary Examination

Uncover the patient's chest and abdominal area so that the motions of the chest and abdominal walls can be observed. Watch the normal respiration pattern and observe differences in the motion of the chest wall and (epigastric) area and note any contraction of the neck muscles and the abdominal muscles.

The epigastric rise and flaring of the lower margin of the rib cage during inspiration indicate that the diaphragm is active. During quiet inspiration, epigastric rise reflects the movement of the diaphragm descending over one intercostal space.[63] In deeper inspiratory efforts, the diaphragm may move across three or more intercostal spaces. The rise on both sides of the linea alba should be symmetric.

An elevation and lateral expansion of the rib cage are indicative of intercostal activity during inspiration (Figs. 4.43–4.46A and B).

Paradoxical breathing is the presence of inward movement of the chest or abdomen during inspiration, and the paradoxical pattern reflects dysfunction of different respiratory muscles. Paradoxical movements of the abdomen reflect diaphragmatic paresis, where the diaphragm elevates and the abdomen pulls inward during inspiratory efforts. Paradoxical inward movements of the chest may be seen in patients with traumatic injuries to the chest.

Measurement

Maximum inspiratory pressure (MIP) is the measurement of strength of inspiratory muscles.

Measurements of MIP and maximal expiratory pressure (MEP) may serve as a means of measuring ventilatory muscle strength, although not the strength of any single muscle. The MIP reflects the strength of the diaphragm and other inspiratory muscles, whereas the MEP reflects the strength of the abdominal muscles and other expiratory muscles.

Equipment: Either a manual pressure gauge (Fig. 4.47) or an electronic pressure gauge (Fig. 4.48) is used. The

FIGURE 4.47

FIGURE 4.48

testing device should include a small (2-mm) air leak to reduce the contribution of the cheek muscles.[64] Place a new cardboard mouthpiece or a clean rubber mouthpiece with flanges on the device for each patient's use.

Maximal Inspiratory Pressure

Position of Patient: Seated in a chair, with a nose clip applied to the nose (Fig. 4.49).

Instructions to Clinician: Stand or sit in front of seated patient so as to read the gauge (see Fig. 4.49; clinician shown at side of patient to better illustrate procedure).

Test: Demonstrate the maneuver, and then have the patient repeat it. Patient first exhales completely and then sucks in as hard as possible. The patient should maintain inspiratory pressure for at least 1.5 seconds; the largest negative pressure sustained for at least 1 second should be recorded. Allow the patient to rest for approximately 1 minute and then repeat the maneuver five times. Provide verbal or visual feedback after each maneuver, but do not allow trunk flexion or extension during the test. The goal is for the variability among measurements to be less than 10 cm H_2O. Measurements should be rounded to the nearest 5 cm H_2O.

Instructions to Patient: "Seal your lips firmly around the mouthpiece, exhale slowly and completely, and then pull in hard, like you are trying to suck up a thick milkshake."

Maximal Expiratory Pressure

Position of Patient: Seated in a chair, with a nose clip applied to the nose.

Instructions to Clinician: Stand or sit in front of seated patient so as to read the gauge.

Test: Demonstrate the maneuver and have the patient repeat it. Patient first inhales completely, then blows out as hard as possible. The patient should maintain expiratory pressure for at least 1.5 seconds. The largest positive pressure sustained for at least 1 second should be recorded. Allow the patient to rest for approximately 1 minute and then repeat the maneuver five times. Provide verbal or visual feedback after each maneuver but do not allow trunk flexion or extension during the test. The goal is for the variability among measurements to be less than 10 cm H_2O. While electronic pressure gauges provide measurements to the nearest 1 cm H_2O, measurements with a manual gauge are less precise and should be rounded to the nearest 5 cm H_2O.

Instructions to Patient: "I want you to inhale completely as you push the mouthpiece firmly against your lips and teeth and then push (or blow) as hard as possible, like you are trying to fill a very stiff balloon."

Grading

A number of participant characteristics can influence expected MIP and MEP normative values, age, sex, and muscularity/fitness level. Additionally, maximal respiratory pressures can differ due to differences in the device setup and test performance, such as a built-in leak, type of mouthpiece, stabilization of the cheeks during testing, and patient understanding, highlighting the importance of test standardization. However, an MIP of ≥80 cm H_2O in men and ≥70 cm H_2O in women usually excludes the presence of inspiratory muscle weakness.[65] Since maximal respiratory tests are unnatural maneuvers and susceptible to influences of learning and effort, they are not recommended for children <6 to 8 years of age.[66]

FIGURE 4.49

Clinical Relevance

Some patients with orofacial muscle weakness may not be able to obtain a good seal with the lips. The use of a flanged mouthpiece can reduce variability with maximal respiratory pressure testing and is recommended for those with oral weakness.[65] It is permissible to allow such patients to use their hands to press their lips against the mouthpiece during each maneuver. Alternatively, the clinician can press the patient's lips against the mouthpiece as necessary to obtain a good seal, or a face mask interface can be substituted.

INTERCOSTALS

There is no method of direct assessment of the strength of the intercostal muscles.

- The scalene muscles, as assessed via needle EMG examination, are active with every inspiratory effort and should be considered a primary muscle of inspiration.[67]

Diaphragm Imaging

Diaphragmatic function can also be measured through ultrasound. This is an examination technique that is not typically included in entry-level education. A machine with a microconvex 2- to 4-MHz probe is used.[68] Two measurements can be used, both of which relate indirectly to the strength of the diaphragm. One is diaphragmatic excursion, measured using an anterior subcostal approach between the anterior axillary and midclavicular lines. A cutoff of less than 25 mm has been suggested as an indicator of severe diaphragmatic dysfunction.[69] The second is the thickening fraction (TF). Inspiratory and expiratory thicknesses are measured where the diaphragm is in contact with the rib cage in the eighth or ninth intercostal space between the mid- and anterior axillary lines. The TF is measured as a percentage of the end-expiratory thickness. A TF less than 20% is likely to indicate severe dysfunction.[70]

Suggested Strength Exercise for Inspiratory Training

Weak inspiratory muscles can be strengthened through targeted inspiratory muscle training. Training principles are similar to those used to increase the strength of any other muscle. Patients either inhale through a mouthpiece with an adjustable diameter opening or using a device with a spring-loaded valve that does not open to allow airflow until a threshold pressure is reached. The use of threshold or electronically-braked trainers, high-intensity training loads (minimum of 50% of maximal inspiratory pressure), low repetitions (five sets of 6 to 8 breaths), and high frequency (one to two times per day, 5 to 7 days per week) are most efficacious for inspiratory strengthening, and benefits can range from improved athletic performance to facilitation of ventilator weaning.[71,72]

In the absence of an available respiratory training device, using abdominal weights to produce resistance can be effective. In this exercise, the patient is supine, and a predetermined weight is placed on the stomach. The goal is to have the patient elevate the weight with each inspiration.[73]

The cough is an essential procedure to maintain airway patency and to clear the pharynx and bronchial tree when secretions accumulate. A cough may be a reflex or voluntary response to irritation anywhere along the airway downstream from the nose. The three phases of cough—inspiration, compression, and forced expiration—are mediated by the muscles of the thorax and abdomen, as well as those of the pharynx, larynx, and tongue. The deep inspiratory effort is supported by the diaphragm, intercostals, and arytenoid abductor muscles (the posterior cricoarytenoids). The palatoglossus and styloglossus elevate the tongue and close off the oropharynx from the nasopharynx. The compression phase requires the lateral cricoarytenoid muscles to adduct and close the glottis.

The strong expiratory movement is augmented by strong contractions of the thorax muscles, particularly the latissimus dorsi and the oblique and transverse abdominal muscles. The abdominal muscles raise intraabdominal pressure, forcing the relaxing diaphragm up and drawing the lower ribs down and medially. Elevation of the diaphragm raises the intrathoracic pressure to approximately 200 mm Hg, and the explosive expulsion phase begins with forced abduction of the glottis.

Coughing often is used as the clinical test for forced expiration. An effective cough requires the use of all muscles of active expiration in contrast to quiet expiration, which is the passive relaxation of the muscles of inspiration. However, it must be recognized that an effective cough may also be due to inspiratory muscle weakness, inadequate laryngeal control, or low vital capacity.

Grading

The usual muscle test grades do not apply here; thus, the following scale to assess the cough is used:

Functional: Normal or only slight impairment:
- Crisp or explosive expulsion of air
- Volume is sharp and clearly audible
- Able to clear airway of secretions

Weak Functional: Moderate impairment that affects the degree of active motion or endurance:
- Decreased volume and diminished air movement
- Appears labored
- May take several attempts to clear airway

Nonfunctional: Severe impairment:
- No clearance of airway
- No expulsion of air
- Cough attempt may be nothing more than an effort to clear the throat

Zero: Cough is absent.

Clinical Relevance

- It is generally accepted that if an individual's forced vital capacity (FVC) is ≥60% of the predicted value, the inspired volume is sufficient to generate a functional, effective cough.[74]
- FVC can be measured with a simple spirometer (Fig. 4.50). A forced expiratory volume ≥60% of the individual's measured FVC should be adequate for sufficiently forceful expulsion.[75]

Cough can also be measured with a portable peak flow device that displays the highest airflow the patient generated through the device. Patients with a peak cough flow rate of <270 L/min typically have a functional cough in their normal state of health but may be at increased risk for respiratory infections.[76] A peak cough flow rate of 160 L/min is highly predictive of successful secretion clearance and subsequent extubation and decannulation in patients with neuromuscular disease.[77]

FIGURE 4.50

Table 4.10 MUSCLES OF QUIET INSPIRATION

I.D.	Muscle	Origin	Insertion	Function
101	Diaphragm	Formed of three parts from the circumference of the thoracic outlet Sternal: Xiphoid Costal: Ribs 7–12 Lumbar: L1-L3 vertebrae	Fibers all converge on central tendon of diaphragm; middle of central tendon is below and partially blended with pericardium	*Inspiration:* Contraction of the diaphragm with the lower ribs fixed draws the central tendon downward and forward during inspiration This increases the vertical thoracic dimensions and pushes the abdominal viscera downward It also decreases the pressure within the thoracic cavity, forcing air into the lungs through the open glottis by the higher pressure of the atmospheric air These events occur along with intercostal muscle action, which elevates the ribs, sternum, and vertebrae, increasing the anteroposterior and transverse thoracic dimensions for the inspiratory effort The diaphragm adds power to expulsive efforts: lifting heavy loads, sneezing, coughing, laughing, parturition, and evacuation of bladder and bowels These activities are preceded by deep inspiration *Expiration:* Passive relaxation allows the half-dome to ascend, thus decreasing thoracic cavity volume and increasing its pressure
102	Intercostales externi (11 pairs)	Ribs 1–11 (lower borders and tubercles; costal cartilages)	Ribs 2–12 (upper margins of rib below; last 2 end in free ends of the costal cartilages) External intercostal membrane	The muscles of respiration are highly coordinated between abdominal and thoracic processes with the diaphragm being the major muscle of inspiration, accounting for about two-thirds of vital capacity The external intercostals are more active in inspiration than expiration but work closely with the internal intercostals to stiffen the chest wall, preventing paradoxical motion during descent of the diaphragm Elevation of ribs in inspiration There are data to support this claim for the upper four or five muscles, but the more dorsal and lateral fibers of the same muscles also are active in early expiration It is possible that the activity of the intercostals during respiration varies with the depth of breathing[78] Depression of the ribs in expiration (supporting data sparse) Rotation of thoracic spine to opposite side (unilateral) Stabilization of rib cage
103	Intercostales interni (11 pairs)	Sternum (anterior) Ribs 1–11 (ridge on inner surface) Costal cartilages of same rib Internal intercostal membrane	Upper border of rib below Fibers run obliquely to the external intercostals	Not as strong as the external intercostals Elevation of ribs in inspiration This may be true at least for the 1st to 5th muscles The more lateral muscle fibers run more obliquely inferior and posterior and are most active in expiration[78] Stabilization of rib cage
104	Intercostales intimi (innermost intercostals) Often absent	Ribs 1–11 (costal groove)	Rib below (upper margin) Fibers run in same pattern as internal intercostals	Presumed to be identical to intercostales interni
107	Levatores costarum (12 pairs)	C7-T11 vertebrae (transverse processes, tip)	Rib below vertebra of origin (external surface)	Elevation of ribs in inspiration (disputed) Lateral bending of spine

Table 4.10 MUSCLES OF QUIET INSPIRATION—cont'd

I.D.	Muscle	Origin	Insertion	Function
80	Scalenus anterior	C3-C6 vertebrae (transverse processes, anterior tubercles)	1st rib (scalene tubercle)	Flexion of cervical spine (both muscles) Elevation of 1st rib in inspiration Rotation of cervical spine to same side Lateral bending of neck to same side
81	Scalenus medius	C2 (axis)-C7 vertebrae (transverse processes, posterior tubercles) C1 (atlas) sometimes	1st rib (superior surface)	Cervical flexion (weak) Lateral bending of cervical spine to same side Elevation of 1st rib in inspiration Cervical rotation to same side
82	Scalenus posterior	C4-C6 vertebrae (transverse processes posterior tubercle, variable)	2nd rib (outer surface)	Cervical flexion (weak) Elevation of 2nd rib in inspiration Lateral bending of cervical spine to same side (accessory) Cervical spine rotation to same side
Others				
131	Pectoralis major (arms fixed)			

The pelvic floor muscles form the "floor" of the pelvis and perform four important functions:

Supportive: by counteracting passive gravitational pull and dynamic intra-abdominal pressures impacting the pelvic viscera in conjunction with the inner core muscles forming the canister of core stabilization.[79]

Sphincteric: by shortening in an anterosuperior direction, these muscles squeeze off the urethra, vagina, and anorectal junction to maintain urinary and fecal continence.[80]

Sexual: by rhythmically contracting during orgasm to enhance sexual satisfaction.

Postural stabilizer: by working with the TA, multifidi, and pulmonary diaphragm, the pelvic floor creates the bottom of the inner core "canister" (Fig. 4.51).

Poor pelvic floor strength is associated with pelvic organ prolapse and urinary or fecal incontinence. One in two women will experience some level of supportive dysfunction in their lifetime, leading to "falling" of the bladder, rectum, uterus, or small intestine.[81] Urinary or fecal incontinence is experienced by more than 60% of women of all ages.[82] Fecal incontinence is thought to be grossly underreported because of the associated social stigma. However, urinary incontinence is amenable to treatment using the Kegel exercise (controlled voluntary contractions used to strengthen the pelvic floor) with good results.[83]

Sexual pain may be related to weak pelvic floor musculature and urinary incontinence.[84,85] The prevalence of sexual dysfunction is estimated to be around 30% to 50% in the general population and increases in women with pelvic floor dysfunction to 50% to 83%.[81]

The pelvic floor muscles can become weakened from childbirth,[81] poor patterns of muscle recruitment, and medical comorbidities such as diabetes, abdominopelvic surgical procedures, constipation, abdominal obesity, chronic cough, hormonal changes, and loss of muscle mass with aging. Because of the frequency of pelvic floor weakness, pelvic floor muscle strength should be routinely assessed to rule out muscle weakness, spasm, or dyscoordination in the presence of lumbopelvic, urologic, gynecologic, sexual, or gastrointestinal dysfunction.

Methods used to assess the strength and function of the pelvic floor muscles include the following:

- Presence of pelvic floor muscle activation: clinical observation, external perineal palpation, vaginal or rectal digital palpation, EMG, and pressure gauges.
- Quantification of pelvic floor muscle strength: manual muscle testing with digital rectal or vaginal palpation, perineometer, vaginal cones, and vaginal or rectal squeeze pressure.[86]
- Additional visualization of the pelvic floor musculature may be done with abdominal or pelvic two-dimensional ultrasound, ultrasound, and magnetic resonance imaging.[86]

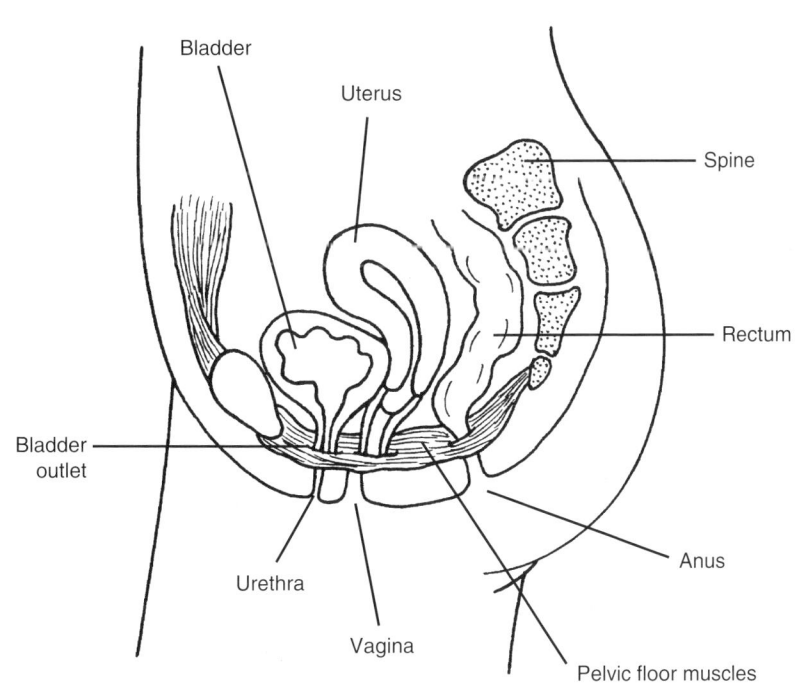

FIGURE 4.51 Pelvic Floor Muscles Serve As a Sling for the Female Organs.

Anatomy of the Pelvic Floor

Muscles of the pelvic floor are difficult to visualize, particularly because most students do not have the opportunity to dissect this region in anatomy class. In both males and females, three layers of urogenital muscles exist that differ in size and disposition in relation to the male and female external genitalia. These five muscles are grouped into superficial, middle, and deep layers. The superficial perineal muscles include the bilateral bulbocavernosus, ischiocavernosus, transverse perineal muscles, and external anal sphincter. The middle layer, or urogenital diaphragm, includes the external urethral sphincter and deep transverse perineal muscles. The deepest layer, also known as the pelvic diaphragm, includes the levator ani (comprised of the pubococcygeus and iliococcygeus), coccygeus, and puborectalis (Fig. 4.52).

The superficial layer is the outermost layer; it resembles a sling and is shaped like a figure eight. Although the superficial layer is relatively thin in terms of mass, it is highly sensitive. This area is responsible for controlling the anal and urethral sphincters, so these muscles play an important role in continence. To work effectively, the sphincters need the support of the rest of the pelvic floor, particularly the connective tissue elements.

The deep layer of the pelvic floor is the real workhorse of the pelvic floor. The deep pelvic floor muscles have the highest resting muscle tone in the body and play a vital role in movement, posture, and breathing. These muscles must continuously support the weight of the pelvic and abdominal organs when the person is upright (see Fig. 4.51). The deep pelvic floor is sometimes called the pelvic diaphragm. Like its companion, "the roof," or the pulmonary diaphragm, it has minimal sensory innervation, and its movement is not felt directly. When it works well, the pelvic floor functions like a well-balanced trampoline and has amazing tensile strength and elasticity. It plays a crucial role in ensuring spinal stability and free locomotion. Deep abdominal muscles in front, the multifidi around the spine, and the pulmonary diaphragm all must work together synergistically with the pelvic diaphragm. Thus, "there is no core without the floor" (Table 4.11).

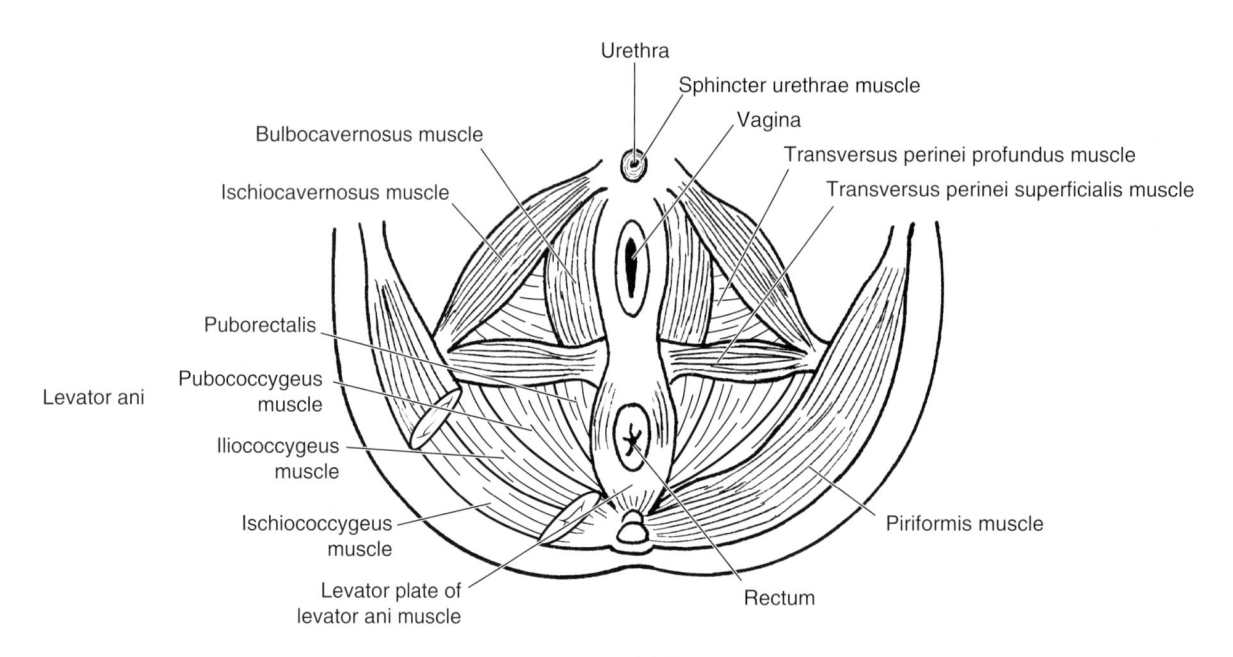

FIGURE 4.52

Table 4.11 **MUSCLES OF FORCED EXPIRATION**

I.D.	Muscle	Origin	Insertion	Function
110	Obliquus externus abdominis	Ribs 5–12 (interdigitating on external and inferior surfaces)	Iliac crest (outer border) Aponeurosis from 9th costal cartilage to ASIS; both sides meet at midline to form linea alba Pubic symphysis (upper border)	Flexion of trunk (bilateral muscles) Tilts pelvis posteriorly Elevates pelvis (unilateral) Rotation of trunk to opposite side (unilateral) Lateral bending of trunk (unilateral) Support and compression of abdominal viscera, counteracting effect of gravity on abdominal contents Assists defecation, micturition, emesis, and parturition (i.e., expulsion of contents of abdominal viscera and air from lungs) Important accessory muscle of forced expiration (during expiration it forces the viscera upward to elevate the diaphragm)
111	Obliquus internus	Iliac crest (anterior two-thirds of intermediate line) Thoracolumbar fascia Inguinal ligament (lateral two-thirds of upper aspect)	Ribs 9–12 (inferior border and abdominis cartilages by digitations that appear continuous with internal intercostals) Ribs 7–9 (cartilages) Aponeurosis to linea alba Pubic crest and pecten pubis	
112	Transversus abdominis	Inguinal ligament (lateral one-third) Iliac crest (anterior two-thirds, inner lip) Thoracolumbar fascia Ribs 7–12 (costal cartilages interdigitate with diaphragm)	Linea alba (blends with broad aponeurosis) Pubic crest and pecten pubis (to form falx inguinalis)	Constricts (flattens) abdomen, compressing the abdominal viscera and assisting in expelling their contents Forced expiration
113	Rectus abdominis	Arise via 2 tendons: Lateral: pubic crest (tubercle) and pecten pubis Medial: symphysis pubis (ligamentous covering)	Ribs 5–7 (costal cartilages) Costoxiphoid ligaments	Flexion of spine (draws symphysis and sternum toward each other) Posterior tilt of pelvis With other abdominal muscles, compresses abdominal contents
103	Intercostales interni	Ribs 1–11 (inner surface) Sternum (anterior) Internal intercostal membrane	Ribs 2–12 (upper border of rib below rib of origin)	Not as strong as the external intercostals Elevation of ribs in inspiration This may be true at least for the 1st to 5th muscles The more lateral muscle fibers run more obliquely inferior and posterior and are most active in expiration[78] Stabilization of rib cage

Table 4.11 MUSCLES OF FORCED EXPIRATION—cont'd

I.D.	Muscle	Origin	Insertion	Function
130	Latissimus dorsi	T6-T12 and all lumbar and sacral vertebrae (spinous processes via supraspinous ligaments) Iliac crest (posterior) Thoracolumbar fascia Ribs 9–12 (interdigitates with external abdominal oblique)	Humerus (floor of intertubercular sulcus) Deep fascia of arm	Extension, adduction, and internal rotation of shoulder Hyperextension of spine (muscles on both sides), as in lifting The muscle is most powerful in overhead activities (such as swimming [downstroke] and climbing), crutch walking (elevation of trunk to arms, i.e., shoulder depression), or swinging Adducts raised arm against resistance (with pectoralis major and teres major) It is very active in strong expiration, as in coughing and sneezing, and in deep inspiration Elevation of pelvis with arms fixed

Other

106	Transversus thoracis			

ASIS, Anterior superior iliac spine.

Testing the Muscles of the Pelvic Floor

Test Description and Procedure

In a separate treatment room, the clinician should explain the pelvic exam in total detail. It is recommended to have patients sign a separate consent form for the pelvic exam prior to beginning the exam. The patient should be advised that they can stop the exam at any time for any reason. After the patient thoroughly understands the exam, the clinician instructs them to disrobe from the waist down, cover themselves with a sheet provided by the clinician, and lie supine on a plinth. The clinician leaves the room while the patient is preparing for the test. After the clinician returns, the patient is asked to roll their legs into external rotation and abduction (hook lying). After the patient is relaxed, the clinician dons sterile gloves that contain no allergens or other potentially irritating material to the patient. The clinician will then apply a nonallergenic lubricant to the gloves for patient comfort. While standing slightly to the side of the patient, the clinician moves the sheet drape aside to locate needed landmarks, replaces the drape, and then slowly inserts the middle finger, index and middle finger, or middle and ring finger, into the vagina or rectum. If a patient has complaints of pelvic pain, usually only one finger is used. Once fingers are in place, the patient is asked to "pull my fingers up and in" a total of three to four times. Contractions are maintained for 1 to 2 seconds (Fig. 4.53).

FIGURE 4.53

Grading

There are several grading scales, but the scale used most commonly is the PERFECT scheme.[87] PERFECT is an acronym representing power, endurance, repetitions, fast, every, contraction, timed. The results of the PERFECT scheme will allow the clinician to develop a pelvic floor muscle exercise regime that will appropriately overload the pelvic floor musculature to produce a training effect in these muscles.

Power refers to muscle strength (MVC) evaluated using the Modified Oxford Scale described later.

Modified Oxford Scale.[88] The Modified Oxford Scale is a six-point scale in which half numbers of + and − can be added when a contraction is considered to fall between two full grades, so that the scale expands to a 15-point scale (when both + and – are used):

0 = Nil (No discernable muscle contraction)

1 = Flicker (Flicker or pulsation is felt under the examiner's finger.)

2 = Weak (An increase in tension is detected, without any discernible lift.)

3 = Moderate (Muscle tension is further enhanced and characterized by lifting of the muscle belly and also elevation of the posterior vaginal or rectal wall. A Grade 3 and stronger can be observed as an indrawing of the perineum and anus.)

4 = Good (Increased tension and a good contraction are present, which are capable of elevating the posterior vaginal wall or rectal wall against resistance.)

5 = Strong (Strong resistance can be applied to the elevation of the posterior vaginal wall or rectal wall; the examining finger is squeezed and drawn into the vagina or rectum [like a hungry baby sucking a finger].)

The Modified Oxford Scale has fair reliability among experienced clinicians.[89] Test accuracy may be enhanced with visual examination during the actual manual muscle test. Visual observation can confirm perineal tightening and whether the fingers are drawn up and in, but most clinicians do not observe the movement for various reasons.

Endurance refers to the amount of time that the MVC assessed with the Modified Oxford Scale can be held for up to 10 seconds before the pelvic floor musculature (PFM) starts to fatigue. Patients should be encouraged to breathe normally during the endurance assessment, and the clinician should ensure that cocontraction.

Repetitions is the number of repetitions recorded at the specific MVC assessed with the Modified Oxford Scale, up to 10 total repetitions. The clinician should allow a 4 second rest between contractions.

Fast refers to the number of one-second MVCs the patient can perform up to 10 repetitions.

Every contraction timed is a reminder to the clinician to time and record each of the assessments listed earlier.

Purpose: The purpose of a digital pelvic examination is to evaluate PFM performance and also to assess for the presence of pain. Many women experience incontinence and/or sexual pain, both of which may be related to pelvic floor weakness.

Position of Patient: Supine on a plinth with the knees flexed and the hips in some abduction.

Test Procedure: After obtaining informed consent for the pelvic examination and permission to begin the examination, a gloved, lubricated finger is inserted into the vagina or rectum. The patient is then asked to perform a pelvic floor muscle contraction, exerting as much force against the inserted finger as possible (squeezing it). The clinician must make sure the patient is *not* holding their breath while performing the pelvic contraction.

Instructions to Patient: "Imagine that you are trying to stop gas from escaping. Squeeze as hard as you can around my finger while doing so."

Scoring Using the PERFECT scheme described earlier, record each assessment. For example, if the patient performs an MVC at a Modified Oxford level of 3, is able to hold that contraction for 5 seconds, repeat that contraction and hold four times, and perform six fast contractions, the scoring would be reported as: 3/5/4/6.

Clinical Relevance

The Kegel (pronounced KAY-gull) exercise is named after Dr. Arnold Kegel, who designed the exercise to strengthen the pelvic floor muscles, especially the pubococcygeal muscles. The goals of strengthening the pelvic floor muscles increases include increasing resting pelvic floor muscle pressure and muscle cross-sectional area, increasing muscle stiffness, and elevating the pelvic floor musculature within the pelvic cavity, thus limiting involuntary urine leakage secondary to stress incontinence. Kegel exercises are often prescribed following surgery to the pelvic region, as part of cancer treatment, and before and after childbirth to address issues with urinary and/or fecal leakage.

Risk Management Considerations

Internal testing of the pelvic floor is typically taught at the post-entry level. Given the sensitivity of this examination, there should be a compelling reason to perform it based on the patient's subjective complaint or previous test findings, and only individuals trained at the post-entry level should perform this assessment on patients. An appropriate level of patient education to ensure informed consent should also be provided. Before engaging in this new area of practice, clinicians should review their state's practice laws to ensure that pelvic floor examination is included within the physical clinician's scope of practice. In addition, each clinician must be able to demonstrate competence through evidence of training specific to pelvic floor rehabilitation, including internal assessment and treatment, before entering this new area of practice.

Table 4.12 MUSCLES OF THE PELVIC FLOOR (PERINEUM)

I.D.	Muscle	Origin	Insertion
120	Bulbocavernosus	Surrounds the orifice of the vagina	Blends with sphincter ani externus
121	Ischiococcygeus	Inner surface of the ischial tuberosity	Tendinous aponeurosis attached to the sides and under surface of the crus clitoridis
118	Transversus perinei superficialis (indistinct, often missing)	Medial/anterior ischial tuberosity	Perineal body
119	Transversus perinei profundus	Inner surface ramus of the ischium	Blends into perineal body and vaginal wall
122	Sphincter urethrae	Superior: encircle lower end of the urethra Inferior: transverse perineal ligament	Interlace with fibers from the opposite side
Others			
115	Puborectalis		
115	Levator ani: Puborectalis Iliococcygeus Pubococcygeus		

1. Balzini L, Vannucchi L, Benvenuti F, et al. Clinical characteristics of flexed posture in elderly women. *J Am Geriatr Soc*. 2003;51(10):1419–1426.

2. Shirazi-Adl A, Sadouk S, Parnianpour M, et al. Muscle force evaluation and the role of posture in human lumbar spine under compression. *Eur Spine J*. 2002;11(6):519–526.

3. Panjabi MM. The stabilizing system of the spine. Part I. Function, dysfunction, adaptation, and enhancement. *J Spinal Disord*. 1992;5:383–389; discussion 397.

4. Panjabi MM. The stabilizing system of the spine. Part II. Neutral zone and instability hypothesis. *J Spinal Disord*. 1992;5:390–396; discussion 397.

5. Okubo Y, Kaneoka K, Imai A, et al. Electromyographic analysis of transversus abdominis and lumbar multifidus using wire electrodes during lumbar stabilization exercises. *J Orthop Sports Phys Ther*. 2010;40(11):743–750.

6. Bergmark A. Stability of the lumbar spine: a study in mechanical engineering. *Acta Orthop Scand Suppl*. 1989;230:1–54.

7. Biering-Sørensen F. Physical measurements as risk indicators for low-back trouble over a one-year period. *Spine*. 1984;9:106–119.

8. Demoulin C, Vanderthommen M, Duysens C, et al. Spinal muscle evaluation using the Sørensen test: a critical appraisal of the literature. *Joint Bone Spine*. 2006;73(1):43–50.

9. Moreau CE, Green BN, Johnson CD, et al. Isometric back extension endurance tests: a review of the literature. *J Manip Physiol Ther*. 2001;24:110–122.

10. Singh DKA, Bailey M, Lee R. Decline in lumbar extensor muscle strength in older adults: correlation with age, gender, and spine morphology. *BMC Muscuolskelet Disor*. 2013;14(1):215.

11. Sinaki M, Nwaogwugwu NC, Phillipls BE, et al. Effect of gender, age, and anthropometry on axial and appendicular muscle strength. *Am J Phys Med Rehabil*. 2001;80(5):330–338.

12. Adedoyin RA, Mbada CE, Farotimi AO, et al. Endurance of low back musculature: normative data for adults. *J Back Musculoskelet Rehabil*. 2011;24:101–109.

13. Luoto S, Heliovaara M, Hurri H, et al. Static back endurance and the risk of low-back pain. *Clin Biomech (Bristol, Avon)*. 1995;10.323–324.

14. Arab AM, Salavati M, Ebrahimi I, et al. Sensitivity, specificity and predictive value of the clinical trunk muscle endurance tests in low back pain. *Clin Rehabil*. 2007;21(7):640–647.

15. Heneghan NR, Lokhaug SM, Tyros I, et al. Clinical reasoning framework for thoracic spine exercise prescription in sport: a systematic review and narrative synthesis. *BMJ Open Sport Exerc Med*. 2020;6:e000713. https://doi.org/10.1136/bmjsem-2019-000713. https://bmjopensem.bmj.com/content/6/1/e000713#ref-11.

16. Steele J, Bruce-Low S, Smith D. A review of the specificity of exercises designed for conditioning the lumbar extensors. *Br J Sports Med*. 2015;49:291–297.

17. Kendall FP, McCreary EK, Provance PG. *Muscles, Testing and Function: With Posture and Pain*. Baltimore, MD: Williams & Wilkins; 1993.

18. Park RJ, Tsao H, Cresswell AG, Hodges PW. Differential activity of regions of the psoas major and quadratus lumborum during submaximal isometric trunk efforts. *J Orthop Res*. 2012;30(2):311–318. https://doi.org/10.1002/jor.21499. Epub 2011 Jul 28. PMID: 21800359.

19. Bordoni B, Varacallo M. Anatomy, abdomen and pelvis, quadratus lumborum 2022 Jul 18. In: *StatPearls*. Treasure Island, FL: StatPearls Publishing; 2022. [Internet] PMID: 30571028.

20. Monfort-Pañego M, Vera-García FJ, Sánchez-Zuriaga D, et al. Electromyographic studies in abdominal exercises: a literature synthesis. *J Manip Physiol Ther*. 2009;32(3):232–244.

21. Hills NF, Graham RB, McLean L. Comparison of trunk muscle function between women with and without diastasis recti abdominis at 1 year postpartum. *Phys Ther*. 2018;98(10):891–901. https://doi.org/10.1093/ptj/pzy083. PMID: 30011041.

22. Escamilla RF, McTaggart MSC, Fricklas EJ, et al. An electromyographic analysis of commercial and common abdominal exercises: implications for rehabilitation and training. *J Orthop Sports Phys Ther*. 2006;36(2):45–57.

23. Cholewicki J, Silfies SP, Shah RA, et al. Delayed trunk muscle reflex responses increase the risk of low back injuries. *Spine*. 2005;30(23):2614–2620.

24. Willson JD, Dougherty CP, Ireland ML, et al. Core stability and its relationship to lower extremity function and injury. *J Am Acad Orthop Surg*. 2005;13(5):316–325.

25. Strand SL, Hjelm J, Schoepe TC, et al. Norms for an isometric muscle endurance test. *J Hum Kinet*. 2014;40:93–102.

26. Brown SH, Haumann ML, Potvin JR. The responses of leg and trunk muscles to sudden unloading of the hands: implications for balance and spine stability. *Clin Biomech (Bristol, Avon)*. 2003;18(9):812–820.

27. Hodges PW, Cresswell AG, Daggfeldt K, et al. Three dimensional preparatory trunk motion precedes asymmetrical upper limb movement. *Gait Posture*. 2000;11(2):92–101.

28. Bliss LS, Teeple P. Core stability: the centerpiece of any training program. *Curr Sports Med Rep*. 2005;4:179e83.

29. Kibler WB, Press J, Sciascia A. The role of core stability in athletic function. *Sports Med*. 2006;36(3):189–198.

30. Liemohn WP, Baumgartner TA, Gagnon LH. Measuring core stability. *J Strength Cond Res*. 2005;19(3):583–586.

31. Cholewicki J, VanVliet 4th JJ. Relative contribution of trunk muscles to the stability of the lumbar spine during isometric exertions. *Clin Biomech (Bristol, Avon)*. 2002;17(2):99–105.

32. McGill SM, Grenier S, Kavcic N, et al. Coordination of muscle activity to assure stability of the lumbar spine. *J Electromyogr Kinesiol*. 2003;13(4):353–359.

33. Jørgensen K. Human trunk extensor muscles physiology and ergonomics. *Acta Physiol Scand Suppl*. 1997;637:1–58.

34. Evans K, Refshauge K, Adams R. Trunk muscle endurance tests: reliability, and gender differences in athletes. *J Sci Med Sport/Sports Med Aus*. 2007;10(6):447–455.

35. Akuhota V, Ferreiro A, Moore T, et al. Core stability exercise principles. *Curr Sports Med Rep*. 2008;7(1):39–44.

36. Stokes IAF, Gardner-Morse MG, Henry SM. Abdominal muscle activation increases lumbar spinal stability: analysis of contributions of different muscle groups. *Clin Biomech (Bristol, Avon)*. 2011;26. 797–798.803.

37. Ikezaki F, Krueger E, de Souza Guerino Macedo C. Performance, reliability and fatigue in prone bridge test and supine unilateral bridge test. *J Bodyw Mov Ther*. 2021;26:238–245. https://doi.org/10.1016/j.jbmt.2020.08.008. Epub 2020 Sep 6. PMID: 33992251.

38. De Blaiser C, De Ridder R, Willems T, et al. Evaluating abdominal core muscle fatigue: assessment of the validity and reliability of the prone bridging test. *Scand J Med Sci Sports*. 2018;28(2):391–399. https://doi.org/10.1111/sms.12919. Epub 2017 Jun 28. PMID: 28544083.

39. Bohannon RW, Steffl M, Glenney SS, et al. The prone bridge test: performance, validity, and reliability among older and younger adults. *J Bodyw Mov Ther*. 2018;22:385–389.

40. Cortell-Tormo JM, García-Jaén M, Chulvi-Medrano I, et al. Influence of scapular position on the core musculature activation in the prone plank exercise. *J Strength Cond Res*. 2017;31(8):2255–2262.

41. Lopes TJA, Simic M, Alves DS, et al. Physical performance measures of flexibility, hip strength, lower limb power, and trunk endurance in healthy navy cadets: normative data and differences between sex and limb dominance. *J Strength Cond Res*. 2018;35(2):458–464.

42. Kavcic N, Grenier S, McGill SM. Determining the stabilizing role of individual torso muscles during rehabilitation exercises. *Spine*. 2004;29:1254–1265.

43. Juker D, McGill S, Kropf P, et al. Quantitative intramuscular myoelectric activity of lumbar portions of psoas and the abdominal wall during a wide variety of tasks. *Med Sci Sports Exerc*. 1998;30:301–310.

44. McGill SM, Childs A, Liebenson C. Endurance times for low back stabilization exercises: clinical targets for testing and training from a normal database. *Arch Phys Med Rehabil*. 1999;80(8):941–944.

45. El-Gohary TM, Abd Elkader SM, Emara HA, et al. Right versus left side bridge static endurance ability among healthy collegiate students at Taibah University. *J Back Musculoskelet Rehabil*. 2018;31(2):231–237. https://doi.org/10.3233/BMR-169538. PMID: 29171976.

46. Oliveira IO, Pilz B, Santos Jr RLG, et al. Reference values and reliability for lumbopelvic strength and endurance in asymptomatic subjects. *Braz J Phys Ther*. 2018;22(1):33–41. https://doi.org/10.1016/j.bjpt.2017.09.008. Epub 2017 Sep 29. PMID: 29031958; PMCID: PMC5816085.

47. Anderson D, Barthelemy L, Gmach R, et al. *Core strength testing: Developing normative data for three clinical tests- Doctor of Physical Therapy Research Papers*, St. Paul, MN: St. Catherine University; 2013. http://sophia.stkate.edu/dpt_papers/21.

48. Juan-Recio C, Prat-Luri A, Galindo A, et al. Is the side bridge test valid and reliable for assessing trunk lateral flexor endurance in recreational female athletes?. *Biology (Basel)*. 2022;11(7):1043. https://doi.org/10.3390/biology11071043. PMID: 36101422; PMCID: PMC9312545.

49. Haff GG, Triplett NT, eds. *Essentials of Strength Training and Conditioning*. 4th ed. Champaign IL: Human Kinetics; 2016.

50. Reiman MP, Krier AD, Nelson JA et al. Comparison of different trunk endurance testing methods in college-aged individuals. *Int J Sports Phys Ther*. N2012;7(5):533–539.

51. Cowley P, Swensen T. Development and reliability of two core stability field tests. *J Strength Cond Res*. 2008;22(2):619–624.

52. Cowley P, Fitzgerald S, Sottung K, et al. Age, weight, and the front abdominal power test as predictors of isokinetic trunk strength and work in young men and women. *J Strength Cond Res*. 2009;23(3):915–925.

53. Butowicz CM, Ebaugh DD, Noehren B, et al. Validation of two clinical measures of core stability. *Int J Sports Phys Ther*. 2016;11(1):15–23.

54. Ekstrom RA, Donatelli RA, Carp KC. Electromyographic analysis of core trunk, hip, and thigh muscles during 9 rehabilitation exercises. *J Orthop Sports Phys Ther*. 2007;37(12):754–755, 762.

55. Calatayud J, Escriche-Escuder A, Cruz-Montecinos C, et al. Tolerability and muscle activity of core muscle exercises in chronic low-back pain. *Int J Environ Res Public Health*. 2019;16(19):3509. https://doi.org/10.3390/ijerph16193509. PMID: 31547140; PMCID: PMC6801665.

56. George SZ, Fritz JM, Silfies SP, et al. Interventions for the management of acute and chronic low back pain: Revision 2021. *J Orthop Sports Phys Ther*. 2021;51(11):CPG1–CPG60. https://doi.org/10.2519/jospt.2021.0304. PMID: 34719942.

57. Imai A, Kaneoka K, Okubo Y, et al. Trunk muscle activity during lumbar stabilization exercises on both a stable and unstable surface. *J Orthop Sports Phys Ther*. 2010;40(6):369–375.

58. Adedoyin RA, Adeleke OE, Fehintola AO, et al. Reference values for chest expansion among adult residents in Ile-Ife. *J Yoga Phys Ther*. 2012;2(3):1000113. https://www.longdom.org/open-access/reference-values-for-chest-expansion-among-adult-residents-in-ileife-4218-0.html.

59. Derasse M, Lefebvre S, Liistro G, Reychler G. Chest expansion and lung function for healthy subjects and individuals with pulmonary disease. *Respir Care*. 2021;66(40):661–668.

60. Sharshar T, Hopkinson NS, Ross ET, et al. Motor control of the costal and crural diaphragm-insights from transcranial magnetic stimulation in man. *Respir Physiol Neurobiol*. 2005;146(1):5–19.

61. Saboisky JP, Gorman RB, De Troyer A, et al. Differential activation among five human inspiratory motoneuron pools during tidal breathing. *J Appl Physiol (1985)*. 2007;102(2):772–780. https://doi.org/10.1152/japplphysiol.00683.2006. Epub 2006 Oct 19. PMID: 17053105.

62. Butler JE, Hudson AL, Gandevia SC. The neural control of human inspiratory muscles. *Prog Brain Res*. 2014;209:295–308.

63. Bain KNS, Kashyap S, Lappin SL. Anatomy, thorax, diaphragm Updated 25 July 2022. In: *StatPearls*. Treasure Island, FL: StatPearls Publishing; 2022 (Internet).

64. Mayos M, Giner J, Casan P, Sanchis J. Measurement of maximal static respiratory pressures at the mouth with different air leaks. *Chest*. 1991;100:364–366. https://doi.org/10.1378/chest.100.2.364.

65. Laveneziana P, Albuquerque A, Aliverti A, et al. ERS statement on respiratory muscle testing at rest and during exercise. *Eur Respir J*. 2019;53(6):1801214. https://doi.org/10.1183/13993003.01214-2018. PMID 30956204.

66. Hull J, Aniapravan R, Chan E, et al. British Thoracic Society guideline for respiratory management of children with neuromuscular weakness. *Thorax*. 2012;67:i1–i40.

67. Bordoni B, Varacallo M. *Anatomy, Head and Neck, Scalenus Muscle*. Treasure Island, FL: StatPearls Publishing; 2022. [Updated 2022 Apr 16]. In: StatPearls [Internet].

68. Le Niendre A, Mongodi S, Philippart F, et al. Thoracic ultrasound: potential new tool for physioclinicians in respiratory management. A narrative review. *J Crit Care*. 2016;31:101–109.

69. Lerolle N, Guérot E, Dimassi S, et al. Ultrasonographic diagnostic criterion for severe diaphragmatic dysfunction after cardiac surgery. *Chest*. 2009;135:401–407.

70. Summerhill EM, El-Sameed YA, Glidden TJ, et al. Monitoring recovery from diaphragmatic paralysis with ultrasound. *Chest*. 2008;133:737–743.

71. HajGhanbari B, Yamabayashi C, Buna TR, et al. Effects of respiratory muscle training on performance in athletes: a systematic review with meta-analyses. *J Strength Cond Res*. 2013;27(6):1643–1663. https://doi.org/10.1519/JSC.0b013e318269f73f.

72. Bissett B, Leditschke IA, Green M, et al. Inspiratory muscle training for intensive care patients: a multidisciplinary practical guide for clinicians. *Aust Crit Care*. 2019;32(3):P249–P255.

73. Watson K, Egerton T, Sheers N, et al. Respiratory muscle training in neuromuscular disease: a systematic review and meta-analysis. *Eur Respir Rev*. 2022;31(166):220065. https://doi.org/10.1183/16000617.0065-2022. PMID: 36450369; PMCID: PMC9724913.

74. Konrad D, Hillegrass E, eds. *Essentials of Cardiopulmonary Physical Therapy*. 4th ed. St. Louis, MO: Elsevier; 2017.

75. Evans JA, Whitelaw WA. The assessment of maximal respiratory mouth pressures in adults. *Respir Care*. 2009;54:1348.

76. Kang S-W, Bach JR. Maximum insufflation capacity. *Chest*. 2000;118(1):P61–P65.

77. Singh RK, Saran S, Baroia AK. The practice of tracheostomy decannulation: a systematic review. *J Intensive Care*. 2017;5:38. https://www.ncbi.nlm.nih.gov/pmc/articles/PMC5477679/.

78. Tang A, Bordoni B. Anatomy, thorax, muscles. In: *StatPearls*. Treasure Island (FL): StatPearls Publishing; 2022. [Internet] [Updated 2022 Jul 25].

79. Neumann P, Grimmer-Somers KA, Gill V, et al. Rater reliability of pelvic floor muscle strength. *Aust N Z Continence J*. 2007;13:9–14.

80. Tim S, Mazur-Bialy AI. The most common functional disorders and factors affecting female pelvic floor. *Life (Basel)*. 2021;11(12):1397. https://doi.org/10.3390/life11121397. PMID: 34947928; PMCID: PMC8704638.

81. Verbeek M, Hayward L. Pelvic floor dysfunction and its effect on quality of sexual life. *Sex Med Rev*. 2019;7(4):559–564.

82. Patel UJ, Godecker AL, Giles DL, Brown HW. Updated prevalence of urinary incontinence in women: 2015–2018 national population-based survey data. *Female Pelvic Med Reconstr Surg*. 2022;28(4):181–187. https://doi.org/10.1097/SPV.0000000000001127.

83. Park S-H, Kang C-B. Effect of Kegel exercises on the management of stress urinary incontinence: a systematic review of randomized controlled trials. *Adv Nurs*. 2014:2014:1–10. Article ID 640262. https://doi.org/10.1155/2014/640262. https://www.hindawi.com/journals/anurs/2014/640262/.

84. Lewis RW, Fugl-Meyer KS, Corona G, et al. Definitions/epidemiology/risk factors for sexual dysfunction. *J Sex Med*. 2010;7(4 Pt 2):1598–1607.

85. Knoepp LR, Shippey SH, Chen CC, et al. Sexual complaints, pelvic floor symptoms, and sexual distress in women over forty. *J Sex Med*. 2010;7:3675–3682.

86. Deegan EG, Stothers L, Kavanagh A, Macnab AJ. Quantification of pelvic floor muscle strength in female urinary incontinence: a systematic review and comparison of contemporary methodologies. *Neurourol Urodyn*. 2018;37(1):33–45. https://doi.org/10.1002/nau.23285. Epub 2017 May 4. PMID: 28471486.

87. Laycock J, Jerwood D. Pelvic floor muscle assessment: the PERFECT scheme. *Physiotherapy*. 2001;87(12):631–642. https://my.instituteofphysicalart.com/media/ipa/pdf2/Laycock2001PERFECTscheme.pdf.

88. Laycock J. Clinical evaluation of the pelvic floor. In: Schussler B, Laycock J, Norton P, et al., eds. *Pelvic Floor Re-education*. London, UK: Springer-Verlag; 1994:42–48.

89. Ferreira CH, Barbosa PB, de Oliveira Souza F, et al. Inter-rater reliability study of the modified Oxford grading scale and the peritron manometer. *Physiotherapy*. 2011;97(2):132–138

5

Testing the Muscles of the Upper Extremity

Shoulder Girdle Strength Testing

   Introduction

Scapular Abduction (Protraction) and Upward Rotation

Scapular Elevation

Scapular Adduction (Retraction)

Scapular Depression and Adduction

Scapular Adduction (Retraction) and Downward Rotation

Latissimus Dorsi

Introduction to Testing the Deltoid

Shoulder Flexion

Shoulder Extension

Shoulder Abduction

Shoulder Horizontal Abduction

Shoulder Horizontal Adduction

Introduction to the Rotator Cuff

Shoulder External Rotation

Shoulder Internal Rotation

Elbow Flexion

Elbow Extension

Forearm Supination

Forearm Pronation

Wrist Flexion

Wrist Extension

Introduction to Testing the Muscles of the Hand

   Extrinsic Muscles

Finger PIP and DIP Flexion

   Combined DIP and PIP Tests

PIP Tests

DIP Tests

Finger MCP Extension

Finger MCP Flexion

   Intrinsic Muscles

Finger Abduction

Finger Adduction

   Thumb Muscles

Thumb MCP and IP Flexion

Thumb IP Flexion

Thumb MCP and IP Extension

Thumb Abduction

   Abductor Pollicis Longus

   Abductor Pollicis Brevis

Thumb Adduction

Opposition (Thumb to Little Finger)

Grip Strength

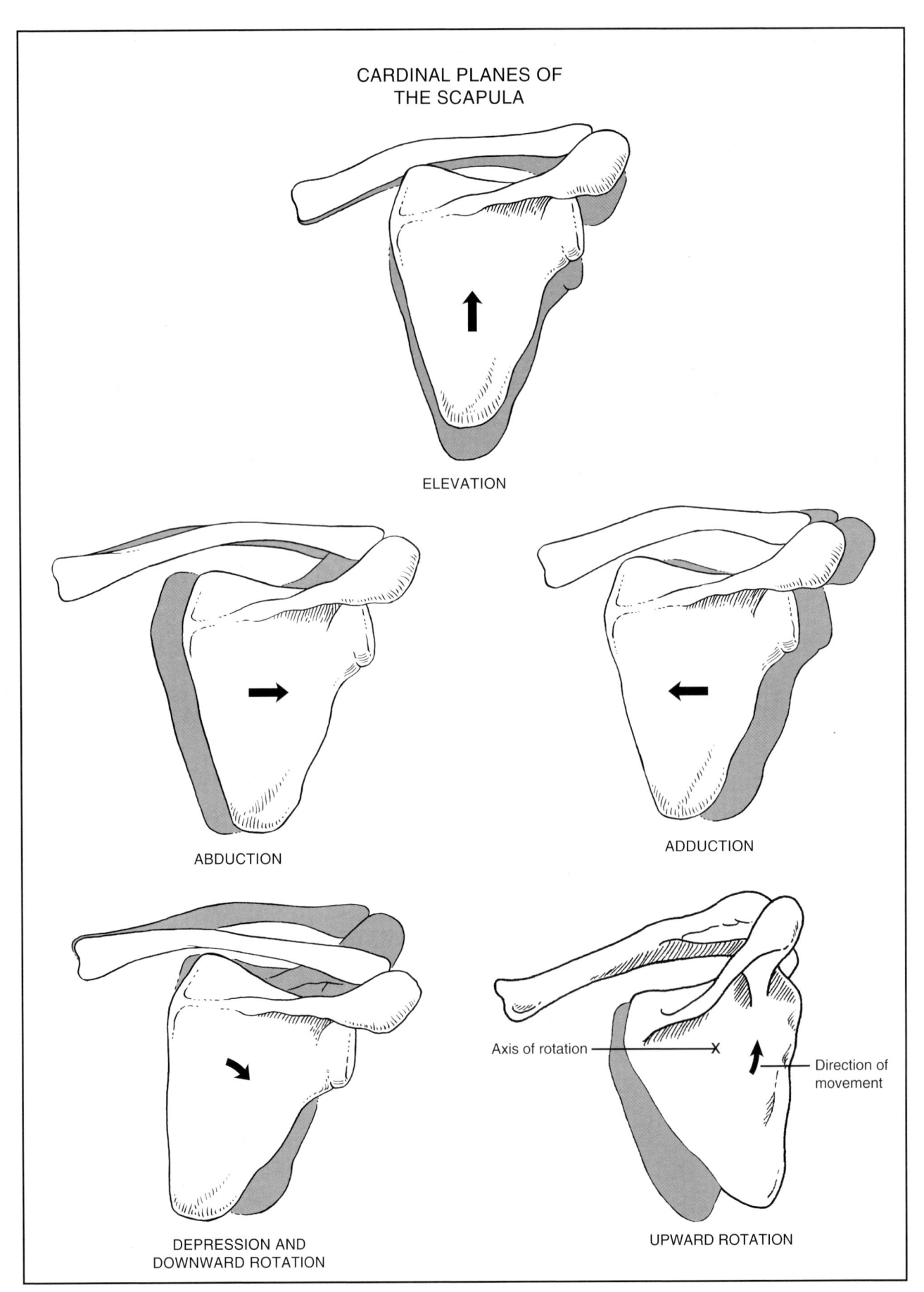

CARDINAL PLANES OF THE SCAPULA

ELEVATION

ABDUCTION

ADDUCTION

DEPRESSION AND
DOWNWARD ROTATION

UPWARD ROTATION

Axis of rotation

Direction of
movement

PLATE 2 Elevation (as in shrugging the shoulders). Abduction (protraction) is forward movement occurring in pushing, thrusting, or reaching. Adduction (retraction) occurs when bracing the shoulders. Depression and downward rotation (medial rotation) when returning scapula to the rest position. Upward rotation (lateral rotation) occurs with shoulder elevation and with protraction of the scapula.

INTRODUCTION

The shoulder girdle is a complex system comprised of 5 distinct joints and at least 16 muscles, many of which have multiple parts and actions. The purpose of scapulohumeral motion is the appropriate positioning of the glenohumeral (G-H) joint in space, while the purpose of scapular stability is to provide a foundation for G-H motion.[1]

The chief muscles that act upon the G-H joint are the deltoid (three parts), the pectorales (two parts), the latissimus dorsi, teres major, and the four rotator cuff muscles (subscapularis, supraspinatus, infraspinatus, and teres minor).[2] The primary muscles acting upon the scapula to properly position the humerus are the serratus anterior and upper and lower trapezius.[2]

Shoulder elevation is any combination of humeral abduction and flexion occurring at the G-H joint that results in raising the arm, and so it is the preferred term used in this text. The most efficient shoulder elevators are the anterior and middle deltoid and the supraspinatus (initially).[1] Shoulder elevation is not to be confused with shoulder girdle elevation, the motion of shrugging the shoulders.

Preliminary Examination

Observation of posture in sitting and standing is important prior to strength testing, noting the natural variability between sides and between individuals. First, examine the sitting patient (with hands in the lap) from the back (posterior view), noting the position of the scapulae at rest, any asymmetry of shoulder height, muscular bulk, position of the G-H joint, and any scapular winging (Figs. 5.1 and 5.2). Some scapular asymmetry is common and has many causes. Handedness, habitual stretch weakness (e.g., rounded shoulders that can accompany the forward head posture [see Fig. 3.14]) and carrying purses or briefcases habitually on one side can all contribute to normal scapular asymmetry.

Position and Symmetry of Scapulae: The normal scapula lies close to the rib cage, with the vertebral border nearly parallel to and from 1 to 3 inches lateral to the spinous processes. The inferior angle is on the chest wall.

The most prominent abnormal posture of the scapula is "winging" in which the vertebral border tilts away from the rib cage, a sign of probable serratus anterior weakness (see Fig. 5.2).

Scapulohumeral Rhythm: Next, observe scapulohumeral rhythm. Scapulohumeral rhythm consists of integrated and simultaneous movements of the G-H, scapulothoracic, acromioclavicular, and sternoclavicular joints. It occurs in sequential fashion to allow full functional motion of the shoulder complex. Although there is normal variability in scapulohumeral rhythm, the overall ratio of G-H to scapulothoracic motion is approximately 2:1 to complete 180° of shoulder elevation but varies throughout the range.[3] Thus, for 180° of shoulder elevation, approximately 120° comes from the G-H abduction and the other 60° from upward rotation of the scapula.

FIGURE 5.1

FIGURE 5.2

Preliminary Examination Continued

Scapular Range of Motion: Total scapular motion increases over the arc of shoulder elevation. G-H and scapular movements occur not as separate motions but as synchronous motions throughout the range. Specifically:

a. The scapula sits against the thorax during the first phase of shoulder abduction and flexion to provide initial stability as the humerus abducts and flexes to 30°. During this first 30°, the scapula's contribution to G-H movement is minimal.

b. From 30° to 90° of elevation, the G-H joint contributes another 30° of motion as the scapula upwardly rotates 30°. During this range, the scapulohumeral rhythm is typically greater than 2:1.[3] The upward rotation is accompanied by clavicular elevation through the sternoclavicular and acromioclavicular joints (Fig. 5.3).

c. The second phase (90° to 120°) is made up of 60° of G-H abduction and flexion and an additional 30° of scapular upward rotation. During this portion of the range, scapulohumeral rhythm declines to approximately 1:1.[3] Scapular rotation is associated with 5° of elevation at the sternoclavicular joint and 25° of rotation at the acromioclavicular joint (see Fig. 5.3).

d. After 120° of shoulder elevation, the scapula rotates approximately 1° for every 1° of shoulder elevation until maximal shoulder elevation is achieved for a total of approximately 35° to 55° of scapular upward rotation.[4]

Observe that the scapula basically remains in its rest position at ranges of less than 30° of shoulder elevation (the position is variable among subjects). To feel upward rotation, palpate the vertebral borders of both scapulae with the thumbs, placing the web of the thumb below the inferior angle and the extended fingers around the axillary borders (see Fig. 5.1), and ask the patient to lift the arm to 180° of shoulder elevation.

If the scapula moves a lot as the G-H joint moves through a range from 0° to 60°—that is, if in this range, they move as a unit—there is limited G-H motion. Above 30° and to about 150° or 160° in both active and passive motions, the scapula moves in concert with the humerus in about a 2:1 ratio.

After assessing the scapular position at rest, ask the patient to raise the test arm above the head in the sagittal plane. If the arm can be raised well above 90° (G-H muscles must be at least Grade 3 to do this), observe the direction and amount of scapular motion that occurs. Normally, the scapula rotates upward in a motion that is controlled by the serratus, and if erratic or "uncoordinated" motion occurs, the serratus is most likely weak. The normal amount of motion from the vertebral border is about the breadth of two fingers (Fig. 5.4). If the patient can raise the arm with simultaneous rhythmical scapular upward rotation, proceed with the test sequence for Grades 5 and 4.

FIGURE 5.3

FIGURE 5.4

Preliminary Examination Continued

Scapula Abnormal Position at Rest: If the scapula is positioned abnormally at rest (i.e., downwardly rotated, abducted, or winging), the patient will not be able to elevate the arm above 90°. Proceed to serratus muscle tests described for Grades 2, 1, and 0. The serratus anterior never can be graded higher than the grade given to shoulder flexion. If the patient has a weak deltoid, the lever for testing is gone, and the arm cannot be used to apply resistance.

Clinical Relevance

Thoracic spine extension is necessary to achieve full shoulder elevation. If a person is kyphotic, shoulder elevation will be sacrificed, and a 10° to 20° deficit of shoulder elevation will be noted.

FIGURE 5.5

FIGURE 5.6

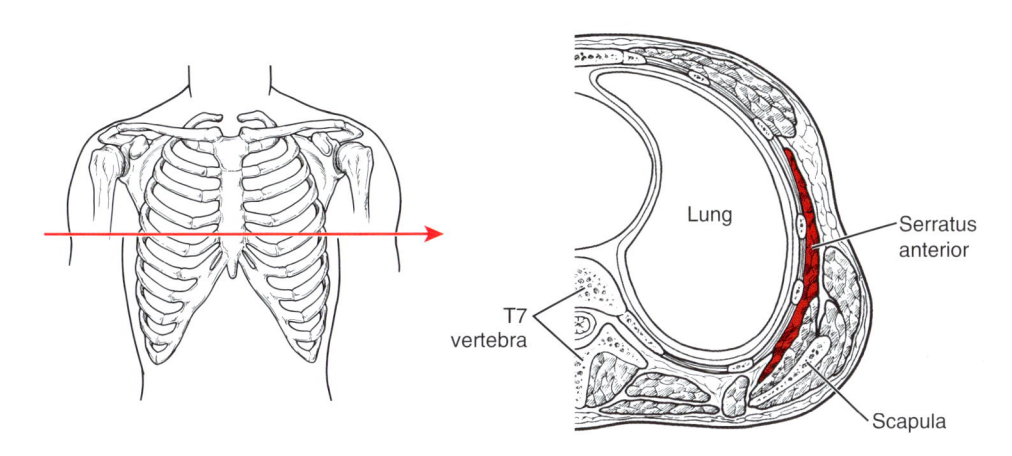

FIGURE 5.7 Arrow indicates level of cross section.

SCAPULAR ABDUCTION (PROTRACTION) AND UPWARD ROTATION

(Serratus anterior)

Range of Motion

Reliable values not available

Table 5.1 SCAPULAR ABDUCTION (PROTRACTION) AND UPWARD ROTATION

I.D.	Muscle	Origin	Insertion	Function
128	**Serratus anterior**	Ribs 1–8 and often 9 and 10 (by digitations along a curved line) Intercostal fascia Aponeurosis of intercostals	Scapula (ventral surface of vertebral border) 1st digitation (superior angle) 2nd–4th digitations (costal surface of entire vertebral border) Lower 4th or 5th digitations (costal surface of inferior angle)	Upward rotation of the scapula (glenoid faces up) • Scapular abduction • Medial border of scapula drawn anteriorly close to the thoracic wall (preventing "winging")
124	Upper and lower trapezius			• Works in conjunction with serratus to produce upward rotation
Other				
129	Pectoralis minor			• Scapular protraction (abduction): scapula moves forward around the chest wall. Works here with serratus anterior • Elevation of ribs in forced inspiration when scapula is fixed by the levator scapulae

The serratus is a prime mover for scapular abduction (protraction), with the pectoralis minor also contributing minimally. Their purpose is to maintain the continuous apposition of the scapula with the humerus. The rhomboids control the rate and range of motion of scapular abduction. As the arm is raised, the serratus helps other muscles to first fix the scapula, then rotate the scapula, allowing the arm to be raised to the vertical. The upper and lower fibers of the trapezius assist with the upward and medial pull of the lateral end of the clavicle and acromion.[1] This simultaneous action of the trapezius has focused attention on the development of exercises that focus on the serratus without simultaneously firing the trapezius. The serratus also works eccentrically in controlling gravity-assisted downward rotation of the scapula, especially if the arm is loaded (weight in hand).

Testing the serratus in the supine position is not recommended at any grade level. The supine position allows too much substitution that may not be noticeable. Lying supine on the table gives added stabilization to the scapula so that it does not "wing" and protraction of the arm may be performed by the clavicular portion of the pectoralis minor. The serratus should always be tested in sitting with shoulder elevation to minimize the synergy with the trapezius.

Grade 5, Grade 4, and Grade 3

Position of the Patient: Short sitting with arm forward flexed to about 130° and then protracted in that plane as far as it can move.

Instructions to Clinician: Stand at test side of patient. Ask patient to protract arm to assess available range and patient's ability to achieve the test position. If successful, position arm as noted earlier. Hand used for resistance grasps the upper arm just above the elbow and gives resistance in a backward direction. The other hand stabilizes the trunk just below the scapula on the same side, thus preventing trunk rotation (Fig. 5.8).

The clinician should select a spot on the wall or ceiling that can serve as a target for the patient to reach toward when the shoulder is at 130° of elevation.

Test: Clinician resists protraction and elevation of the arm at about 130° of flexion. Patient holds against maximal resistance.

Instructions to Patient: "Hold your arm here. Don't let me move it."

Grading

Grade 5: Scapula maintains its abducted and rotated position against maximal resistance (see Fig. 5.8).

Grade 4: Scapular muscles "give" or "yield" against maximal resistance. The G-H joint is normally held rigid in the presence of a strong deltoid, but if the serratus yields, the scapula moves in the direction of adduction and downward rotation.

Grade 3: Scapula moves through full range of motion without winging and without resistance other than the weight of the arm (Fig. 5.9).

FIGURE 5.8

FIGURE 5.9

(Serratus anterior)

Grade 2

Position of the Patient: Short sitting with arm flexed above 90° and supported by clinician.

Instructions to Clinician: Stand at test side of patient. One hand supports patient's arm at the elbow, maintaining the arm above the horizontal (Fig. 5.10). The other hand is placed at the inferior angle of the scapula with the thumb positioned along the axillary border and the fingers along the vertebral border (see Fig. 5.10).

Test: Clinician monitors scapular motion by using a light grasp on the scapula at the inferior angle. Clinician must be sure not to restrict or resist motion. The scapula is observed for winging.

Instructions to Patient: "Hold your arm in this position" (i.e., above 90°). "Let it relax. Now hold your arm up again. Let it relax."

Grading

Grade 2: If the scapula abducts and rotates upward as the patient attempts to hold the arm in the elevated position, the weakness is in the G-H muscles. If the scapula does not smoothly abduct and upwardly rotate without the weight of the arm or if the scapula moves toward the vertebral spine, the weakness is in the serratus and should be graded a 2.

FIGURE 5.10

(Serratus anterior)

Grade 1 and Grade 0

Position of Patient: Short sitting with arm forward flexed to above 90° (supported by clinician).

Instructions to Clinician: Stand in front of and slightly to one side of patient. Support the patient's arm at the elbow, maintaining it above 90° (Fig. 5.11). Use the other hand to palpate the serratus, with the tips of the fingers just in front of the inferior angle along the axillary border (see Fig. 5.11).

Test: Patient attempts to hold the arm in the test position.

Instructions to Patient: "Try to hold your arm in this position."

Grading

Grade 1: Muscle contraction is palpable.

Grade 0: No discernable palpable contraction.

Alternate Test for the Serratus Anterior[7]

This test may detect winging of the scapula.

Position of the Patient: Short sitting with arm flexed 90° to 100°, with elbow held in full extension and fingers in a fist.

Instructions to Clinician: Stand at test side and front of patient. Ask patient to protract arm, reaching forward. Place one hand over the serratus. The hand used for resistance is placed over the patient's fist, with open hand (Fig. 5.12).

Test: Clinician resists the patient's push into a position of retraction and internal rotation (IR).

Instructions to Patient: "Push into me. Don't let me move it."

Clinical Relevance

- The highest level of serratus anterior electromyography (EMG) activity is achieved below 90° of humeral elevation and with resistance in an inferior direction.[5,6]
- If a patient has a painful elbow (e.g., tennis elbow or epicondylitis), resistance may be applied above the painful joint, on the proximal arm.
- The serratus anterior directs the movements of posterior tilt and external rotation of the upwardly rotating scapula during elevation of the arm, which may increase or at least maintain the amount of subacromial space.[7]
- The serratus can be tested with the patient in supine, but it is difficult to palpate the serratus in this position.

FIGURE 5.11

FIGURE 5.12 Alternate test for the serratus anterior.

SCAPULAR ABDUCTION (PROTRACTION) AND UPWARD ROTATION

(Serratus anterior)

Suggested Exercises for Serratus Anterior

- Push-up progression
- Least muscle demand: wall push-up
- Moderate muscle demand: push-up on knees
- Highest muscle demand: push-up with feet elevated.[8]
- Push-up plus[a] (produces minimal upper trapezius activation and maximum activation of the serratus)[9]
- Dynamic hug[9]
- Diagonal exercise flexion (D1[8,10] and D2,[8] D2 diagonal pattern extension)[8]
- Bench press, seated (using a weight machine) with upper trapezius[10]
- Isometric low row (with lower trapezius)[9]
- Lawnmower rows (with lower trapezius)[9]

[a]Push-up plus is a classic push-up with extended arms and a narrow hand width. On fully extended arms, lift the back toward the ceiling. Then, drop the trunk down, bending elbows 30°; then, raise trunk again, lifting the back toward the ceiling at the end of the movement (it is a small movement, just a couple of inches).

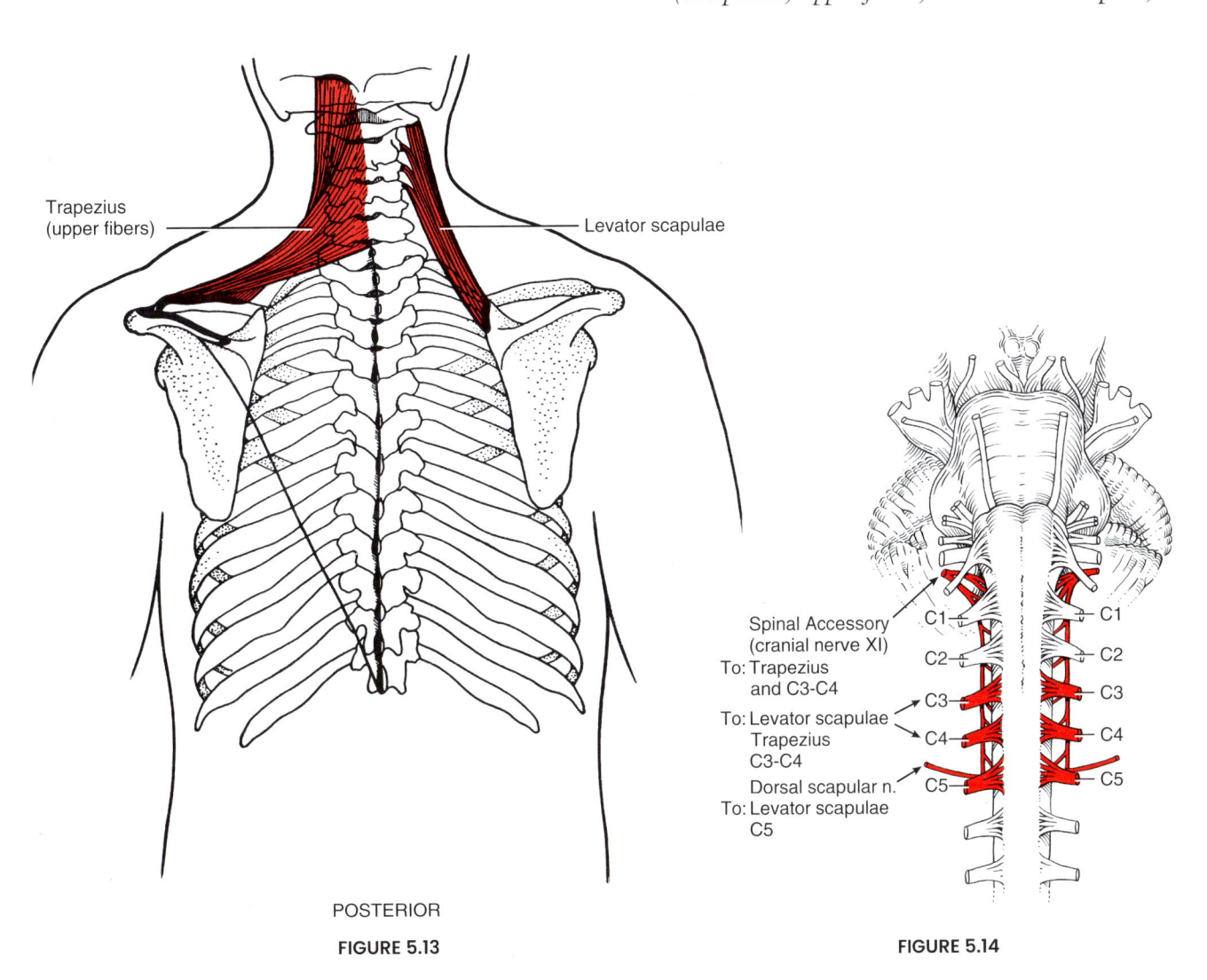

POSTERIOR

FIGURE 5.13

FIGURE 5.14

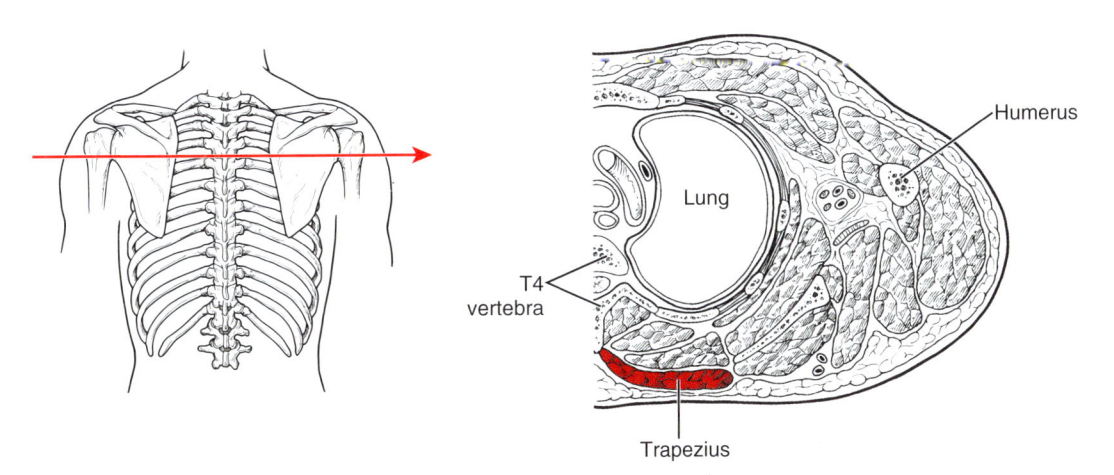

FIGURE 5.15 Arrow indicates level of cross section.

SCAPULAR ELEVATION

(Trapezius, upper fibers, and Levator scapula)[11]

Range of Motion

Reliable data not available.

Table 5.2 SCAPULAR ELEVATION

I.D.	Muscle	Origin	Insertion	Function
124	**Trapezius (upper fibers)**	Occiput (external protuberance and superior nuchal line, medial one-third) Ligamentum nuchae C7 vertebra (spinous process)	Clavicle (posterior border of lateral one-third)	Upper: • Elevation of shoulder girdle ("shrugging") (with levator scapulae) • Rotation of head to opposite side (one) • Capital extension (both) Upper and Lower: • Rotation of the scapula so glenoid faces up (inferior angle moves laterally and forward); occurs only if contracting in conjunction with serratus anterior • Cervical extension (both)
127	Levator scapulae	C1-C4 vertebrae (transverse processes)	Scapula (vertebral border between superior angle and root of scapular spine)	• Elevates and adducts scapula • Scapular downward rotation (glenoid faces down) • Lateral bending of cervical spine to same side (one) • Cervical rotation to same side (one) • Cervical extension (both assist)
Others				
125	Rhomboid major	See Table 5.3		
126	Rhomboid minor	See Table 5.5		

Elevation of the scapula and point of the shoulder, as in shrugging the shoulders, is generated by the trapezius acting on the lateral clavicle, acromion, and spine of the scapula, with some assistance from the levator scapula. In the intact muscle, elevation should be a straight "up" movement.

Grade 5, Grade 4, and Grade 3

Position of the Patient: Short sitting over end or side of table in erect posture. Hands relaxed in lap.

Instructions to Clinician: Stand behind seated patient. Ask patient to elevate (shrug) the shoulders (Grade 3). If range is full and symmetrical, apply resistance. Contour hands over top of both shoulders to give resistance in a downward direction. This muscle is quite strong, so the clinician's arms should be nearly straight, transferring the clinician's body weight through the arms to provide enough resistance. If unilateral weakness is suspected (rare), testing each side separately may be indicated.

Test: Patient elevates (shrugs) shoulders. The test is almost always performed on both sides simultaneously (Fig. 5.16).

Instructions to Patient: "Shrug your shoulders" OR "Raise your shoulders toward your ears. Hold it. Don't let me push them down."

FIGURE 5.16

Grade 5, Grade 4, and Grade 3 Continued

Grading

Grade 5: Holds test position against maximal resistance (Fig. 5.17).

Grade 4: Patient holds test position against strong to moderate resistance. The shoulder muscles may "give" at the end point.

Grade 3: Elevates shoulders through full available range without resistance.

Grade 2, Grade 1, and Grade 0

Position of the Patient: Prone, fully supported on table. Head may be turned away from test side for patient comfort and to reduce the potential contribution of the levator scapulae (Fig. 5.18).

Instructions to Clinician: Stand at test side of patient. Support test shoulder in palm of one hand. The other hand palpates the upper trapezius near its insertion above the clavicle. A second site for palpation is the upper trapezius just adjacent to the cervical vertebrae.

Test: With the clinician supporting the shoulder, the patient elevates the shoulder (usually done unilaterally) toward the ear.

Instructions to Patient: "Raise your shoulder toward your ear (shrug)."

Grading

Grade 2: Patient completes full range of motion in gravity-minimized position.

Grade 1: Upper trapezius fibers can be palpated at clavicle or neck. The levator muscle lies deep and is more difficult to palpate in the neck (between the sternocleidomastoid and the trapezius). It can be felt at its insertion on the vertebral border of the scapula superior to the scapular spine when the head is turned toward the side being tested.

Clinical Relevance

- If the patient cannot assume the sitting position for testing for any reason, the tests for Grade 5 and Grade 4 in the supine position will be quite inaccurate. If the Grade 3 test is done in the supine position, it will require manual resistance because gravity is neutralized.
- If the prone position is not comfortable, the tests for Grades 2, 1, and 0 may be performed with the patient supine, but palpation in such cases will be less than optimal.
- Injury to the spinal accessory nerve may cause paralysis or marked weakness of both the sternocleidomastoid and trapezius muscles.
- Isolated weakness of the trapezius typically results in a "drooping" of the shoulder girdle with excessive downward rotation of the scapula.[12]
- No difference in mean electromyography (EMG) activity was found between the shoulder shrug test (Fig. 5.16), resisted shoulder flexion, and resisted shoulder abduction with resisted neck side bending to the same side.[6]

Suggested Exercises for the Upper Trapezius

- Shoulder shrug with retraction[12]
- Overhead shrug[12]
- Abduction to 45°, 90°, and 120° (decreases middle trapezius activity)
- Low row (decreases serratus anterior activity)
- Prone horizontal abduction at 135° with external rotation (ER) (thumb up) (optimizes upper trapezius and decreases serratus anterior activity)[8]

FIGURE 5.17

FIGURE 5.18

(Trapezius, middle fibers)

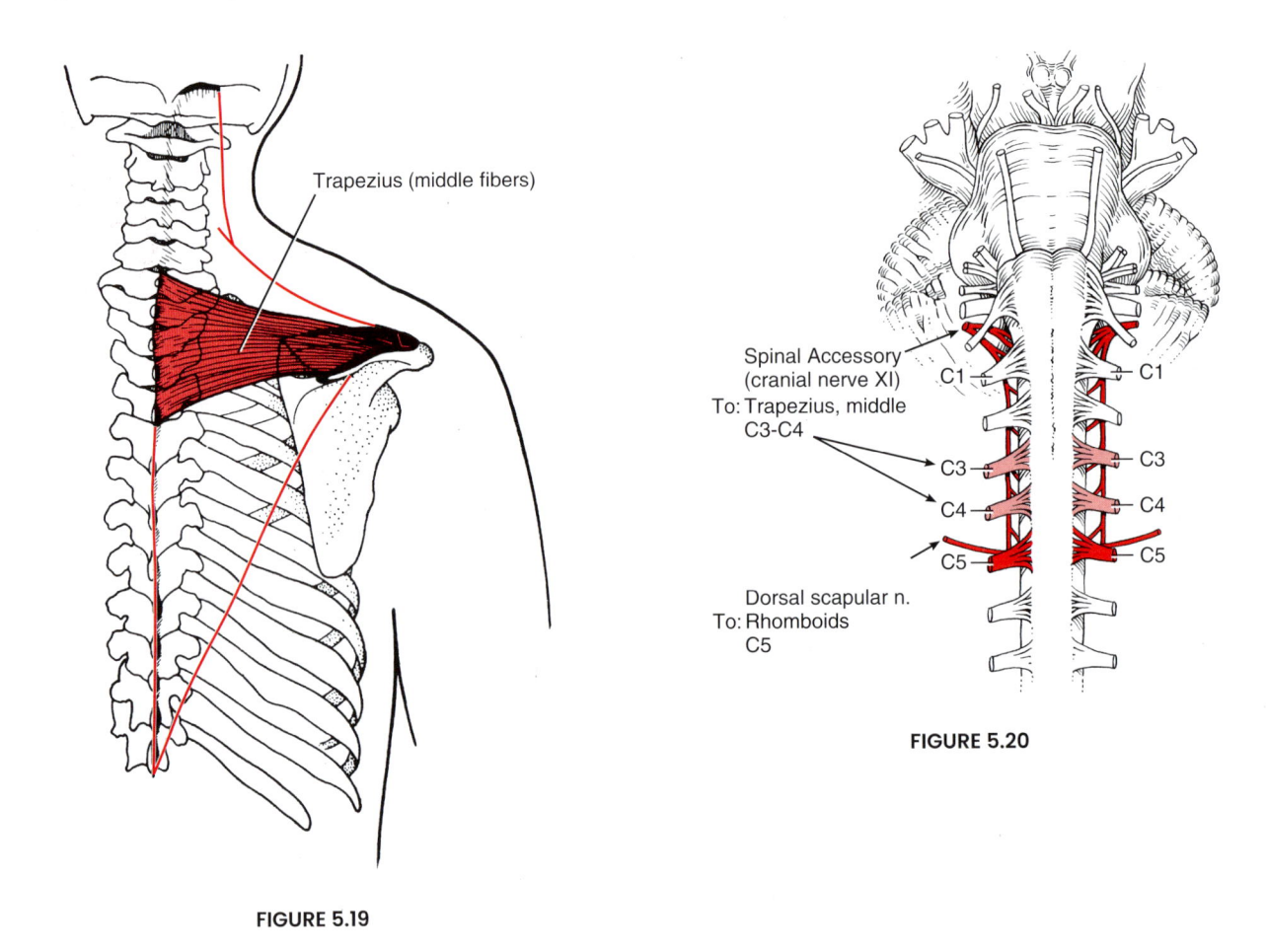

Trapezius (middle fibers)

Spinal Accessory
(cranial nerve XI)
To: Trapezius, middle
C3-C4

Dorsal scapular n.
To: Rhomboids
C5

C1   C1
C3   C3
C4   C4
C5   C5

FIGURE 5.20

FIGURE 5.19

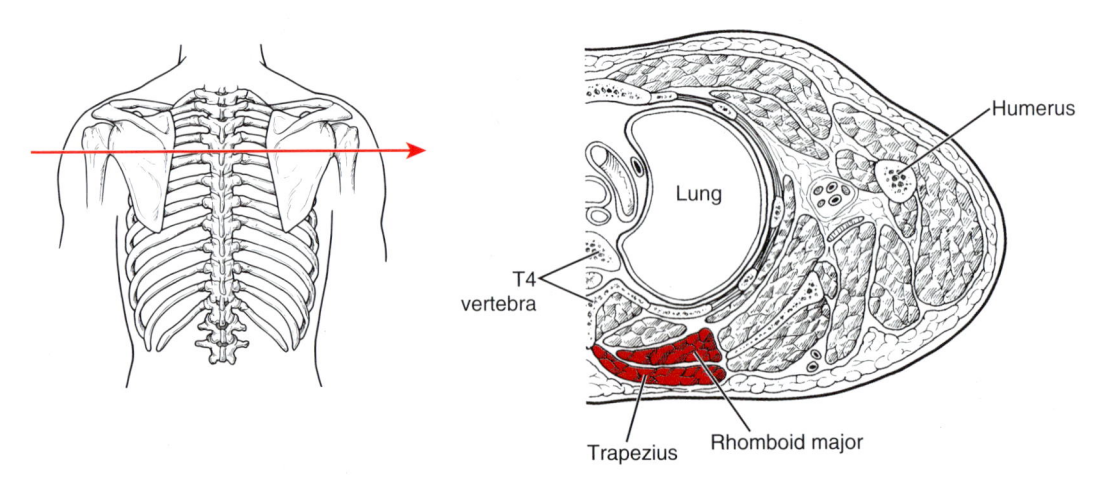

Humerus

Lung

T4
vertebra

Trapezius   Rhomboid major

FIGURE 5.21 Arrow indicates level of cross section.

Table 5.3 SCAPULAR ADDUCTION (RETRACTION)

I.D.	Muscle	Origin	Insertion	Function
124	**Trapezius (middle fibers)**	T1-T5 vertebrae (spinous processes) Supraspinous ligaments	Scapula (medial acromial margin and superior lip of crest on scapular spine)	Scapular adduction (retraction) (with rhomboids)
125	Rhomboid major	T2-T5 vertebrae (spinous processes) Supraspinous ligaments	Scapula (vertebral border between root of spine and inferior angle)	Scapular adduction Downward rotation of scapula (glenoid faces down) Scapular elevation
Others				
126	Rhomboid minor	See Table 5.5	See Table 5.5	
124	Trapezius (upper and lower)	See Tables 5.3 and 5.4		
127	Levator scapulae	See Table 5.2	See Plate 3	

Grade 5, Grade 4, and Grade 3

Position of the Patient: Prone with shoulder at edge of table. Shoulder is abducted to 90°. Elbow is flexed to a right angle with forearm and hand hanging off table (Fig. 5.22). Head may be turned to either side for comfort.

Instructions to Clinician: Stand at test side close to patient's arm. Stabilize the contralateral scapular area to prevent trunk rotation. Ask the patient to lift elbow toward the ceiling (Grade 3). If able to complete full range, proceed to apply resistance in the test position in a downward direction (Fig. 5.23). Palpate the middle fibers of the trapezius at the spine of the scapula from the acromion to the vertebral column with the fingers of the other hand, as necessary.

Test: Patient horizontally abducts arm and adducts scapula.

FIGURE 5.22

FIGURE 5.23

SCAPULAR ADDUCTION (RETRACTION)

(Trapezius, middle fibers)

Grade 5, Grade 4, and Grade 3 Continued

Instructions to Patient: "Lift your elbow toward the ceiling. Hold it. Don't let me push it down."

Grading

Grade 5: Holds test position against maximal resistance.

Grade 4: Holds test position against strong to moderate resistance.

Grade 3: Completes available range without manual resistance (Fig. 5.24).

Grade 2, Grade 1, and Grade 0

Position of Patient and Clinician: Same as for Grade 5 test except that the clinician uses one hand to cradle the patient's shoulder and arm, thus supporting the arm's weight (Fig. 5.25), and the other hand for palpation.

Test: Same as that for Grades 5 to 3.

Instructions to Patient: "Try to lift your elbow toward the ceiling."

Grading

Grade 2: Completes full range of motion without the weight of the arm.

Grade 1 and Grade 0: A Grade 1 muscle exhibits contractile activity or slight movement. There will be neither motion nor discernable palpable contractile activity in the Grade 0 muscle.

Substitutions

By the rhomboids: The rhomboids can partially substitute for the middle trapezius in adduction of the scapula, but if that should happen, adduction occurs simultaneously with scapular downward rotation.

Clinical Relevance

When the posterior deltoid muscle is weak, support the patient's shoulder with the palm of one hand and allow the patient's elbow to flex. Passively move the scapula into adduction via horizontal abduction of the arm (see Fig. 5.25). Have the patient hold the scapula in adduction as the clinician slowly releases the shoulder support. Observe whether the scapula maintains its adducted position. If it does, the muscle is a Grade 3.

Suggested Exercises for Middle Trapezius

- Prone external rotation (ER)[10]
- Prone horizontal abduction[12]
- Overhead retraction[12]
- Side-lying ER[10]
- Row with elbows extended

FIGURE 5.24

FIGURE 5.25

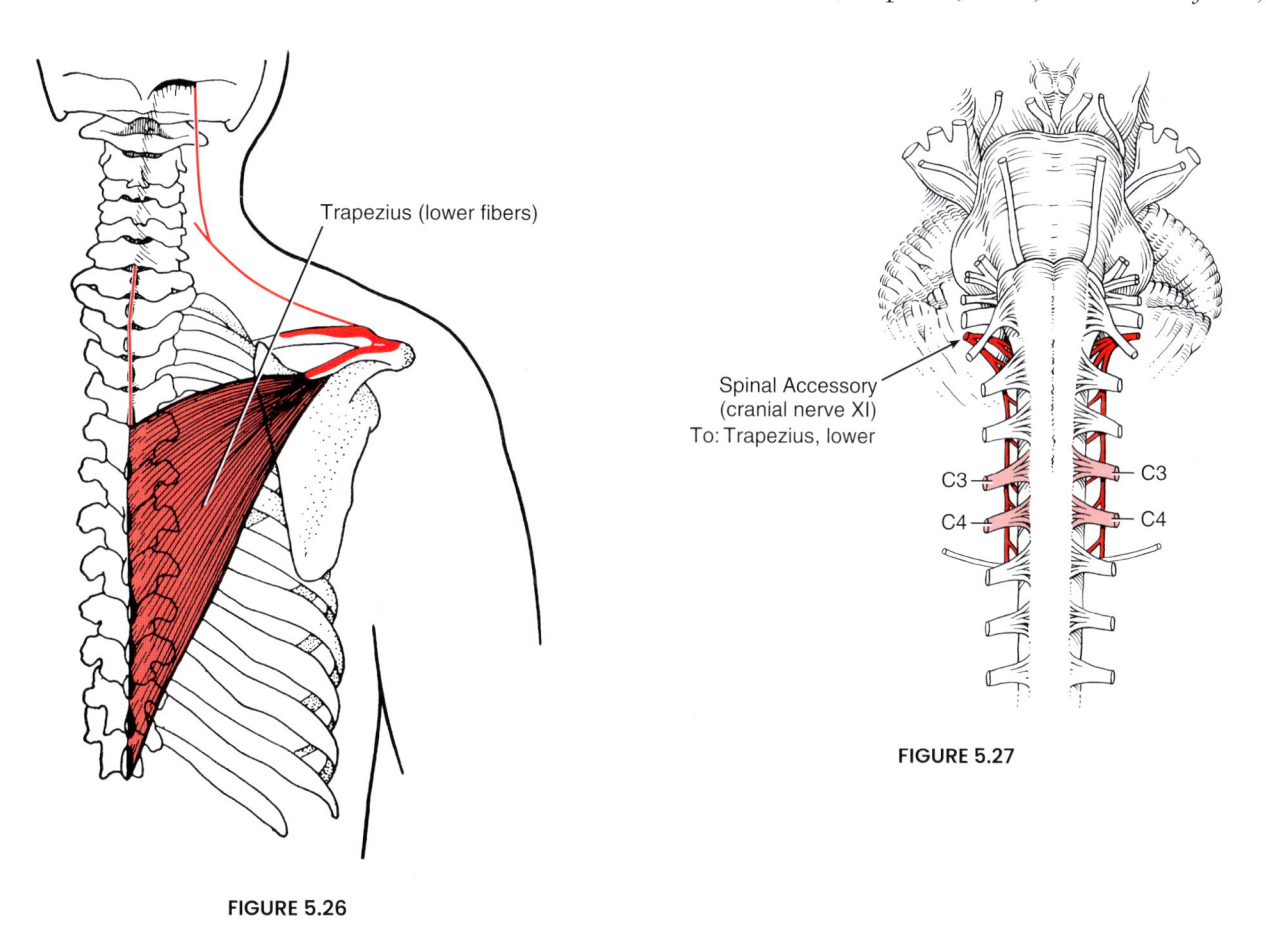

Trapezius (lower fibers)

FIGURE 5.26

Spinal Accessory
(cranial nerve XI)
To: Trapezius, lower

C3 — C3
C4 — C4

FIGURE 5.27

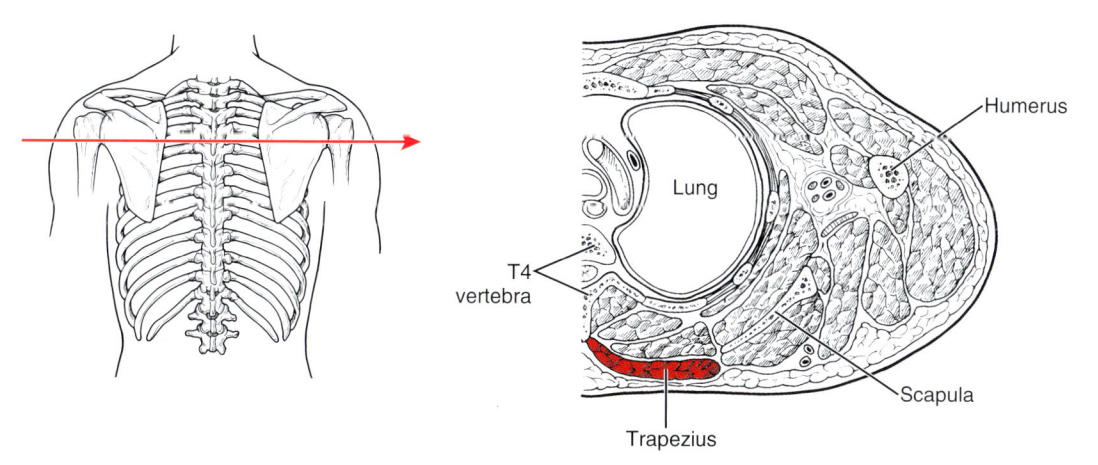

Humerus

Lung

T4
vertebra

Scapula

Trapezius

FIGURE 5.28 Arrow indicates level of cross section.

Range of Motion

Reliable data not available.

SCAPULAR DEPRESSION AND ADDUCTION

(Trapezius, lower, and middle fibers)

Table 5.4 SCAPULAR DEPRESSION AND ADDUCTION

I.D.	Muscle	Origin	Insertion	Function
124	**Trapezius (middle and lower fibers)**	T1-T5 vertebrae (spinous processes) Supraspinous ligaments T6-T12 vertebrae (spinous processes)	Scapula (spine, medial end, and tubercle at lateral apex via aponeurosis)	*Middle*: • Scapular adduction (retraction) (with rhomboids) *Lower*: • Scapular adduction and depression
130	Latissimus dorsi	Spines of the 6 lower thoracic vertebrae, thoracolumbar fascia, crest of the ilium, lowest 4 ribs	Anterior humerus, lower margin of the intertubercular sulcus	• Scapular depression if the arms are fixed • Extension, adduction, and internal rotation of shoulder • Hyperextension of spine (muscles on both sides), as in lifting • The muscle is most powerful in overhead activities (such as swimming [downstroke] and climbing), crutch walking, elevation of trunk to arms, i.e., shoulder depression, or swinging[13]
Others				
131	Pectoralis major	Sternal half of clavicle, entire anterior surface of the sternum	Lateral lip of the intertubercular sulcus of anterior humerus	
129	Pectoralis minor	Ribs 3–5, intercostal cartilage	Coracoid process	

Grade 5, Grade 4, and Grade 3

Position of Patient: Prone with test arm over head to about 145° of shoulder elevation and abduction (in line with the fibers of the lower trapezius). Forearm is in midposition (neutral rotation) with the thumb pointing toward the ceiling. Head should be turned to the test side.

Instructions to Clinician: Stand at test side. Ask patient to raise the arm from the table as high as possible (Grade 3) (Fig. 5.29). If full range is present, provide resistance.

Hand giving resistance is contoured over the distal forearm, just above wrist (Fig. 5.30). Resistance will be given straight downward (toward the floor). Fingertips of the opposite hand palpate below the spine of the scapula and

FIGURE 5.29

FIGURE 5.30

Grade 5, Grade 4, and Grade 3 Continued

across to the thoracic vertebrae, following the muscle as it curves down to the lower thoracic vertebrae. If patient cannot hold the test position with resistance given on the forearm, apply resistance over distal humerus, above elbow (Grade 4).

Instructions to Patient: "Hold your arm. Don't let me push it down."

Grading

Grade 5: Holds test position against strong resistance applied over the forearm.

Grade 4: Holds test position against strong resistance applied over the distal humerus or light resistance over the forearm.

Grade 3: Patient raises arm from the table in test position against gravity, but patient cannot tolerate manual resistance (see Fig. 5.29).

Grade 2, Grade 1, and Grade 0

Position of Patient: Same as for Grade 5.

Instructions to Clinician: Stand at test side. Support patient's arm under the elbow (Fig. 5.31).

FIGURE 5.31

Test: Patient attempts to lift the arm from the table. If the patient is unable to lift the arm because of a weak posterior and middle deltoid, the examiner should lift and support the weight of the arm. In the presence of a weak lower trapezius, the patient may substitute the middle trapezius and rhomboids, causing a lowering of the arm into an abducted position.

Instructions to Patient: "Try to lift your arm from the table past your ear."

Grading

Grade 2: Completes full scapular range of motion without the weight of the arm.

Grade 1: Contractile activity can be palpated in the triangular area between the root of the spine of the scapula and the lower thoracic vertebra (T7-T12), that is, the course of the fibers of the lower trapezius.

Grade 0: No discernable palpable contractile activity.

Clinical Relevance

- The lower trapezius will not be active with shoulder elevation of less than 120°, so if the patient does not have sufficient glenohumeral (G-H) range to assume the test position, the lower trapezius is nearly impossible to test as the scapulae adduct and the rhomboids take over. If the patient cannot isolate this test or substitutes away from test position, the grade is 0 (zero), or clinician should document, "Unable to assume test position."
- Examiners are reminded of the test principle that the same lever arm must be used in sequential testing (over time) for valid comparison of results.

Suggested Exercises for Lower Trapezius

- Prone rowing[8]
- Prone flexion with thumb up[10]
- Modified prone cobra[14]
- D2 diagonal pattern flexion with elastic tubing[8]
- Prone horizontal abduction at 90° and 125°[8]

(Rhomboids)

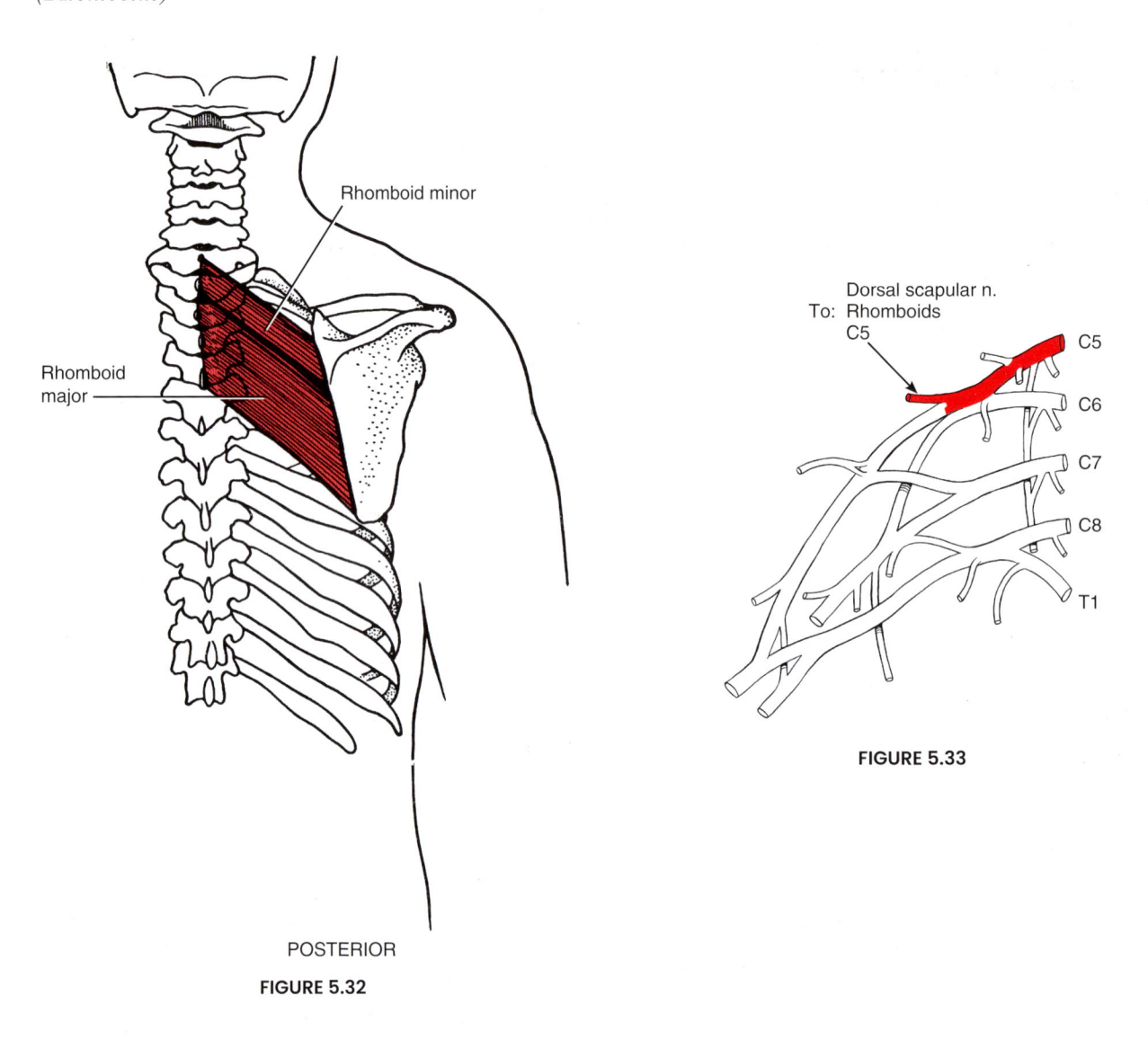

POSTERIOR

FIGURE 5.32

FIGURE 5.33

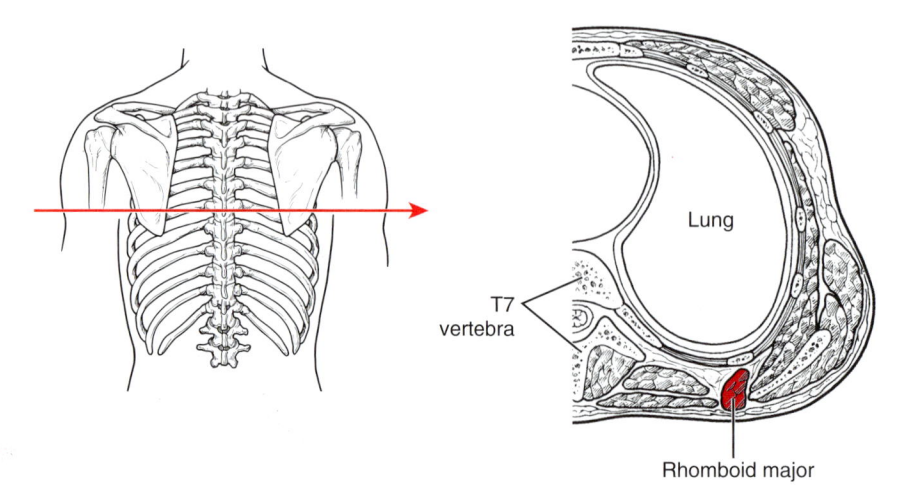

FIGURE 5.34 Arrow indicates level of cross section.

(Rhomboids)

Table 5.5 SCAPULAR RETRACTION AND DOWNWARD ROTATION

I.D.	Muscle	Origin	Insertion	Function
125	Rhomboid major	T2-T5 vertebrae (spinous processes) Supraspinous ligaments	Scapula (upper vertebral border)	• Scapular adduction • Downward rotation of scapula (glenoid faces down)
126	Rhomboid minor	C7-T1 vertebrae (spinous processes) Ligamentum nuchae (lower)	Scapula (lower vertebral margin)	Scapular adduction Scapular downward rotation (glenoid faces down)
Other				
127	Levator scapulae	See Table 5.2		

The test for the rhomboid muscles has become the focus of some clinical debate. Kendall and coworkers claim, with good evidence, that these muscles frequently are underrated; that is, they are too often graded at a level less than their available performance.[15] At issue also is the confusion that can occur in separating the function of the rhomboids from those of other scapular or shoulder muscles, particularly the trapezius and the pectoralis minor. Because the rhomboids are innervated only by one nerve root (C5), a test for the rhomboids, correctly conducted, can confirm or rule out a nerve root lesion at this level. With these issues in mind, the authors present first their method and then, with the generous permission of Mrs. Kendall, her rhomboid test as another method of assessment.

Grade 5, Grade 4, and Grade 3

Position of Patient: Prone. Head may be turned to either side for comfort. Shoulder is internally rotated, and the arm is adducted across the back with the elbow flexed and hand resting on the back (Fig. 5.35).

Instructions to Clinician: Stand at test side. Ask patient to place hand at the small of the back and lift it several inches away from the back (Grade 3). If patient can successfully place the hand in this position, apply resistance in the test position. When the patient's shoulder extensor muscles are Grade 3 or higher, the hand used for resistance is placed on the humerus just above the elbow, and resistance is given in an outward and downward direction (Fig. 5.36).

FIGURE 5.35

FIGURE 5.36

SCAPULAR ADDUCTION (RETRACTION) AND DOWNWARD ROTATION

(Rhomboids)

Grade 5, Grade 4, and Grade 3 Continued

When the shoulder extensors are weak, place the hand for resistance along the axillary border of the scapula (Fig. 5.37). Resistance is applied in a downward and outward direction.

The fingers of the hand used for palpation are placed deep under the vertebral border of the scapula.

Test: Patient lifts the hand off the back, maintaining the arm position across the back. At the same time, the examiner is applying resistance above the elbow in an outward direction. With strong muscle activity, the clinician's fingers will "pop" out from under the edge of the scapular vertebral border (see Fig. 5.35.)

Instructions to Patient: "Lift your hand. Hold it. Don't let me push it down."

Grading

Grade 5: Completes available range and holds against maximal resistance (Fig. 5.38). The fingers will "pop out" from under the scapula when strong rhomboids contract.

Grade 4: Completes range and holds against strong to moderate resistance. Fingers usually will "pop out."

Grade 3: Completes range but tolerates no manual resistance at either the humerus or scapula (Fig. 5.39).

FIGURE 5.37

FIGURE 5.38

FIGURE 5.39

SCAPULAR ADDUCTION (RETRACTION) AND DOWNWARD ROTATION

(Rhomboids)

Grade 2, Grade 1, and Grade 0

Position of Patient: Short sitting with shoulder internally rotated and arm extended and adducted behind back (Fig. 5.40).

Instructions to Clinician: Stand at test side; support arm by grasping the wrist. The fingertips of one hand palpate the muscle under the vertebral border of the scapula.

Test: Patient attempts to move hand away from back.

Instructions to Patient: "Try to move your hand away from your back."

Grading

Grade 2: Completes range of scapular motion.

Grade 1 and Grade 0: A Grade 1 muscle has palpable contractile activity. A Grade 0 muscle shows no discernable palpable contractile activity.

FIGURE 5.40

Alternate Rhomboid Test after Kendall[15]

As a preliminary to this rhomboid test, the shoulder adductors should be tested and found sufficiently strong to allow the arm to be used as a lever.

Position of Patient: Prone with head turned to side of test. Non-test arm is abducted with elbow flexed. Test arm is near the edge of the table. Arm (humerus) is fully adducted and held firm to the side of the trunk in external rotation (ER) and some extension with elbow fully flexed. In this position, the scapula is in adduction, elevation, and downward rotation (glenoid down).

Instructions to Clinician: Stand at test side. Hand used for resistance is cupped around the flexed elbow. The resistance applied by this hand will be in the direction of scapular abduction and upward rotation (out and up; Fig. 5.41). The other hand is used to give resistance simultaneously. It is contoured over the shoulder joint and gives resistance caudally in the direction of shoulder depression.

Test: Examiner tests the ability of the patient to hold the scapula in its position of adduction, elevation, and downward rotation (glenoid down).

Instructions to Patient: "Hold your arm as I have placed it. Do not let me pull your arm out and forward" OR "Hold the position you are in; keep your shoulder blade against your spine as I try to pull it away."

Clinical Relevance

- The rhomboid test, where the resistance is applied to the humerus in an outward motion, should not be confused with the lift-off test, a diagnostic test for a subscapular muscle tear.
- When the rhomboid test is performed with the hand behind the back, never allow the patient to lead the lifting motion with the elbow because this will activate the humeral extensors.
- Using needle electromyography (EMG) on 11 male subjects, Smith and colleagues[11] found the posterior deltoid manual muscle test produced more rhomboid EMG activity (30%) than the muscle test shown in Fig. 5.38. The manual muscle test described in Fig. 5.38 produced very high EMG activity in the latissimus dorsi and levator scapula muscles and equal activation in the middle trapezius, posterior deltoid, and rhomboids.
- The sitting position used in the posterior deltoid muscle test position described by Smith and colleagues[11] requires the rhomboids to function as a scapular rotator and scapular retractor as opposed to the prone position, which only requires the rhomboids to act as a scapular retractor.[16]
- The Kendall test (see Fig. 5.41) demonstrated greater rhomboid EMG activity (78%) maximum voluntary contraction (MVC) than the rhomboid test shown in Fig. 5.38 (52% MVC), although the differences were not statistically significant.[17]

Suggested Exercises for Rhomboids

- D2 diagonal pattern flexion and extension[8]
- Lat pulldown with pronated wide grip in front of body[16,18]
- Prone row[8]
- Modified prone cobra (prone, arms extended at sides, lift trunk up, retracting scapulas, and pulling hands towards feet).

FIGURE 5.41

This large, broad muscle is anatomically complex, contributing to many movements at the humerus, scapula, and pelvis. It is the only muscle connecting the arms to the spine. Literally, it was our "swinging from the trees" muscle. It does not have a singular prime action. Rather, its actions are dependent on the fixation of the humerus or pelvis. For example, when the humerus is fixed, the latissimus dorsi can lift the pelvis, which occurs during pressure relief in a wheelchair and during a sliding transfer (see Fig. 5.46). It is the main muscle used when we participate in the chin-up/pull-up exercise. When the pelvis is fixed, the latissimus dorsi acts on the arm in three ways:

1. Shoulder extension
2. Shoulder adduction
3. Shoulder medial rotation

The latissimus can also depress the humerus and internally rotate, adduct, and extend the shoulder, particularly from a position of flexion. The student will find the latissimus dorsi part of multiple muscle actions, described in several places in this chapter, further supporting the importance and complexity of this muscle.

The latissimus dorsi also assists in the act of breathing, with forced expiration as well as deep inspiration of breath from the lungs.

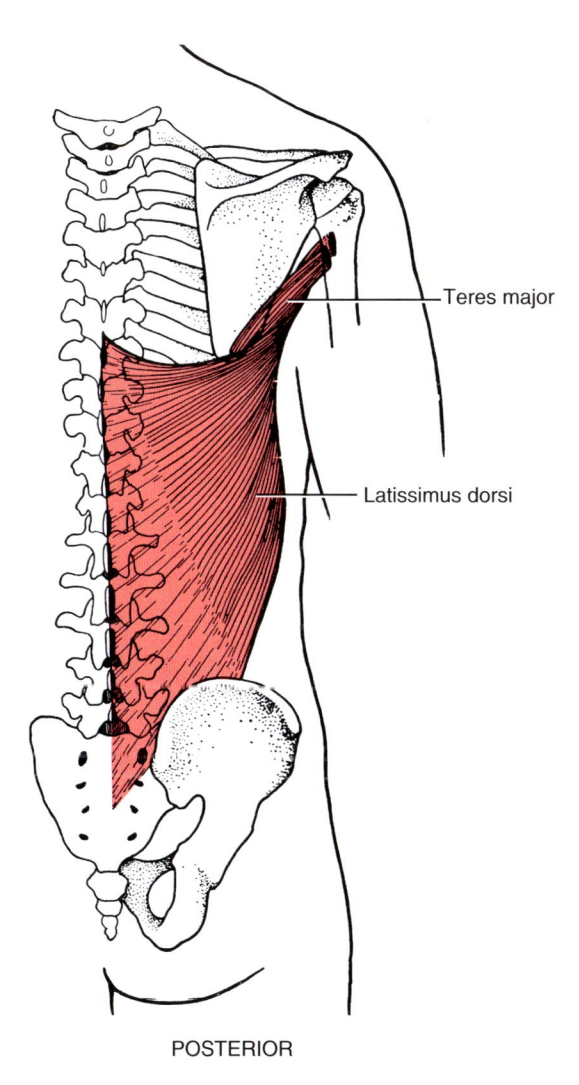

Teres major

Latissimus dorsi

POSTERIOR

FIGURE 5.42

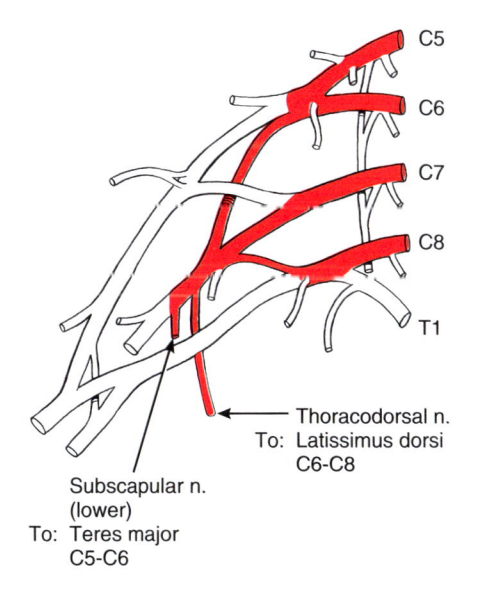

C5

C6

C7

C8

T1

Thoracodorsal n.
To: Latissimus dorsi
C6-C8

Subscapular n.
(lower)
To: Teres major
C5-C6

FIGURE 5.43

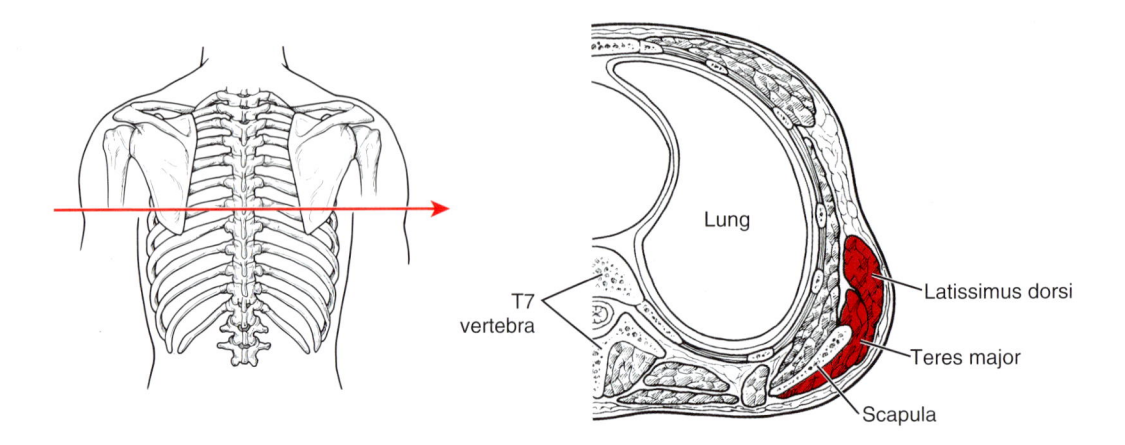

FIGURE 5.44

Table 5.6 **LATISSIMUS DORSI**

I.D.	Muscle	Origin	Insertion	Function
130	Latissimus dorsi	Spines of the 6 lower thoracic vertebrae, thoracolumbar fascia, crest of the ilium, lowest 4 ribs	Anterior humerus, lower margin of the intertubercular sulcus	Shoulder extension, adduction and internal (medial) rotation Hyperextension of the spine Strong expiration and deep inspiration Elevation of the pelvis with arms fixed

Grade 5, Grade 4, Grade 3, Grade 2, and Grade 1

Position of the Patient: Prone with head turned to test side; arms at sides, and test shoulder internally rotated (palm up).

Instructions to Clinician: Stand at test side. Ask patient to lift arm into shoulder extension and adduction (keeping arm close to trunk) (Grade 3). If full range is present, apply appropriate resistance. With shoulder in extension and adduction and elbow extended, apply resistance with hand over medial forearm above patient's wrist in direction of abduction and slight flexion (outwards and down) (Fig. 5.45). No stabilization is needed because of the prone position.

Test: Patient lifts arm into extension and adduction (close to trunk).

Instructions to Patient: "Hold your arm. Don't let me move it."

Grading

Grade 5: Patient holds test position against maximal resistance (see Fig. 5.45).

Grade 4: Patient holds test position against moderate resistance.

Grade 3: Completes range but tolerates no resistance.

Grade 2: Movement observable but range is limited.

Grade 1: Muscle activity is palpable.

Grade 0: No movement and no discernable muscle contraction occurs.

FIGURE 5.45

Alternate Test for Latissimus Dorsi

As explained earlier, with the upper limb fixed, elevation of the trunk and pelvis is possible through the action of the latissimus dorsi, such as in crutch walking or buttock pressure releases in sitting.

Position of Patient: Short sitting, arms adducted to trunk with hands flat on table adjacent to hips (Fig. 5.46).

If the patient's arms are too short to assume this position, provide a push-up block for each hand.

Instructions to Clinician: Stand behind patient. Fingers are used to palpate fibers of the latissimus dorsi on the lateral aspect of the thoracic wall (bilaterally) just above the waist (see Fig. 5.46).

Test: Patient pushes down on hands (or blocks) and lifts buttocks from table (see Fig. 5.46).

Instructions to Patient: "Lift your bottom off the table. Keep your arms into your sides."

Grading

Grade 3, Grade 4, and Grade 5: Patient can lift buttocks clear of table.

FIGURE 5.46

Suggested Exercises for the Latissimus Dorsi

- Pull-ups[19]
- Lat pulldowns[19]
- Inverted row[19]
- Press up[8]
- Standing extension from 90° to 0° with elastic tubing[8]

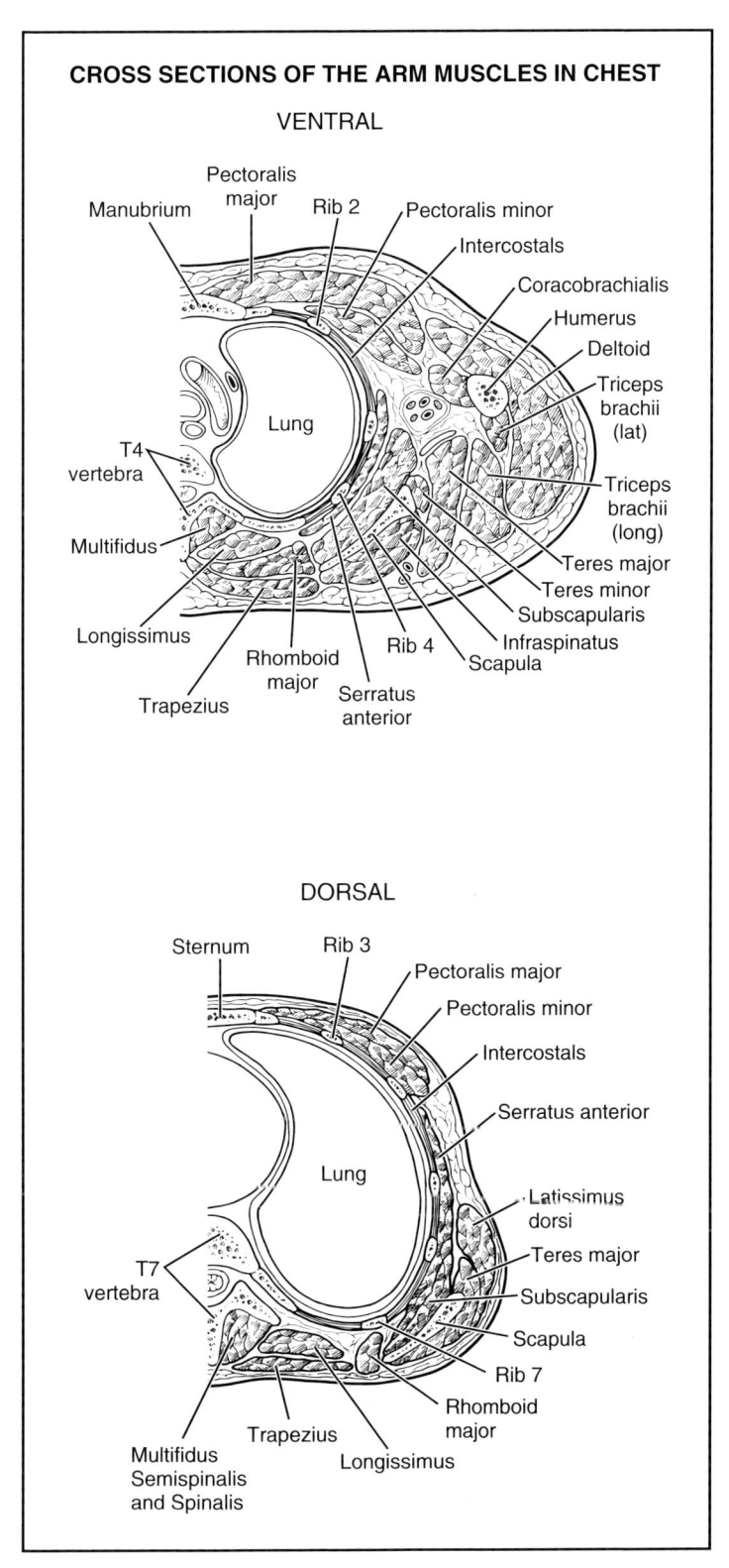

PLATE 3 Cross sections of the arm muscles in chest.

The deltoid muscle, made of three parts (anterior, middle, and posterior), has multiple functions of mobility and stabilization of the head of the humerus into the glenoid fossa. The deltoid can act in part or as a whole. Together, the three parts allow swinging of the arm and prevent downward dislocation of the humeral head when carrying an object in the hanging hand.[20] The three parts work together to produce abduction of the shoulder joint. The anterior part has a flexion and IR function, and the posterior part has an extension and ER function.[1] The anterior part acts with the rotator cuff to raise the arm in both flexion and abduction. The middle part is a strong shoulder abductor, while the posterior part is a strong extensor (with the latissimus dorsi and teres major) and, to a lesser degree, a horizontal abductor. The deltoid is capable of extending the humerus beyond the midline, whereas the latissimus dorsi is not.

(Anterior deltoid, Rotator cuff, Clavicular portion of pectoralis major, and Coracobrachialis[a])

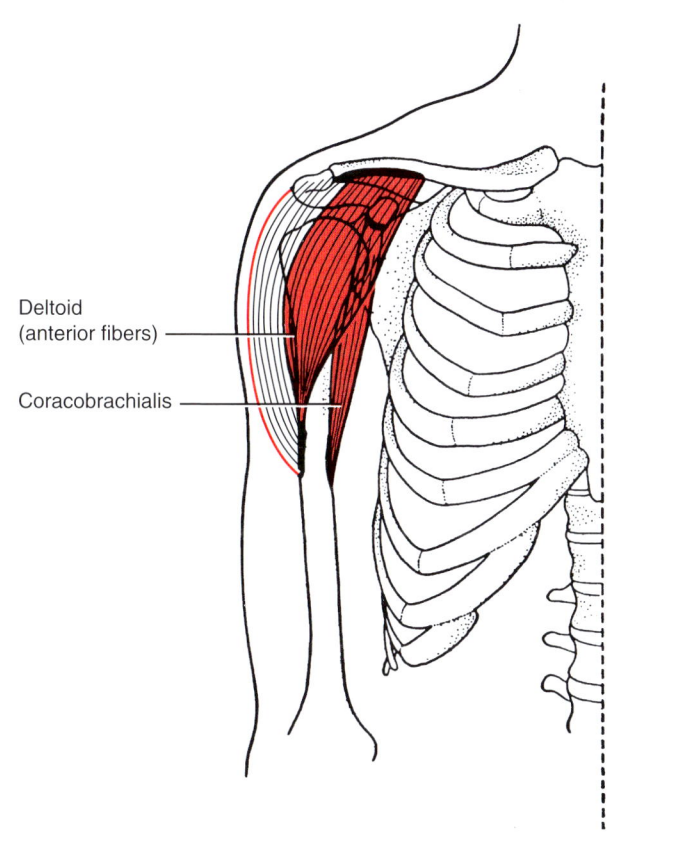

Deltoid
(anterior fibers)

Coracobrachialis

ANTERIOR

FIGURE 5.47

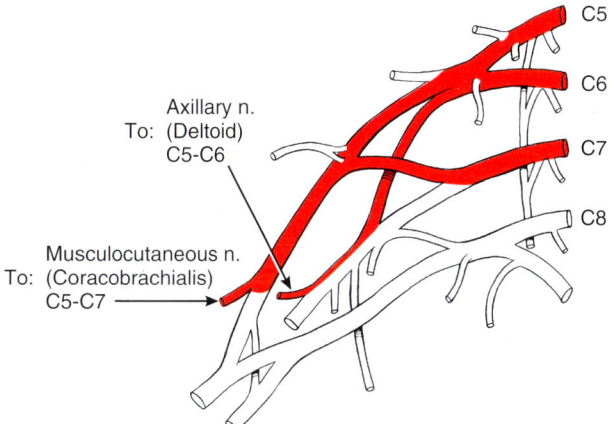

Axillary n.
To: (Deltoid)
C5-C6

Musculocutaneous n.
To: (Coracobrachialis)
C5-C7

C5
C6
C7
C8

FIGURE 5.48

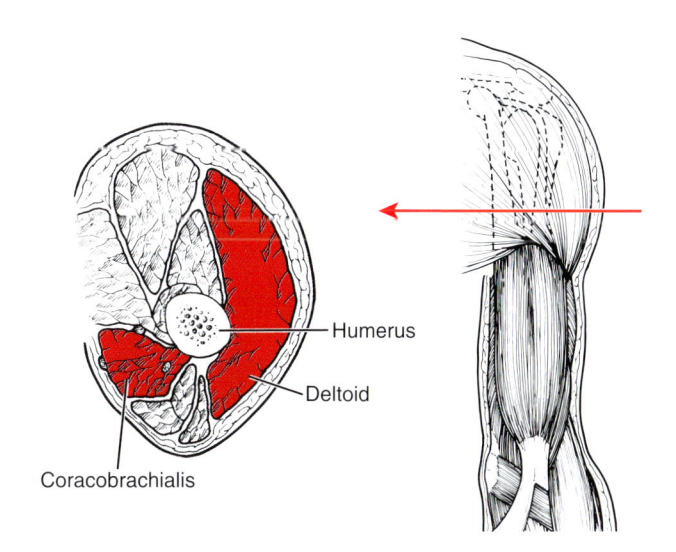

Humerus

Deltoid

Coracobrachialis

FIGURE 5.49

[a] The coracobrachialis muscle cannot be isolated, nor is it really palpable. It has no unique function. It is included here because classically it is considered a shoulder flexor and adductor.

SHOULDER FLEXION

(Anterior deltoid, Rotator cuff, Clavicular portion of pectoralis major, and Coracobrachialis

Range of Motion
0°–180°

Table 5.7 **SHOULDER FLEXION**

I.D.	Muscle	Origin	Insertion	Function
133	**Deltoid (anterior)**	Clavicle (anterior superior border of lateral one-third of shaft)	Humerus (deltoid tuberosity on shaft)	Flexion and internal rotation of shoulder (anterior fibers) The deltoid tends to displace the humeral head upward Shoulder horizontal adduction (anterior fibers)
139	Coracobrachialis	Scapula (coracoid process at apex)	Humerus (shaft, medial surface at middle one-third)	Flexion of arm Adduction of shoulder
131	Pectoralis major (clavicular fibers)	See Table 5.11		*Clavicular fibers*: Flexion of shoulder Horizontal shoulder adduction Internal rotation of shoulder
Others				
135	Supraspinatus	Scapula (supraspinous fossa, medial two-thirds) Supraspinatus fascia	Humerus (greater tubercle, highest facet) Articular capsule of G-H joint	Maintains humeral head in glenoid fossa (with other rotator cuff muscles) Shoulder flexor Abduction of shoulder External rotation of shoulder
	Long and short head of biceps	See Table 5.14		

G-H, Glenohumeral.

(Anterior deltoid, Rotator cuff, Clavicular portion of pectoralis major, and Coracobrachialis)

Due to the increasing moment arm with abduction, the anterior deltoid is more effective as a shoulder abductor in higher abduction angles (120°), with its greatest force production above the horizontal,[21] in contrast to the supraspinatus, which is a more effective shoulder abductor at lower abduction ranges. The supraspinatus has a role as a humeral head depressor during shoulder flexion.[2] The middle deltoid also provides G-H stabilization with greater amounts of shoulder flexion.

Grade 5, Grade 4, and Grade 3

Position of the Patient: Short sitting with arms at sides, elbow slightly flexed, forearm pronated.

Instructions to Clinician: Stand at test side. Ask patient to raise arm forward to shoulder height (90°) in the sagittal plane, keeping elbow straight and with hand pronated. If full range is present (Grade 3), position arm in test position (90°) and apply appropriate resistance. Clinician's hand giving resistance is contoured over the distal humerus just above the elbow. The other hand may stabilize the shoulder (Fig. 5.50).

Test: Patient flexes shoulder to 90° with elbow straight without rotation or horizontal movement (see Fig. 5.50). The scapula should be allowed to abduct and upwardly rotate.

Instructions to Patient: "Hold your arm. Don't let me push it down."

Grading

Grade 5: Holds test position (90°) against maximal resistance.

Grade 4: Holds test position against strong to moderate resistance.

Grade 3: Completes test range (90°) without resistance (Fig. 5.51)

FIGURE 5.50

FIGURE 5.51

SHOULDER FLEXION

(Anterior deltoid, Rotator cuff, Clavicular portion of pectoralis major, and Coracobrachialis)

Grade 2, Grade 1, and Grade 0

Position of the Patient: Side-lying position (test side up).

Instructions to Clinician: With patient side lying to minimize gravity, stand behind patient and cradle the test arm at the elbow to avoid shoulder adduction. Then, ask patient to flex the shoulder. (A powder board may also be used.)

Test: Patient attempts to flex shoulder.

Instructions to Patient: "Try to raise your arm."

Grade 1 and Grade 0

Instructions to Clinician: Stand behind patient. Fingers used for palpation are placed over the superior and anterior surfaces of the deltoid over the shoulder joint (Fig. 5.52).

Grading

Test for Grade 2, Grade 1, and Grade 0:
Grade 2: Completes full range of motion in gravity-minimized position.

Grade 1: Clinician feels or sees contractile activity in the anterior deltoid, but no motion occurs.

Grade 0: No discernable palpable contractile activity.

Substitutions

- In the absence of a deltoid, the patient may attempt to flex the shoulder with the biceps brachii by first externally rotating the shoulder (Fig. 5.53). To avoid this, the arm should be kept in the mid-position between internal and external rotation.
- Attempted substitution by the upper trapezius results in shoulder elevation.
- Attempted substitution by the pectoralis major results in horizontal adduction. It should be noted that substitution by the pectoralis major as a shoulder flexor can only occur up to about 70°.
- The patient may lean backward or try to elevate the shoulder girdle to assist in flexion.

FIGURE 5.53

FIGURE 5.52

Suggested Exercises for Anterior Deltoid and Supraspinatus

- Push up (40% to 50% maximum voluntary contraction [MVC])[22]
- Pressing incline activities between 28° and 90°,[23,24] such as dumbbell press
- Plyometric push-up (clapping) (60% to 70% MVC)[22]
- Full and empty can.[9,25,26] Full can produces less deltoid activity.
- Slow, controlled shoulder flexion at 90° and 125°[25]
- Prone horizontal abduction at 100° with external rotation [9]
- Upright row[27]

(Posterior deltoid, Latissimus dorsi, Teres major, and Long head of triceps)

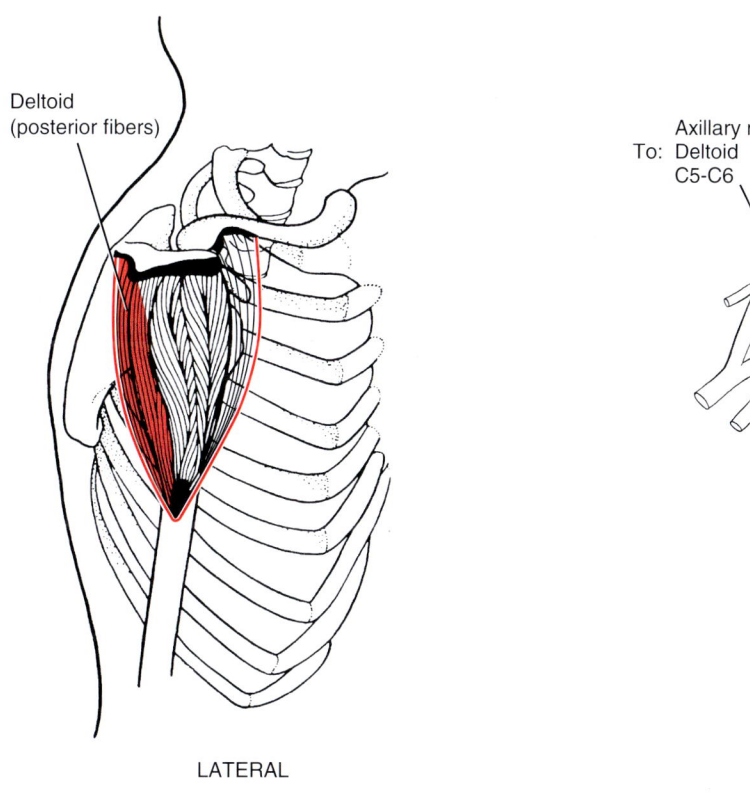

Deltoid
(posterior fibers)

LATERAL

FIGURE 5.54

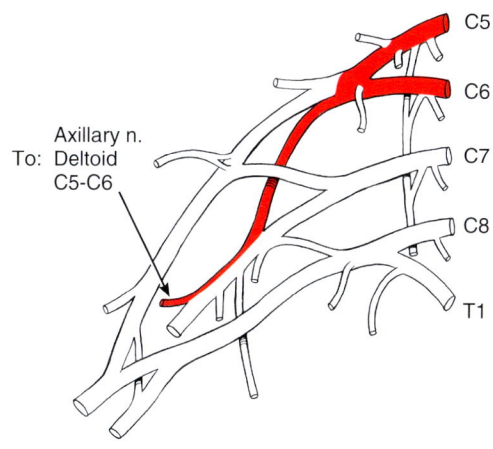

C5

C6

C7

C8

T1

Axillary n.
To: Deltoid
C5-C6

FIGURE 5.55

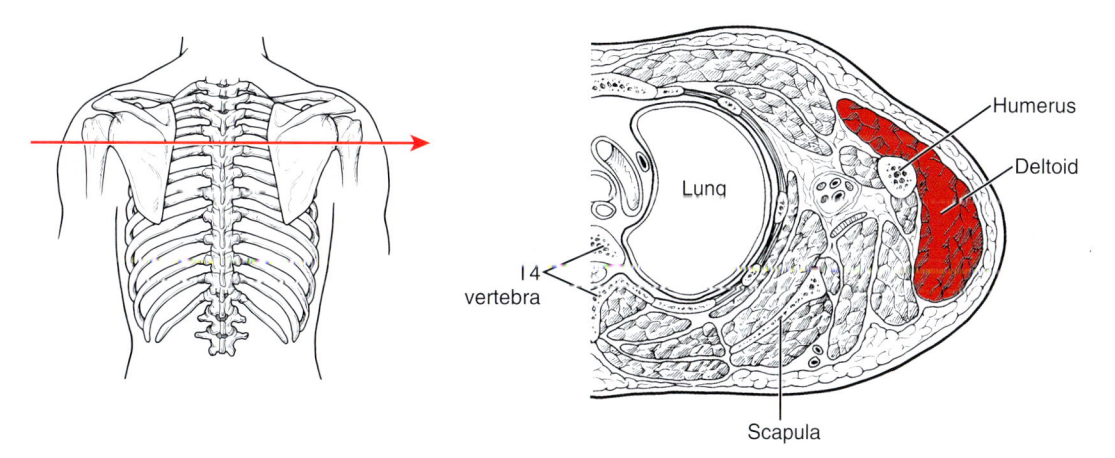

Humerus

Deltoid

Lung

I 4
vertebra

Scapula

FIGURE 5.56 Arrow indicates level of cross section.

SHOULDER EXTENSION

(Posterior deltoid, Latissimus dorsi, Teres major, and Long head of triceps)

Range of Motion
0°–45° (up to 60°)

Table 5.8 **SHOULDER EXTENSION**

I.D.	Muscle	Origin	Insertion	Function
133	**Deltoid (posterior)**	Scapula (spine on lower lip of lateral and posterior borders)	Humerus (deltoid tuberosity on midshaft via humeral tendon)	Extension and external rotation. The posterior fibers of the deltoid tends to displace the humeral head upward. Shoulder horizontal abduction
130	Latissimus dorsi	T6-T12, L1-L5, and sacral vertebrae (spinous processes) Supraspinous ligaments Ribs 9–12 (by slips interdigitating with obliquus abdominis externus) Ilium (crest, posterior) Thoracolumbar fascia	Humerus (intertubercular sulcus, floor) Deep fascia of arm	Shoulder extension (from a position of flexion) adduction, and internal rotation
138	Teres major	Scapula (dorsal surface of inferior angle)	Humerus (intertubercular sulcus, medial lip)	Extension of shoulder from a flexed position Internal rotation of shoulder Adduction and extension of shoulder
Other				
142	Triceps brachii (long head)			

(Posterior deltoid, Latissimus dorsi, Teres major, and Long head of triceps)

The posterior deltoid is a stronger shoulder extensor throughout the range with the greatest contribution when the arm is below horizontal. Its peak moment arm is at 30° of flexion. The posterior deltoid is the primary shoulder hyperextensor because neither the pectoralis major nor the latissimus dorsi extends the shoulder beyond anatomical neutral. This hyperextension function allows the patient to reach behind the body to the gluteal area and beyond.[20] The posterior deltoid opposes the anterior deltoid in the sagittal (flexion) plane and acts as a strong external rotator (up to 80% when elevated into the plane of the scapula).[1]

Grade 5, Grade 4, Grade 3, and Grade 2

Position of the Patient: Prone with arms at sides and shoulder internally rotated (palm up) (Fig. 5.57).

Instructions to Clinician: Stand at test side. Ask patient to lift arm as high as possible. If full range is available (Grade 3), position arm in test position near end range and apply appropriate resistance. The hand used for resistance is contoured over the posterior arm just above the elbow (Fig. 5.58).

Test: Patient raises arm off the table, keeping the elbow straight (Fig. 5.59).

Instructions to Patient: "Lift your arm as high as you can. Hold it. Don't let me push it down."

Grading

Grade 5: Holds test position against maximal resistance.

Grade 4: Holds test position against strong resistance.

Grade 3: Completes available range of motion with no manual resistance (see Fig. 5.59).

Grade 2: Completes partial range of motion.

FIGURE 5.58

FIGURE 5.57

FIGURE 5.59

SHOULDER EXTENSION

(Posterior deltoid, Latissimus dorsi, Teres major, and Long head of triceps)

Grade 1 and Grade 0

Position of the Patient: Prone with arms at sides and shoulder internally rotated (palm up).

Instructions to Clinician: Stand at test side. Fingers for palpation are placed on the posterior aspect of the upper arm (posterior deltoid) (Fig. 5.60).

Palpate over the posterior shoulder just superior to the axilla for posterior deltoid fibers. Palpate the teres major on the lateral border of the scapula just below the axilla. The teres major is the lower of the two muscles that enter the axilla at this point; it forms the lower posterior rim of the axilla.

Test and Instructions to Patient: Patient attempts to lift arm from table.

Grading

Grade 1: Palpable contractile activity in any of the participating muscles but no movement of the shoulder.

Grade 0: No palpable contractile response in participating muscles.

FIGURE 5.60

> ### Suggested Exercises for the Middle and Posterior Deltoid
>
> - D1 diagonal pattern extension[8]
> - D2 diagonal pattern flexion[8]
> - Push-ups[8]
> - Prone shoulder elevation (arm raised overhead in line with lower trapezius fibers)[8,25]
> - Extension with internal rotation (IR)[25] shoulder abduction 30° with elbow extended. Arm extended and IR
> - Side-lying external rotation (ER) at 0° abduction[8]
> - Empty can[25]
> - 45° incline row

(Middle deltoid and Supraspinatus)

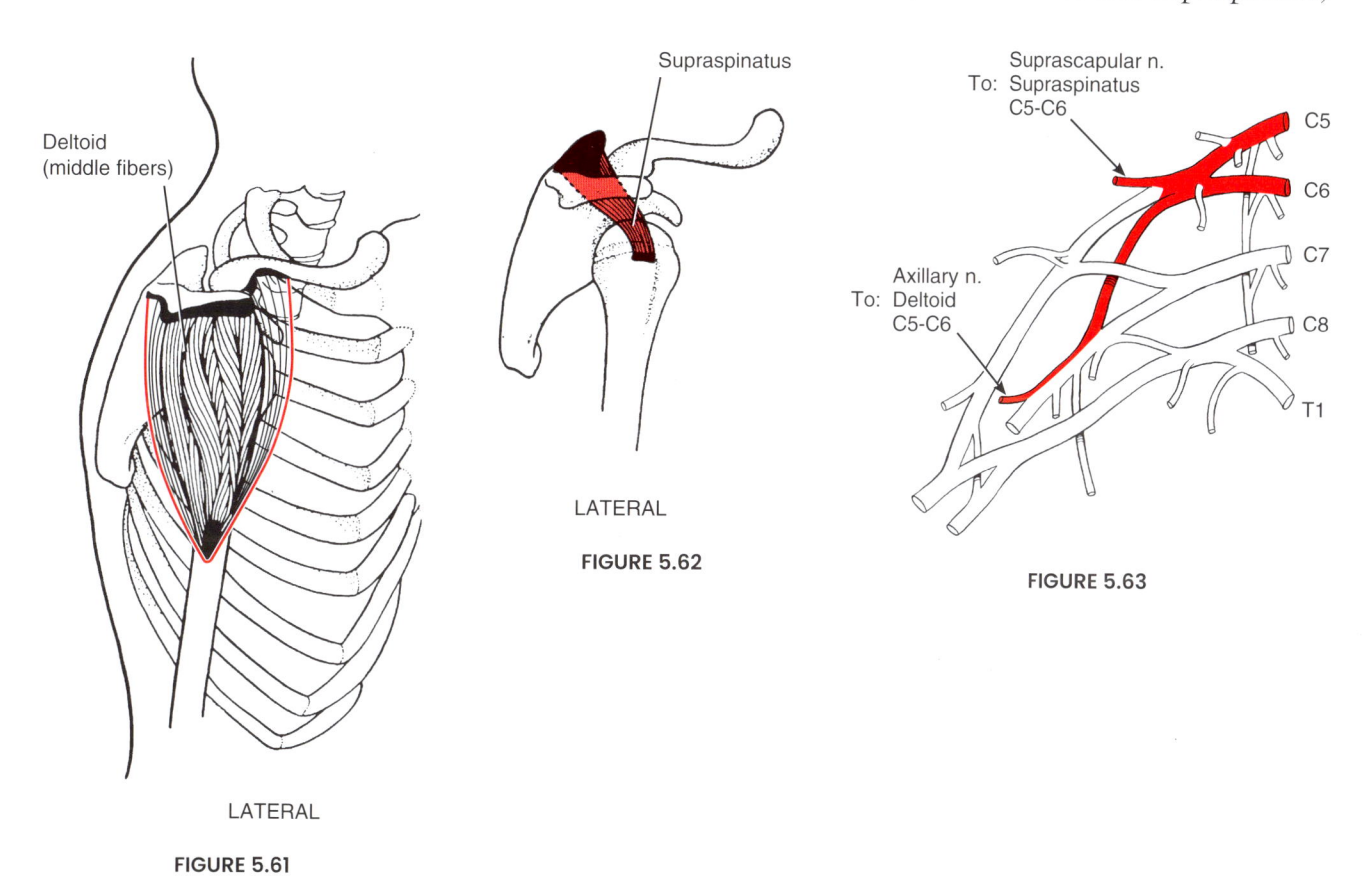

LATERAL

FIGURE 5.61

LATERAL

FIGURE 5.62

FIGURE 5.63

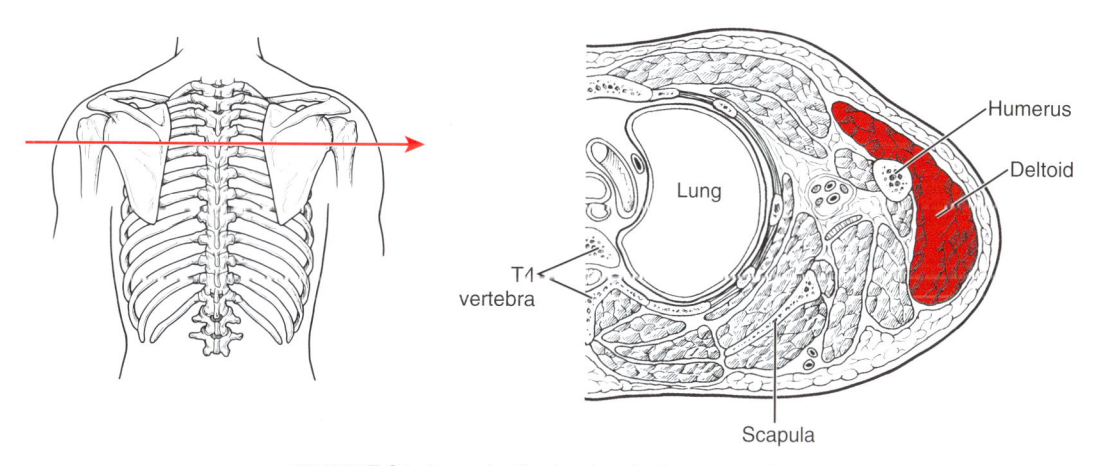

FIGURE 5.64 Arrow indicates level of cross section.

Range of Motion
0°–180°

SHOULDER ABDUCTION

(Middle deltoid and Supraspinatus)

Table 5.9 **SHOULDER ABDUCTION**

I.D.	Muscle	Origin	Insertion	Function
133	**Deltoid (middle fibers)**	Scapula (acromion, lateral margin, superior surface, and crest of spine)	Humerus (deltoid tuberosity on shaft via humeral tendon)	Abduction of shoulder (G-H joint): primarily the acromial middle fibers. The anterior and posterior fibers in this motion stabilize the limb in its cantilever position
135	Supraspinatus	Scapula (supraspinous fossa, medial two-thirds) Supraspinatus fascia	Humerus (greater tubercle, highest facet) Articular capsule of G-H joint	Maintains humeral head in glenoid fossa (with other rotator cuff muscles) Abduction of shoulder External rotation of shoulder
Other		Long head of biceps (if humerus externally rotated		
		Remaining cuff muscles: Infraspinatus, teres minor, subscapularis		Depresses head of humerus

G-H, Glenohumeral.

In the frontal plane, the middle deltoid performs shoulder abduction. It also performs horizontal abduction with the posterior deltoid. It has the largest cross-sectional area of the three deltoids. The supraspinatus and other rotator cuff muscles stabilize the humeral head against the elevating effect of the middle deltoid.[28]

Testing the Supraspinatus

Much controversy exists regarding the diagnosis of supraspinatus pathology. Two tests used to examine the supraspinatus muscle are the empty can test (also known as the Jobe test) and the full can test. In the full can test, the arm is externally rotated (thumb pointed up); in the empty can test, the arm is internally rotated (thumb pointed down). In both tests, the shoulder is in abduction but with 30° of flexion included. In a comparison of the empty can and full can tests by magnetic resonance imaging (MRI) validated by surgery, both tests had poor specificities of 58.8% and 47.1% respectively.[29] Furthermore, the empty can (thumb pointed down) and full can (thumb pointed up) positions were not statistically different in their performance of identifying pathology, probably because the supraspinatus generates abduction torque in neutral rotation.[30]

(Middle deltoid and Supraspinatus)

Grade 5, Grade 4, and Grade 3

Position of Patient: Short sitting with arm at side and elbow slightly flexed.

Instructions to Clinician: Stand behind patient. Ask patient to lift arm out to the side to shoulder level (test position) with arm in neutral rotation and elbow straight. If sufficient range is present, proceed to test Grade 5. Clinician's hand giving resistance is contoured over arm just above elbow (Fig. 5.65). Resistance is given in a downward direction.

Test: Patient abducts arm to 90°.

Instructions to Patient: "Lift your arm out to the side to shoulder level. Hold it. Don't let me push it down."

Grading

Grade 5: Holds test position against maximal resistance.

Grade 4: Holds test position against strong resistance.

Grade 3: Completes range of motion to 90° without resistance (Fig. 5.66).

FIGURE 5.65

FIGURE 5.66

SHOULDER ABDUCTION

(Middle deltoid and Supraspinatus)

Grade 2

Position of Patient: Supine. Arm at side supported on table in neutral rotation (thumb pointed outward) (Fig. 5.67).

Instructions to Clinician: Stand at test side of patient (clinician is shown on opposite side of test in figure to clearly illustrate test procedure). Hand used for palpation is positioned over the middle deltoid, lateral to acromial process on the superior aspect of the shoulder.

Test: Patient attempts to abduct shoulder by sliding arm on table without rotating it (see Fig. 5.67). A powder board or towel under the arm may be used to decrease friction.

Instructions to Patient: "Take your arm out to the side."

Grading

Grade 2: Completes full range of motion in this gravity-minimized position or cannot raise shoulder to 90° with elbow straight (cannot lift the weight of the extended arm)

Grade 1 and Grade 0

Position of Patient: Supine with arm at side and elbow slightly flexed.

Clinician Instructions: Stand at side of table at a place where the deltoid can be reached. Palpate deltoid on the lateral surface of the upper third of the arm (Fig. 5.68).

Grade 1: Palpable or visible contraction of deltoid with no movement.

Grade 0: No discernable palpable contractile activity.

FIGURE 5.67

FIGURE 5.68

Substitution by Biceps Brachii

When a patient uses the biceps to substitute, the shoulder will externally rotate, and the elbow will flex. The arm will be raised but not by the action of the abductor muscles. To avoid this substitution, begin the test with the arm in a few degrees of elbow flexion, but do not allow active contraction of the biceps during the test.

Suggested Exercises for Middle Deltoid and Supraspinatus (Combined)

- Flexion at 125°[25]
- Prone horizontal abduction at 100° with full external rotation[9,26]
- Standing external rotation[26]

Clinical Relevance

- Turning the face to the opposite side and extending the neck will put the trapezius on slack and make the supraspinatus more accessible for palpation.
- The deltoid and supraspinatus work in tandem; when one is active in abduction, the other also will be active. Only when supraspinatus weakness is suspected is it necessary to palpate.
- Do not allow shoulder elevation or lateral flexion of the trunk to the opposite side because these movements can create an illusion of abduction.
- The tendon of the supraspinatus is the most frequently injured of all the rotator cuff muscles because of its vulnerable position between the humeral head and acromion.[2]
- The supraspinatus is activated first when the patient abducts the arm from a neutral position of hanging at the side.[2] It functions to prevent the deltoid from superiorly translating the humeral head during abduction.
- Peak activation of the supraspinatus is at 90° of abduction, which corresponds with the largest shoulder joint compressive loads, generating forces 20× greater than the weight of the load.[2]

(Posterior deltoid)

POSTERIOR

FIGURE 5.69

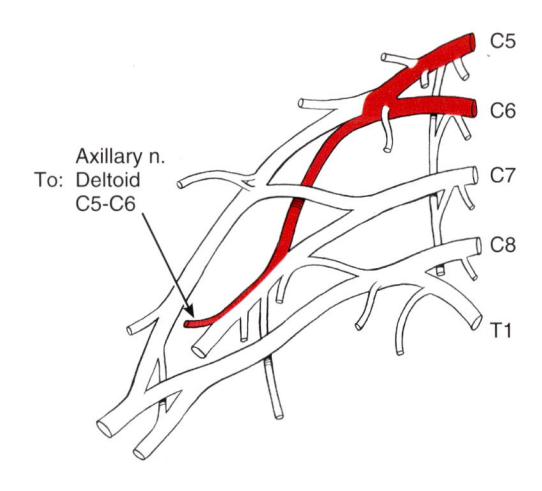

FIGURE 5.70

> ## Range of Motion
>
> 0°–90° (range, 90°) when starting from a position of 90° of forward flexion
>
> −40° to 90° (range, 130°) when starting with the arm in full horizontal adduction

Table 5.10 SHOULDER HORIZONTAL ABDUCTION

I.D.	Muscle	Origin	Insertion	Function
133	**Deltoid (posterior fibers)**	Scapula (spine on lower lip of crest)	Humerus (deltoid tuberosity via humeral tendon)	Shoulder horizontal abduction Extension and external rotation: posterior fibers
	Deltoid (middle fibers)	See Table 5.9		
Others				
136	Infraspinatus			
137	Teres minor			
125	Rhomboid major			
124	Trapezius (middle)			

(Posterior deltoid)

Grade 5, Grade 4, and Grade 3

Position of the Patient: Prone. Shoulder abducted to 90° and forearm off edge of table with elbow straight.

Instructions to Clinician: Stand at test side. Ask patient to lift elbow up toward the ceiling. If full range is present (Grade 3), apply appropriate resistance. Clinician's hand giving resistance is contoured over posterior arm just above the elbow (Fig. 5.71).

Test: Patient horizontally abducts shoulder. Care should be taken to not allow the humerus to drop (lower), allowing substitution of the rhomboids.

Instructions to Patient: "Lift your arm up toward the ceiling. Hold it. Don't let me push it down."

Grading

Grade 5: Holds test position against maximal resistance.

Grade 4: Holds test position against strong to moderate resistance.

Grade 3: Completes range of motion without manual resistance (Fig. 5.72). Note that the elbow can be flexed for a Grade 3.

FIGURE 5.71

FIGURE 5.72

(Posterior deltoid)

Grade 2, Grade 1, and Grade 0

Position of the Patient: Short sitting.

Instructions to Clinician: Stand at test side. Support forearm under volar aspect (Fig. 5.73) and palpate over the posterior surface of shoulder just superior to the axilla.

Test: Patient attempts to horizontally abduct shoulder. Take care not to allow the patient to drop the arm, substituting the rhomboids.

Instructions to Patient: "Try to move your arm backward."

FIGURE 5.73

Alternate Test for Grade 2, Grade 1, and Grade 0

Position of the Patient: Short sitting with arm supported on table (smooth surface) in 90° of abduction; elbow partially flexed. A powder board can be used.

Instructions to Clinician: Stand behind patient. Stabilize by contouring one hand over the superior aspect of shoulder and the other over the scapula (Fig. 5.74). Palpate the fibers of the posterior deltoid below and lateral to the spine of the scapula and on the posterior aspect of the proximal arm adjacent to the axilla.

Test: Patient slides (or tries to move) the arm across the table in horizontal abduction.

Instructions to Patient: "Slide your arm backward."

Grading

Grade 2: Moves through full range of motion.

Grade 1: Palpable contraction; no motion.

Grade 0: No discernable palpable contractile activity.

FIGURE 5.74

Clinical Relevance

If the scapular muscles are weak, the clinician must manually stabilize the scapula to avoid scapular abduction.

Substitution by Triceps Brachii (Long Head)

Maintain the elbow in flexion to avoid substitution by the long head of the triceps.

Suggested Exercises for Posterior Deltoid

- Bent over rear deltoid raise
- Prone rear deltoid raise
- Prone horizontal abduction at 100° with full external rotation[26]
- Prone external rotation at 90° of abduction[26]

(Pectoralis major)

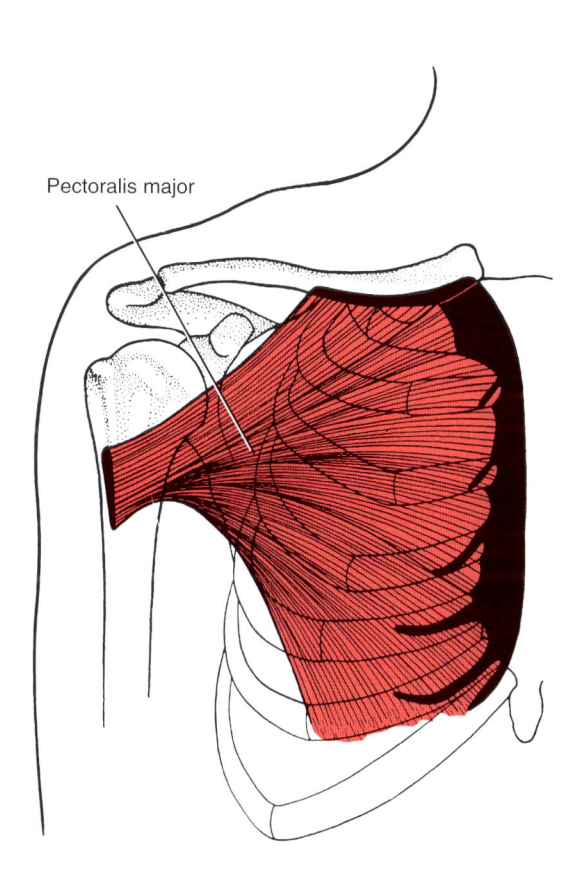

Pectoralis major

FIGURE 5.75

Lateral pectoral n.
To: Pectoralis major
(Clavicular part)
C5-C6

C5
C6
C7
C8
T1

Medial pectoral n.
To: Pectoralis major
(Sternocostal part)
C6-T1

FIGURE 5.76

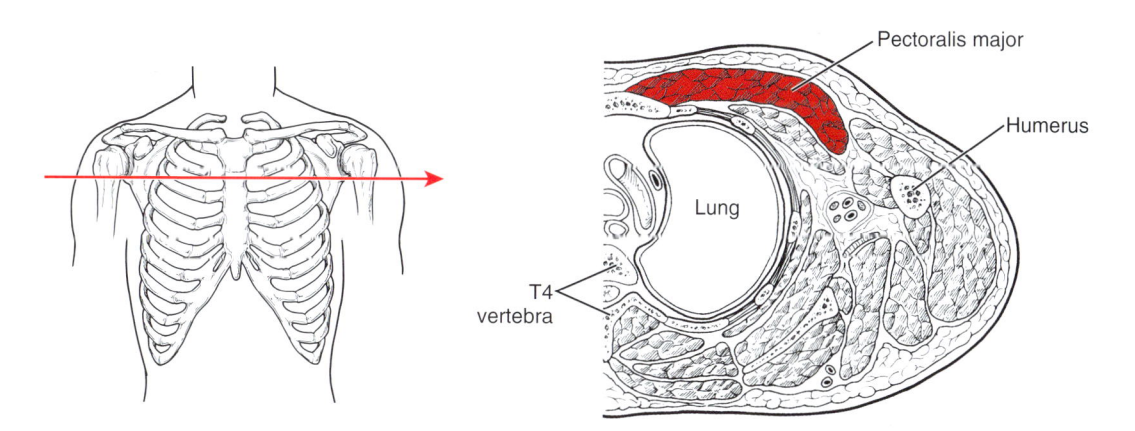

Pectoralis major

Humerus

Lung

T4
vertebra

FIGURE 5.77 Arrow indicates level of cross section.

(Pectoralis major)

<table>
<tr><td colspan="2" style="background:red;color:white">Range of Motion</td></tr>
<tr><td>0°–130°</td></tr>
<tr><td>When starting from a position of 90° of forward flexion: 0° to −40° (range, 40°)</td></tr>
<tr><td>When starting with the arm in full horizontal abduction: 0° passing across the midline to −40° (range, 130°)</td></tr>
</table>

Table 5.11 SHOULDER HORIZONTAL ADDUCTION

I.D.	Muscle	Origin	Insertion	Function
131	Pectoralis major			
	Clavicular part	Clavicle (sternal half of anterior surface)	Humerus (intertubercular sulcus, lateral lip)	Internal rotation of shoulder Flexion of shoulder Horizontal shoulder adduction
	Sternal part	Sternum (anterior surface down to rib 6) Ribs 2–7 (costal cartilages) Aponeurosis of obliquus externus abdominis	Both parts converge on a bilaminar common tendon	Horizontal shoulder adduction Extension of shoulder Draws trunk upward and forward in climbing
Other				
133	Deltoid (anterior fibers)	See Table 5.7		

The two parts of the pectoralis major muscle can work separately or together. Together, they adduct the arm across the body and medially rotate the shoulder. The clavicular portion acts with the anterior fibers of the deltoid to swing the extended arm forward and medially.[1] If the arm is fixed, such as gripping a branch overhead, the pectoralis major draws the trunk up and forward.[1]

Grade 5 and Grade 4

Position of the Patient:

Whole Muscle: Supine. Shoulder abducted to 90°; elbow flexed to 90°.

Clavicular Head: Patient begins test with shoulder in 60° of abduction with elbow flexed. Patient then is asked to horizontally adduct the shoulder in a slightly upward diagonal direction.

Sternal Head: Patient begins test with shoulder in about 120° of abduction with elbow flexed. Patient is asked to horizontally adduct the shoulder in a slightly downward diagonal direction.

Instructions to Clinician: Stand at side of shoulder to be tested. Ask the patient to move the arm with elbow flexed in horizontal adduction, keeping it parallel to the floor without rotation, checking the range of motion. If the arm moves across the body in a diagonal motion, test the sternal and clavicular heads of the muscle separately. If full range is present in a horizontal adducted direction (Grade 3), test the whole muscle together.

Clinician's hand used for resistance is contoured around upper arm, just proximal to elbow, allowing the forearm to hang free. Resistance is applied in the direction opposite the trunk in the transverse plane.

Grade 5 and Grade 4 Continued

Clavicular Head: Resistance is applied above the elbow in a downward direction (toward floor) and outward (i.e., opposite to the direction of the fibers of the clavicular head, which moves the arm diagonally up and inward) (Fig. 5.78).

Sternal Head: Resistance is applied above the elbow in an up and outward direction (Fig. 5.79) (i.e., opposite to the motion of the sternal head, which is diagonally down and inward).

Test: When the *whole muscle* is tested, the patient horizontally adducts the shoulder in the transverse plane through the available range of motion (Fig. 5.80).

When the *clavicular head* is tested, the patient's motion begins at 60° of abduction and moves up and in across the body.

When the *sternal head* is tested, the motion begins at 120° of shoulder abduction and moves diagonally down and in toward the patient's opposite hip.

Instructions to Patient:
Both Heads: "Move your arm across your chest. Hold it. Don't let me pull it back."

Clavicular Head: "Move your arm up and in."

Sternal Head: "Move your arm down and in."

Grading

Grade 5: Holds test position against maximal resistance.

Grade 4: Holds test position with strong to moderate resistance, but muscle exhibits some "give" at end of range.

Grade 3: Completes available range of motion in all three tests (if appropriate) with no resistance other than the weight of the extremity.

FIGURE 5.79

FIGURE 5.78

FIGURE 5.80

SHOULDER HORIZONTAL ADDUCTION

(Pectoralis major)

Grade 2, Grade 1, and Grade 0

Position of the Patient: Supine. Arm is supported in 90° of abduction with elbow flexed to 90°.

Alternate Position: Patient is seated with test arm supported on table (at level of axilla) with arm in 90° of abduction midway between flexion and extension and elbow slightly flexed (Fig. 5.81). Friction of the table surface should be minimized (as with a powder board).

Instructions to Clinician: Stand at side of shoulder to be tested or behind the seated patient. If the patient is supine, support the full length of the forearm and hold the limb at the wrist (see Fig. 5.78).

For both tests, palpate the pectoralis major muscle on the anterior aspect of the chest medial to the shoulder joint (Fig. 5.82.)

Test: Patient attempts to horizontally adduct the shoulder. The use of the alternate test position, in which the arm moves across the table, precludes individual testing for the two heads.

Instructions to Patient: "Try to move your arm across your chest." In seated position: "Move your arm in toward your body."

Grading

Grade 2: Patient horizontally adducts shoulder through available range of motion with the weight of the arm supported by the clinician or the table.

Grade 1: Palpable contractile activity.

Grade 0: No discernable palpable contractile activity.

Clinical Relevance

Testing both heads of the pectoralis major separately should be routine in any patient with cervical spinal cord injury because of their different nerve root innervation.

Suggested Exercises for Pectoralis Major, Pectoralis Major, and Teres Major

- Push-up with narrow hand placement[31]
- Push-up plus[32]
- D2 diagonal[32]

FIGURE 5.81

FIGURE 5.82

(Pectoralis major)

The rotator cuff is made up of the four tendons of the subscapularis, supraspinatus, infraspinatus, and teres minor muscles. However, the teres minor, parts of the infraspinatus, and most of the subscapularis do not have tendons, so the term rotator cuff is a misnomer.[1] However, it is a familiar term and will be used in this discussion. The teres major has an important role in stabilizing the head of the humerus into the glenoid when the arm is elevated over 90° and is often considered a part of the rotator cuff.[1] The rotator cuff functions to provide a compressive force in all positions of the arm at the shoulder. The infraspinatus and teres minor act as an external rotator, and the subscapularis and teres major act as an internal rotator. The supraspinatus initiates and assists with abduction and assists with ER when the shoulder is abducted. The shoulder with a poorly performing rotator cuff is quite impaired because of the importance of humeral stabilization.[1]

Resistance applied in tests of shoulder rotation should be administered gradually and carefully because of the inherent instability of the shoulder and in the presence of pain, muscle tears, or instability.

(Infraspinatus and Teres minor)

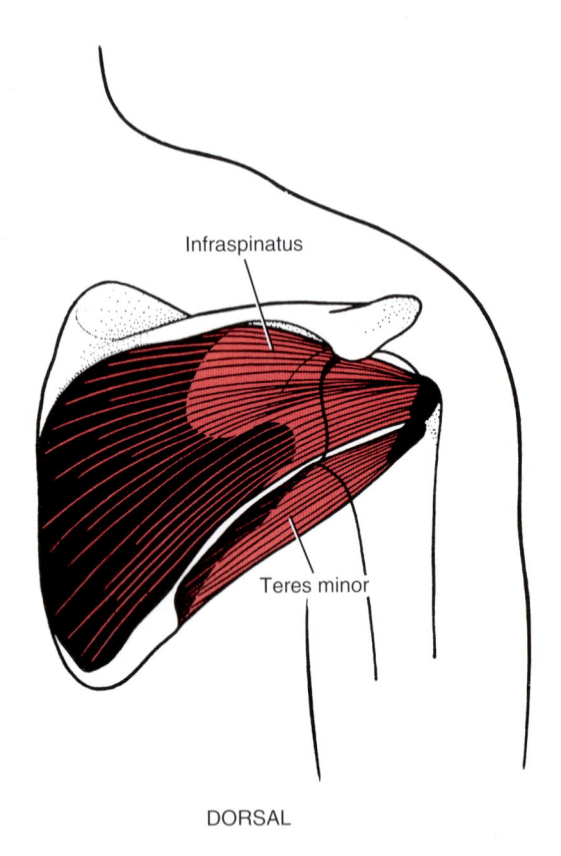

DORSAL

FIGURE 5.83

Suprascapular n.
To: Infraspinatus
C5-C6

C5

C6

C7

C8

T1

Axillary n.
To: Teres minor
C5-C6

FIGURE 5.84

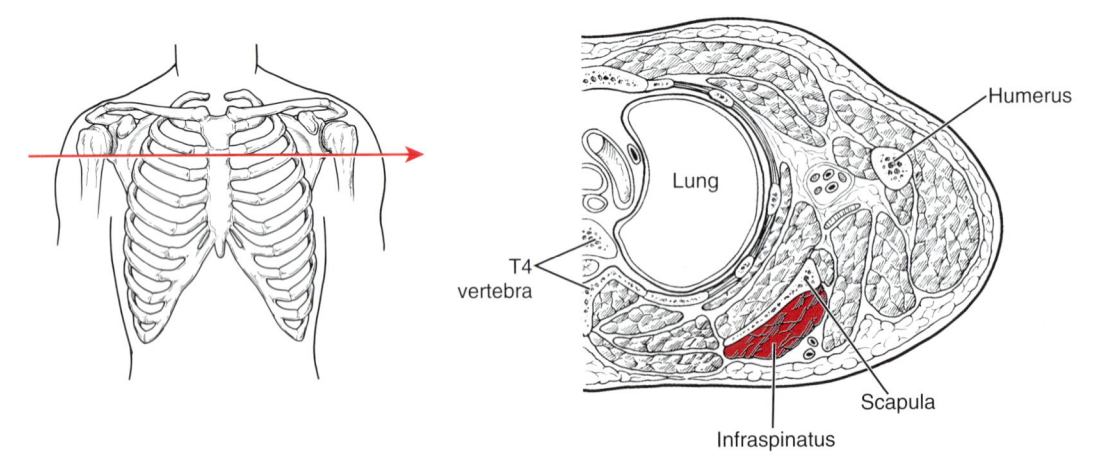

Humerus

Lung

T4
vertebra

Scapula

Infraspinatus

FIGURE 5.85 Arrow indicates level of cross section.

Table 5.12 SHOULDER EXTERNAL ROTATION

I.D.	Muscle	Origin	Insertion	Function
136	**Infraspinatus**	Scapula (infraspinous fossa, medial two-thirds) Infraspinous fascia	Humerus (greater tubercle, middle facet)	External rotation of shoulder Stabilizes shoulder joint by depressing humeral head in glenoid fossa
137	Teres minor	Scapula (lateral border, superior two-thirds)	Humerus (greater tubercle, lowest facet) Humerus (shaft, distal to lowest facet) Capsule of G-H joint	External rotation of shoulder Maintains humeral head in glenoid fossa, thus stabilizing the shoulder joint
Other				
135	Supraspinatus	See Table 5.9		
133	Deltoid (posterior)	See Table 5.10		

G-H, Glenohumeral.

SHOULDER EXTERNAL ROTATION

(Infraspinatus and Teres minor)

Grade 5, Grade 4, and Grade 3

Position of the Patient: Short sitting, with elbow flexed to 90° and forearm in neutral rotation, perpendicular with patient's trunk.

Instructions to Clinician: Stand in front of patient. Ask patient to move the forearm away from the trunk. If full range is available (Grade 3), apply appropriate resistance. One hand stabilizes the medial aspect of the elbow, and the other hand provides resistance at the dorsal (extensor) surface of the forearm just proximal to the wrist to avoid eliciting the wrist extensors (Fig. 5.86). Resistance is given on the outside of the forearm toward the trunk. Because this is not an antigravity position, maximal resistance should be used, if appropriate.

Test: Patient externally rotates arm, pushing forearm away from trunk.

Instructions to Patient: "Push your forearm away. Hold it. Don't let me move it."

Grade 3: Instructions to Patient:
"Move your forearm away from your stomach" (Fig. 5.87).

Grading

Grade 5: Holds test position against maximal resistance.

Grade 4: Holds test position against strong resistance with some yield.

Grade 3: Completes available range of motion without manual resistance.

FIGURE 5.86

FIGURE 5.87

Grade 2, Grade 1, and Grade 0

Position of Patient: Short sitting with elbow flexed to 90° and forearm in neutral rotation with hand facing forward, supported on table with friction minimized by clinician (Figs. 5.88 and 5.89), powder board, or other means.

Instructions to Clinician: Sit or stand on a low stool at test side of patient at shoulder level (picture shows clinician on opposite side to avoid obstructing view). One hand stabilizes the forearm, while the other hand palpates for the tendon of the infraspinatus over the body of the scapula below the spine in the infraspinous fossa. Palpate the teres minor on the inferior margin of the axilla and along the axillary border of the scapula (see Fig. 5.89). Supination may occur instead of the requested ER during the testing of Grades 2 and 1. This motion can be mistaken for ER.

Test: Patient attempts to move forearm away from the trunk (see Fig. 5.89).

Instructions to Patient: "Try to push your forearm away from your stomach."

Grading

Grade 2: Completes available range in this gravity-eliminated position.

Grade 1: Palpation of either or both muscles reveals contractile activity but no motion.

Grade 0: No discernable palpable contractile activity.

FIGURE 5.88

FIGURE 5.89

SHOULDER EXTERNAL ROTATION

(Infraspinatus and Teres minor)

Alternate Position for Grade 5, Grade 4, and Grade 3

Position of Patient: Prone with head turned toward test side. Shoulder abducted to 90° with arm fully supported on table; forearm is hanging vertically over edge of table. Place a folded towel under the arm or use the clinician's hand to cushion the arm if the table has a sharp edge (Fig. 5.90).

Instructions to Clinician: Stand at test side at level of patient's waist (see Fig. 5.90). Use one hand to give resistance over the forearm, as near the wrist as possible, for Grades 5 and 4. The other hand supports the elbow to provide some counterpressure at the end of the range. Note: Resistance will be much less than in the sitting position, and care should be taken in this vulnerable position.

Test: Patient moves forearm upward through the range of ER.

Instructions to Patient: "Raise your arm to the level of the table. Hold it. Don't let me push it down." Clinician may need to demonstrate the desired motion.

Grading

Grade 5: Holds test position against strong resistance.

Grade 4: Holds test position, but end range yields or gives way with strong resistance.

Grade 3: Completes available range of motion without manual resistance (Fig. 5.91).

Clinical Relevance

- The optimal manual muscle test (MMT) position for the infraspinatus is in 0° abduction, where the least activation of the supraspinatus muscle occurs (see Fig. 5.86).[33]
- Range of motion for individuals over 60 years old is less than younger adults and averages 71° to 72° for men and women.[34]
- Range of motion averages for children and adolescents are 93° to 99°.[34]

Suggested Exercises for the Infraspinatus

- Prone horizontal abduction at 100° with ER and IR
- Side-lying ER with 0° abduction[8,26] (minimizes upper trapezius activity)
- D1 and D2 diagonal pattern flexion (may elicit upper trapezius)
- Standing ER at 90° abduction (full can)[8]

Suggested Suggested Exercises for the Teres Minor

- Flexion above 120° with ER (thumb up)[8]
- Standing scapular rows at various degrees of flexion (45°, 90°, and 135°)[8]
- Side-lying ER at 0° abduction[8]
- Prone horizontal abduction at 90°[8]
- Abduction with ER (thumb up and down)[8]

FIGURE 5.90

FIGURE 5.91

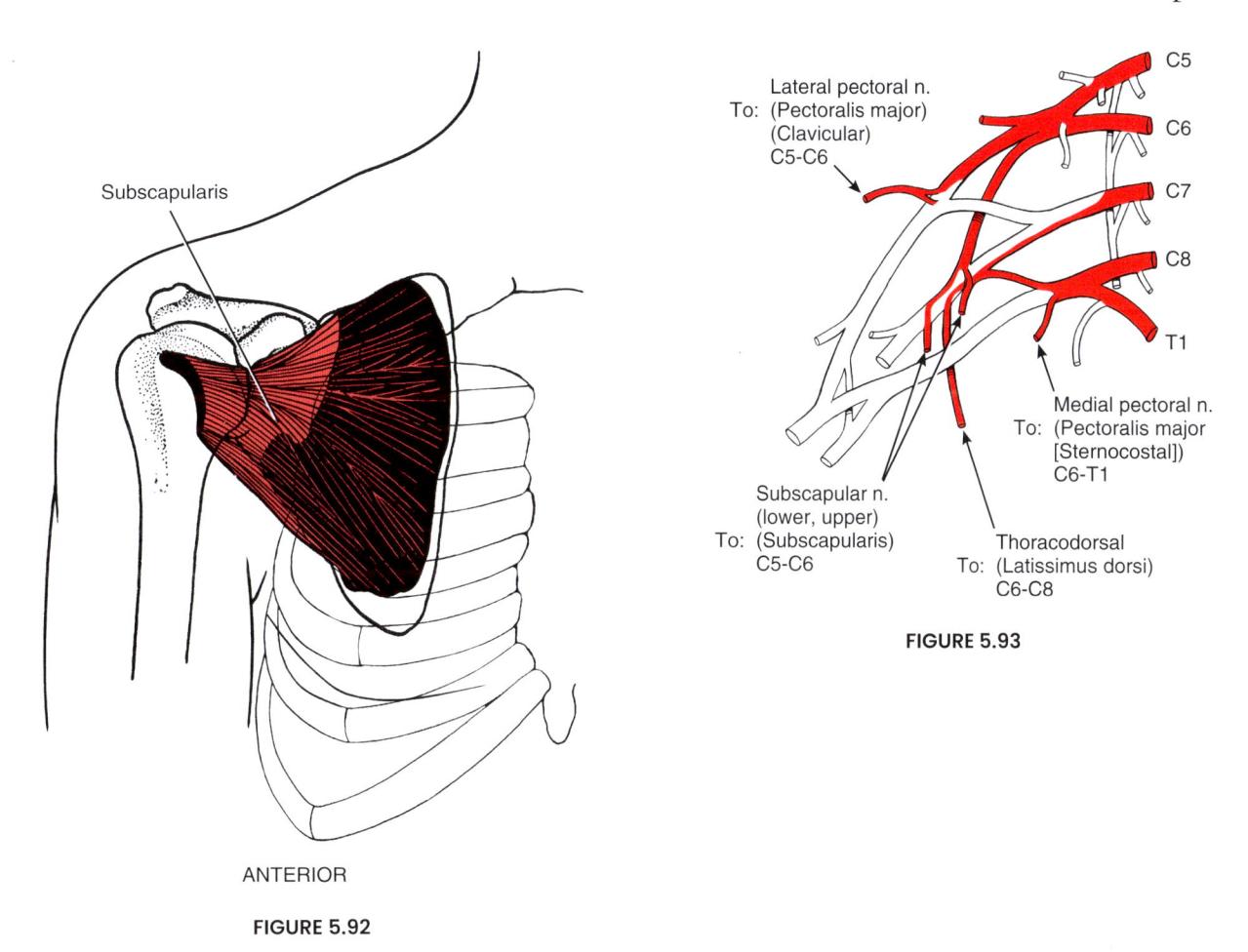

Subscapularis

ANTERIOR

FIGURE 5.92

Lateral pectoral n.
To: (Pectoralis major)
(Clavicular)
C5-C6

C5

C6

C7

C8

T1

Medial pectoral n.
To: (Pectoralis major
[Sternocostal])
C6-T1

Subscapular n.
(lower, upper)
To: (Subscapularis)
C5-C6

Thoracodorsal
To: (Latissimus dorsi)
C6-C8

FIGURE 5.93

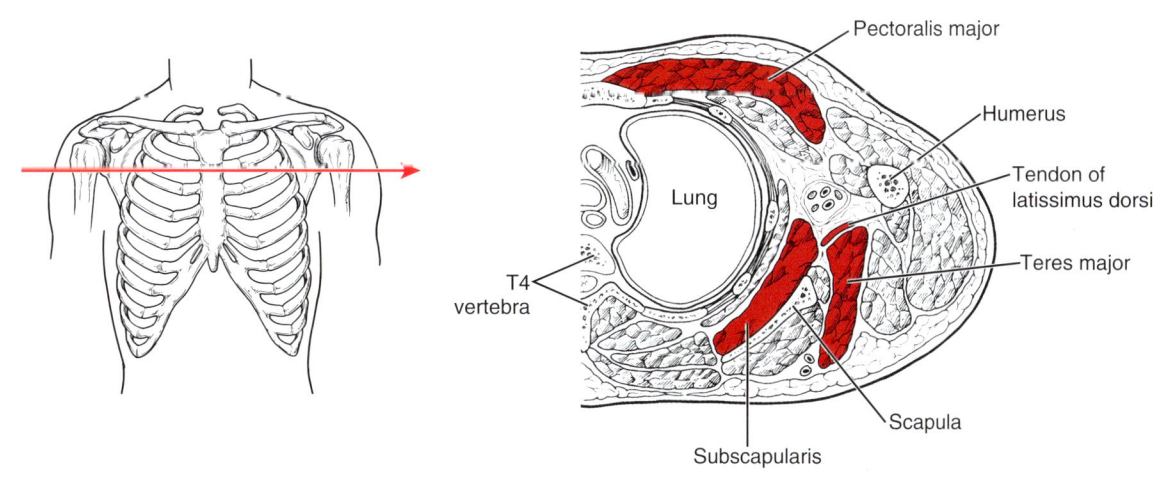

Pectoralis major

Humerus

Tendon of
latissimus dorsi

Teres major

Lung

T4
vertebra

Scapula

Subscapularis

FIGURE 5.94 Arrow indicates level of cross section.

SHOULDER INTERNAL ROTATION

(Subscapularis)

<table>
<tr><td>**Range of Motion**</td></tr>
<tr><td>0°–60°</td></tr>
</table>

Table 5.13 SHOULDER INTERNAL ROTATION

I.D.	Muscle	Origin	Insertion	Function
134	**Subscapularis**	Scapula (fills fossa on costal surface) Intermuscular septa Aponeurosis of subscapularis	Humerus (lesser tubercle) Capsule of G-H joint (anterior)	Internal rotation of shoulder Maintains humeral head in glenoid fossa (with other rotator cuff muscles) Abduction of shoulder
138	Teres major	Scapula (dorsal surface of inferior angle)	Humerus (intertubercular sulcus, medial lip)	Internal rotation of shoulder Adduction and extension of shoulder Extension of shoulder from a flexed position
131	Pectoralis major	Sternal half of clavicle, entire anterior surface of the sternum	Lateral lip of the intertubercular sulcus of anterior humerus	
	Clavicular part	Clavicle (sternal half of anterior surface)	Humerus (intertubercular sulcus, lateral lip)	*Clavicular fibers*: Internal rotation of shoulder Flexion of shoulder Horizontal shoulder adduction
130	Latissimus dorsi	T6-T12, L1-L5, and sacral vertebrae (spinous processes) Supraspinous ligaments Ribs 9–12 (by slips that interdigitate with obliquus externus abdominis) Ilium (crest, posterior) Thoracolumbar fascia	Humerus (floor of intertubercular sulcus) Deep fascia of arm	Internal rotation of shoulder

G-H, Glenohumeral.

Grade 5, Grade 4, and Grade 3

Position of Patient: Short sitting with elbow flexed to 90°, forearm in neutral rotation, perpendicular to the trunk.

Instructions to Clinician: Stand in front of patient and ask patient to pull forearm toward the trunk. If full range is present (Grade 3), apply resistance. Stabilize the outside of the elbow with one hand while the other hand provides resistance at the volar (flexor) surface of the forearm, just proximal to the wrist (Fig. 5.95) so as not to elicit wrist flexors. Resistance is given on the volar surface in the direction away from the trunk. As in the tests for ER, this is a gravity-minimized position, so maximal resistance is used, if appropriate.

Test: Patient internally rotates arm, pulling forearm toward trunk.

Instructions to Patient: "Pull your forearm toward your stomach. Hold it. Don't let me pull it out."

Grading

Grade 5: Holds test position against maximum resistance.

Grade 4: Holds test position against strong resistance. Some yield is felt.

Grade 3: Completes available range without manual resistance.

FIGURE 5.95

SHOULDER INTERNAL ROTATION

(Subscapularis)

Grade 2, Grade 1, and Grade 0

Position of Patient: Short sitting or sitting at a table, with elbow flexed and forearm in neutral rotation.

Instructions to Clinician: Stand at test side or sit on low stool. One hand stabilizes the forearm, while the other hand palpates for the tendon of the subscapularis, deep in the axilla (Fig. 5.96). Note: The hand of the clinician under the patient's hand will eliminate friction in the Grade 2 test if a flat surface is being used (Fig. 5.97). Alternatively, a powder board can be used.

Test: Patient attempts to internally rotate arm, pulling forearm toward trunk.

Instructions to Patient: "Try to pull your forearm toward your stomach."

Grading

Grade 2: Is not able to complete available range.

Grade 1: Palpable contraction occurs.

Grade 0: No discernable palpable contractile activity.

FIGURE 5.96

FIGURE 5.97

Alternate Test for Grade 5, Grade 4, and Grade 3

Used if patient cannot sit.

Position of Patient: Prone with head turned toward test side. Shoulder is abducted to 90° with folded towel placed under distal arm and forearm hanging vertically over edge of table.

Instructions to Clinician: Stand at test side. Hand giving resistance is placed on the volar side of the forearm just above the wrist. The other hand provides counterforce at the elbow (Fig. 5.98). The resistance hand applies resistance in a downward and forward direction; the counterforce is applied backward and slightly upward. Stabilize the scapular region if muscles are weak or perform test in the supine position. Note: Resistance will be much less than in the sitting position.

Test: Patient moves arm through available range of internal rotation (backward and upward).

Instructions to Patient: "Move your forearm up and back. Hold it. Don't let me push it down." Demonstrate the desired motion to the patient.

FIGURE 5.98

(Subscapularis)

Alternate Test for Grade 5, Grade 4, and Grade 3 Continued

Grading

Grade 5: Holds test position firmly against strong resistance.

Grade 4: Holds test position, but there is a give against strong resistance.

Grade 3: Completes available range with no manual resistance (Fig. 5.99).

FIGURE 5.99

Clinical Relevance

- Internal rotation is a stronger motion than external rotation. This is largely a factor of muscle mass.
- No clinical test for subscapularis tendon tears, including the lift-off test, the belly test, and the bear hug test, has a pooled sensitivity/specificity of 0.80 or greater; however, the bear hug test holds the most promise.[35]
- The belly press test was found to activate the upper subscapularis muscle more than the lift-off test, whereas the lift-off test was found to activate the lower subscapularis muscle more than the belly press test.[36]
- The upper portion (innervated by the upper subscapularis nerve) is a more effective internal rotator at lower abduction angles compared with higher abduction angles. The lower subscapularis muscle activity (innervated by the lower subscapularis nerve) is unaffected by abduction angle.
- Performing internal rotation (IR) at 0° abduction produces similar amounts of upper and lower subscapularis activity.[37]

Suggested Exercises for the Subscapularis

- Push-up or palm press[8,25]
- Internal rotation at 0°[25,32]
- Standing high, mid-, and low scapular rows
- Flexion above 120° with ER (thumb up).[8]
- Push-up plus exercise[32]
- D2 diagonal[32]
- Dynamic hug[32]

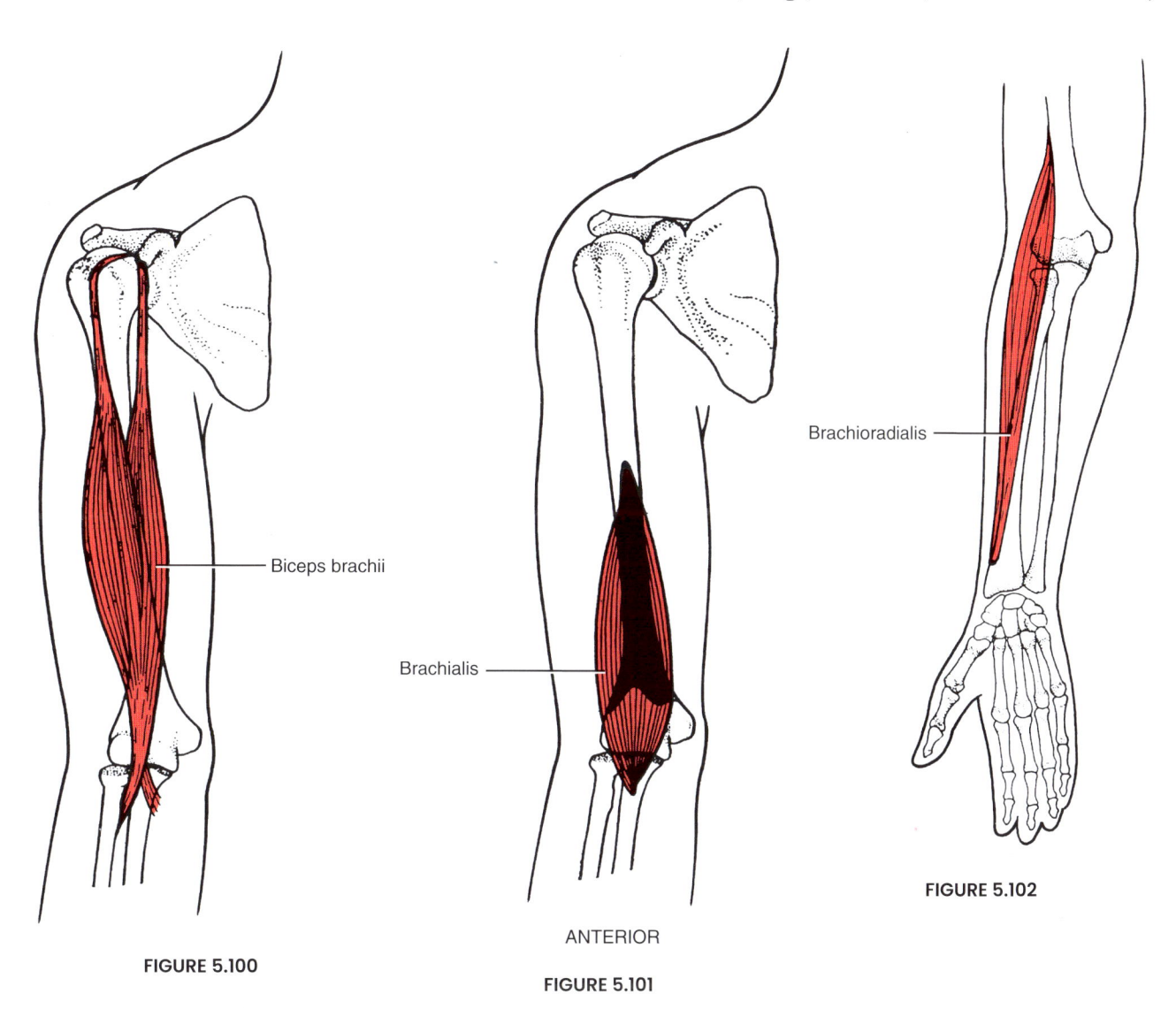

Biceps brachii

FIGURE 5.100

Brachialis

ANTERIOR

FIGURE 5.101

Brachioradialis

FIGURE 5.102

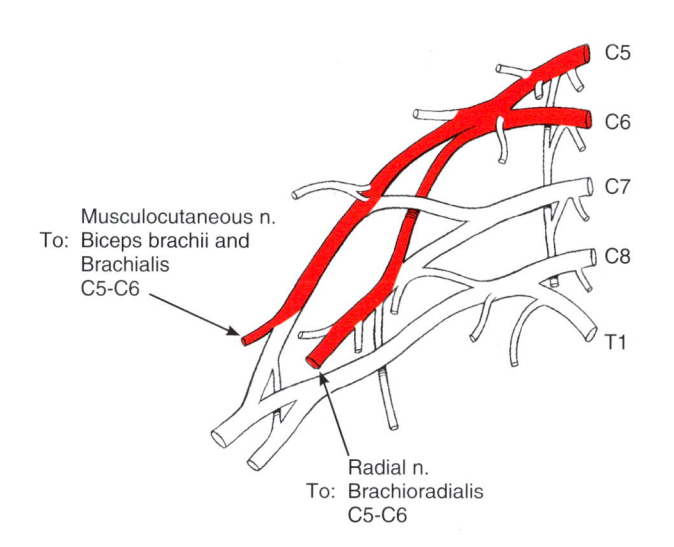

C5
C6
C7
C8
T1

Musculocutaneous n.
To: Biceps brachii and
Brachialis
C5-C6

Radial n.
To: Brachioradialis
C5-C6

FIGURE 5.103

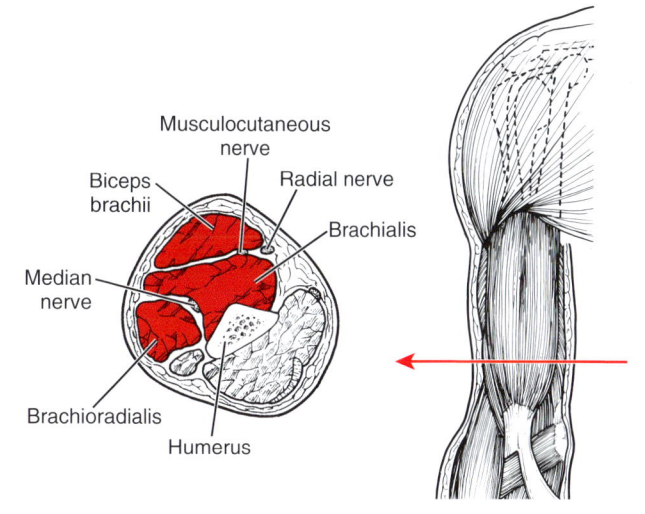

Musculocutaneous
nerve
Biceps
brachii
Radial nerve
Brachialis
Median
nerve
Brachioradialis
Humerus

FIGURE 5.104 Arrow indicates level of cross section.

ELBOW FLEXION

(Biceps, Brachialis, and Brachioradialis)

Table 5.14 ELBOW FLEXION

I.D.	Muscle	Origin	Insertion	Function
141	**Brachialis**	Humerus (shaft anterior, distal one-half) Intermuscular septa (medial)	Ulna (tuberosity and coronoid process)	Flexion of elbow, forearm supinated or pronated
140	Biceps brachii Short head Long head	Scapula (coracoid process, apex) Scapula (supraglenoid tubercle) Capsule of G-H joint and glenoid labrum	Radius (radial tuberosity) Bicipital aponeurosis	*Both heads*: Flexion of elbow Supination of forearm (powerful) *Long head*: Stabilizes and depresses humeral head in glenoid fossa during deltoid activity
143	Brachioradialis	Humerus (lateral supracondylar ridge, proximal two-thirds) Lateral intermuscular septum	Radius (distal end just proximal to styloid process)	Flexion of elbow
Others				
146	Pronator teres	See Table 5.17		
148	Extensor carpi radialis longus	See Table 5.19		
151	Flexor carpi radialis	See Table 5.18		
153	Flexor carpi ulnaris	See Table 5.18		

G-H, Glenohumeral.

The two heads of the biceps work together to accomplish flexion of the elbow. As in the three heads of the triceps, the multiple heads are considered reserves, as both work together to flex the elbow.

Grade 5, Grade 4, and Grade 3

Position of the Patient: Short sitting with arms at sides. The biceps brachii and brachialis cannot be differentiated, as both flex and supinate the elbow.[38]

Biceps Brachii and Brachialis: Shoulder in neutral position with <u>forearm in supination</u> and elbow flexed to midrange (Fig. 5.105).

FIGURE 5.105

Grade 5, Grade 4, and Grade 3 Continued

Brachioradialis: Shoulder in neutral position with forearm in midposition between pronation and supination (Fig. 5.106). The muscle can be palpated and easily seen during maximum effort, as it stands out or "bowstrings" across the elbow.

Instructions to Clinician: Stand in front of patient toward the test side. Ask patient to bend elbow with shoulder in 0° flexion. If full elbow range is present (Grade 3), apply appropriate resistance. Clinician's hand giving resistance is contoured over the volar (flexor) surface of the forearm proximal to the wrist (see Fig. 5.106). The other hand is placed on the posterior aspect of the upper arm, just above the elbow and applies counterforce by resisting any upper arm movement.

FIGURE 5.106

FIGURE 5.107

No resistance is given in a Grade 3 test. The test elbow is cupped by the clinician's hand for support (Fig. 5.107, biceps illustrated at end range).

Test (Both Forearm Positions): Patient flexes elbow through range of motion.

Instructions to Patient (All Three Tests)
Grade 5 and Grade 4: "Bend your elbow. Hold it. Don't let me pull it down."

Grade 3: "Bend your elbow."

Grading

Grade 5: Holds test position against maximal resistance.

Grade 4: Holds test position against strong to moderate resistance, but the end point may not be firm.

Grade 3: Completes available range with each forearm position.

ELBOW FLEXION

(Biceps, Brachialis, and Brachioradialis)

Grade 2

Position of the Patient:
Both Elbow Flexors: Short sitting with shoulder flexed to 90° and internally rotated (to minimize gravity) and supported by clinician (Fig. 5.108). Forearm is supinated (biceps), pronated (brachialis), and in midposition (brachioradialis).

Alternate Position for Patients Unable to Sit: Patient is side lying with arm supported at the elbow in 90° flexion to minimize gravity. Elbow is flexed to about 45° with forearm supinated (biceps and brachialis), and in midposition (for brachioradialis; Fig. 5.109, biceps illustrated).

Instructions to Clinician:
Both Flexors: Stand in front of patient and support flexed arm under the elbow and wrist if necessary. Palpate the tendon of the biceps in the antecubital space (see Fig. 5.108). On the arm, the muscle fibers may be felt on the anterior surface of the middle two-thirds of the biceps with the short head lying medial to the long head.

FIGURE 5.108

FIGURE 5.109

Palpate the brachialis in the distal arm medial to the tendon of the biceps. Palpate the brachioradialis on the lateral surface of the neutrally positioned forearm, where it forms the lateral border of the cubital fossa.

Test: Patient attempts to flex the elbow.

Instructions to Patient: "Try to bend your elbow."

Grading

Grade 2: Completes range of motion with gravity minimized (in each of the muscles tested).

Grade 1 and Grade 0

Position of Patient: Side lying for all three muscles with clinician standing at test side. All other aspects are the same as for the Grade 2 test.

Test: Patient attempts to bend elbow with hand supinated and in midposition.

Grading

Grade 1: Clinician can palpate a contractile response in each of the three muscles for which a Grade 1 is given.

Grade 0: No discernable palpable contractile activity.

Clinical Relevance

- The patient's wrist flexor muscles should remain relaxed throughout the test because strongly contracting wrist flexors may assist in elbow flexion. The clinician's hand position above the patient's hand that is providing resistance is key to this. Recall that the wrist flexors originate above the elbow joint axis on the distal humerus.
- Only the brachioradialis contributes to pronation with elbow flexion.[39]
- During resisted shoulder flexion with the elbow straight, both heads of the biceps are always active.[40]
- Basmajian[40] noted that the three elbow flexors work together without a lot of predictability of one muscle's action over the others when lifting a load. Generally, they are 20% to 25% stronger in elbow flexion with supination than pronation.[2]
- The brachialis is considered the workhorse of the elbow flexors, as it is active in isometric flexion and eccentric extension. The other two flexors are not as active in eccentric extension.[40]
- The biceps brachii is composed of 60% type II fibers.[41]

Suggested Exercises for Biceps, Brachialis and Brachioradialis

- Dumbbell biceps curl and inclined dumbbell curl (shoulder extended) elicited the same maximal muscle activation (>40% MVC) concentrically and eccentrically throughout range.[42]

ELBOW EXTENSION

(Triceps brachii)

POSTERIOR

FIGURE 5.110

Radial n.
To: (Triceps brachii)
C6-C8

FIGURE 5.111

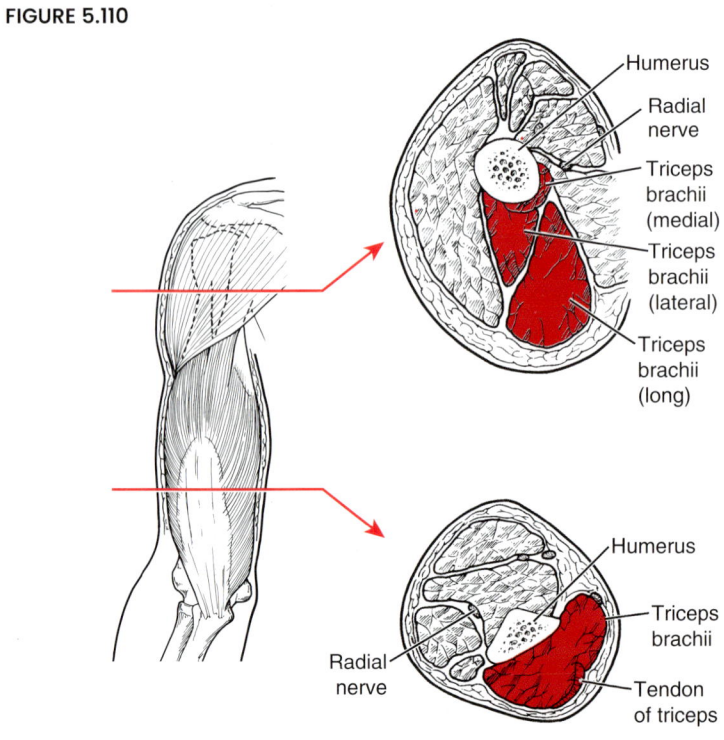

FIGURE 5.112 Arrow indicates level of cross section.

Range of Motion

150° to −5° (many people, especially females, will have hyperextension of the elbow)

Table 5.15 ELBOW EXTENSION

I.D.	Muscle	Origin	Insertion	Function
142	Triceps brachii		All heads have a common tendon to:	Extension of elbow *head*: Extension and adduction of shoulder (assist)
	Long head	Scapula (infraglenoid tuberosity and capsule of G-H joint)	Ulna (olecranon process, upper surface)	*Long and lateral heads*: Especially active in resisted extension, otherwise minimally active[25] *Long head*: Extension and adduction of shoulder (assist)
	Lateral head	Humerus (shaft: oblique ridge, posterior surface) Lateral intermuscular septum	Blends with antebrachial fascia Capsule of elbow joint	*Long and lateral heads*: Especially active in resisted extension, otherwise minimally active
	Medial head	Humerus (shaft: entire length of posterior surface) Medial and lateral intermuscular septa		*Medial head*: Active in all forms of extension

G-H, Glenohumeral.

ELBOW EXTENSION

(Triceps brachii)

As in the biceps, all heads of the triceps brachii work together to extend the elbow. The triceps can fixate the elbow joint when the forearm and hand are used for fine movement (e.g., when writing). The triceps have a greater proportion of type II muscle fibers. The lateral head is used for movements requiring occasional high-intensity force, while the medial head enables precise, low-force movements.

Grade 5, Grade 4, and Grade 3

Position of Patient: Prone on table. The test is begun with the shoulder in 90° of abduction and the elbow flexed to 90° and in neutral rotation (forearm hanging over the side of the table) (Fig. 5.113).

Instructions to Clinician: Stand to the side of patient. Ask patient to straighten the elbow. If full range is present (Grade 3), apply appropriate resistance. Provide support with one hand underneath the arm, just above the elbow. The other hand is used to apply downward resistance on the distal dorsal surface of the extended forearm just proximal to the wrist (Fig. 5.114 illustrates end position). Be sure to have the elbow in minimal flexion so as not to allow the patient to "lock out" the elbow. This is especially important if hyperextension exists.

Test: Patient straightens elbow.

Instructions to Patient: "Hold it. Don't let me bend it."

Grading

Grade 5: Holds test position firmly against maximal resistance.

Grade 4: Holds test position against strong resistance, but there is a "give" to the resistance at the end range.

Grade 3: Completes available range with no manual resistance (Fig. 5.115).

FIGURE 5.115

FIGURE 5.113

FIGURE 5.114

Grade 2, Grade 1, and Grade 0

Position of Patient: Short sitting. The shoulder is abducted to 90° and neutral rotation with the elbow flexed to about 45° to minimize gravity. The entire limb is parallel to the floor (Fig. 5.116).

Instructions to Clinician: Stand at test side of patient. For the Grade 2 test, support the limb at the elbow. For a Grade 1 or 0 test, support the limb under the forearm and palpate the triceps on the posterior surface of the arm just proximal to the olecranon process (Fig. 5.117).

Test: Patient attempts to extend the elbow.

Instructions to Patient: "Try to straighten your elbow."

Grading

Grade 2: Completes available range with gravity minimized.

Grade 1: Clinician can feel tension in the triceps tendon just proximal to the olecranon (see Fig. 5.117) or contractile activity in the muscle fibers on the posterior surface of the arm.

Grade 0: No discernable palpable muscle activity.

FIGURE 5.116

FIGURE 5.117

ELBOW EXTENSION

(Triceps brachii)

Substitutions

- Via external rotation. With the patient sitting with the arm abducted, elbow extension can be accomplished with a Grade 0 triceps (Fig. 5.118) when the patient externally rotates the shoulder, thus dropping the arm below the forearm. As a result, the elbow literally falls into extension. This can be prevented by using a table or powder board to support the arm.
- Via horizontal adduction. This substitution can accomplish elbow extension and is done purposefully by patients with a cervical cord injury and a Grade 0 triceps. With the distal segment fixed (as when the clinician stabilizes the hand or wrist), the patient horizontally adducts the arm and the thrust pulls the elbow into extension (Fig. 5.119). The clinician, therefore, should provide support at the elbow for testing purposes rather than at the wrist.

FIGURE 5.118

FIGURE 5.119

Clinical Relevance

- Give resistance in Grade 5 and Grade 4 tests with the elbow slightly flexed to avoid enabling the patient to "lock" the elbow joint by hyperextending it.
- Although elbow extension is tested in the prone position, the clinician must be aware that with the shoulder horizontally abducted, the two-joint muscle is less effective, and the test grade may be lower than it should be.[15]
- An alternate position for Grades 5, 4, and 3 is with the patient short sitting. The clinician stands behind the patient, supporting the arm in 90° of abduction just above the flexed elbow (Fig. 5.120). The patient straightens the elbow against the resistance given just proximal to the wrist.
- Triceps strength is usually the limiting factor in pressing-type movements such as pushups.

FIGURE 5.120

Suggested Exercises for Triceps Brachii

- Exercises that challenge the triceps close to full extension (lockouts) are likely to be highly beneficial.
- Close grip bench press
- Suspended push-ups elicited more activity than conventional push-ups[43]
- Standard push-ups with narrow base hand position[44]
- Dips
- Triceps extension overhead
- Triceps press down using rope

FOREARM SUPINATION

(Supinator and Biceps brachii)

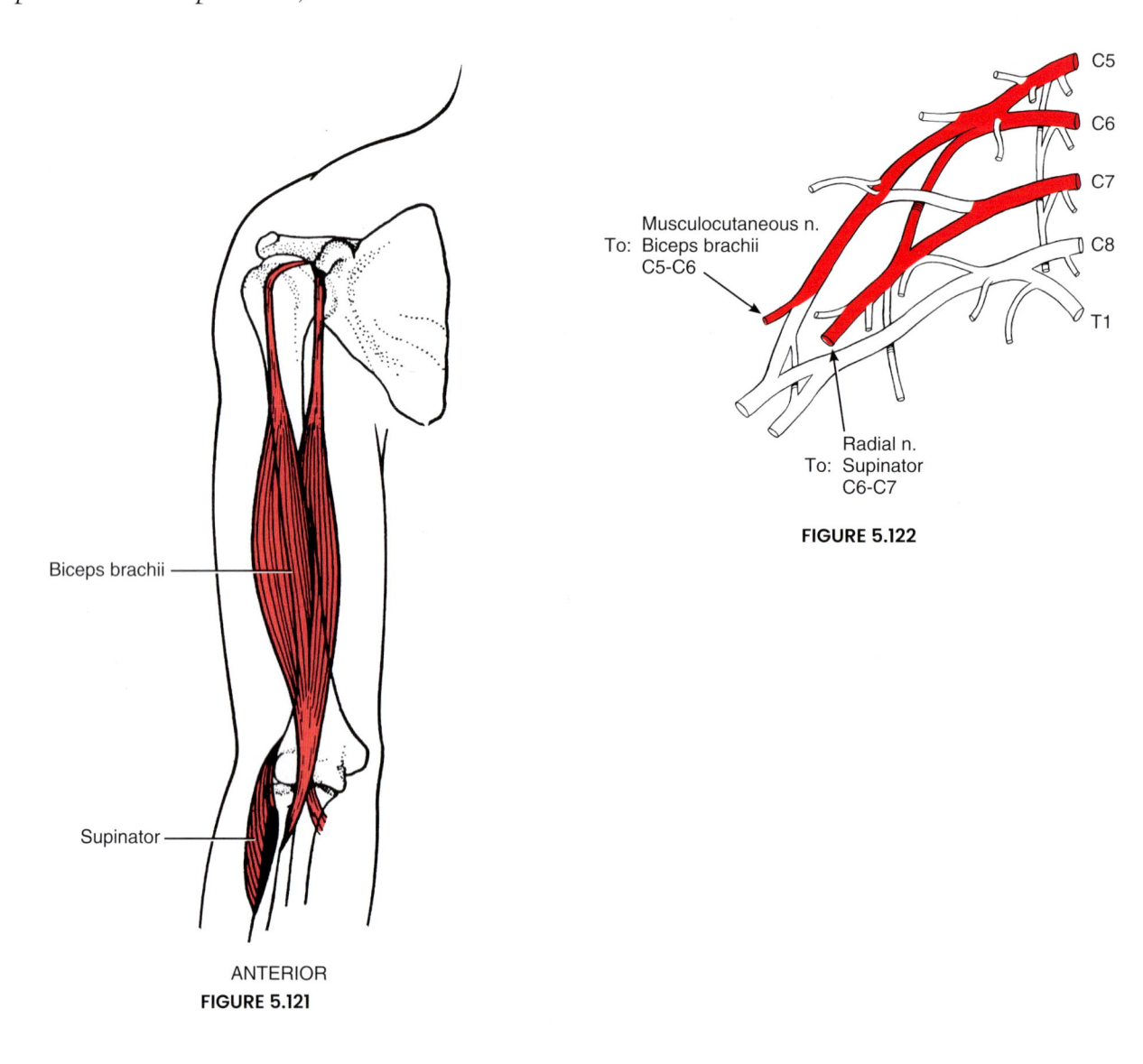

Biceps brachii

Supinator

Musculocutaneous n.
To: Biceps brachii
C5-C6

C5
C6
C7
C8
T1

Radial n.
To: Supinator
C6-C7

FIGURE 5.122

ANTERIOR
FIGURE 5.121

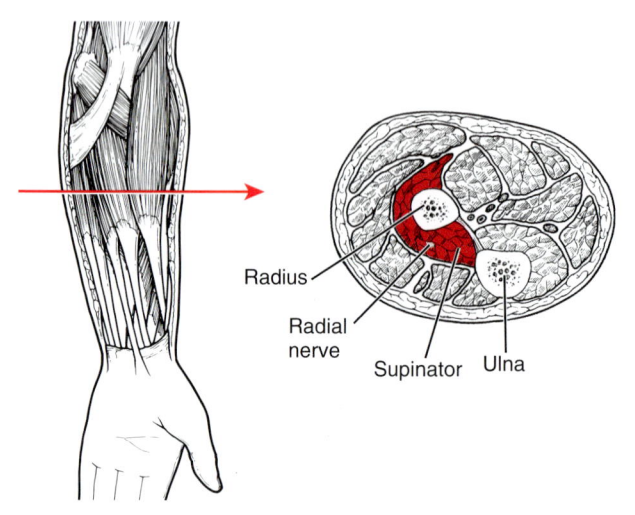

Radius

Radial nerve

Supinator   Ulna

FIGURE 5.123 Arrow indicates level of cross section.

(Supinator and Biceps brachii)

Range of Motion
0°–80°

Table 5.16 FOREARM SUPINATION

I.D.	Muscle	Origin	Insertion	Function
140	Biceps brachii Both heads			Flexion of elbow Supination of forearm (powerful) if combined with elbow flexion
145	Supinator	Humerus (lateral epicondyle) Ulna (supinator crest) Radial collateral ligament of elbow joint Annular ligament of radioulnar joint Aponeurosis of supinator	Radius (shaft, lateral aspect of proximal one-third)	Supination of forearm (pure)

Grade 5, Grade 4, Grade 3, and Grade 2

Position of Patient: Short sitting; arm at side and elbow flexed to 90°; forearm in full pronation to neutral. Alternatively, patient may sit at a table with elbow supported.

Instructions to Clinician: Stand at side or in front of patient. Ask patient to turn the palm up as if holding soup in the hand. If sufficient range is present, proceed to apply resistance. One hand supports the elbow. Apply resistance with the heel of clinician's hand over the dorsal (extensor) surface at the wrist, being careful not to grip the flexor surface of the forearm (Fig. 5.124).

Test: Patient begins in pronation and supinates the forearm until the palm faces the ceiling. Clinician resists motion in the direction of pronation.

Alternate Test: Grasp patient's hand as if shaking hands; cradle the elbow and resist via the hand grip (Fig. 5.125). This test is used if the patient has Grade 5 or 4 wrist and hand strength. It should not be used if there is wrist instability.

FIGURE 5.124

FIGURE 5.125

FOREARM SUPINATION

(Supinator and Biceps brachii)

Grade 5, Grade 4, Grade 3, and Grade 2 Continued

Instructions to Patient: "Turn your palm up. Hold it. Don't let me turn it down. Keep your wrist and fingers relaxed."

For Grade 3: "Turn your palm up."

Grading

Grade 5: Holds test position against maximal resistance.

Grade 4: Holds test position against strong to moderate resistance.

Grade 3: Completes available range of motion without resistance (Fig. 5.126, showing end range).

Grade 2: Completes partial range of motion.

FIGURE 5.126

Grade 1 and Grade 0

Position of Patient: Short sitting. Arm and elbow are flexed as for the previous tests.

Instructions to Clinician: Support the forearm just distal to the elbow. Palpate the supinator distal to the head of the radius on the dorsal aspect of the forearm (Fig. 5.127).

Test: Patient attempts to supinate the forearm.

Instructions to Patient: "Try to turn your palm so it faces the ceiling."

Grading

Grade 1: Slight contractile activity but no limb movement.

Grade 0: No discernable palpable contractile activity.

FIGURE 5.127

Substitution

Patient may externally rotate and adduct the arm across the body (Fig. 5.128) as forearm supination is attempted. When this occurs, the forearm rolls into supination with no activity of the supinator muscle.

FIGURE 5.128

Clinical Relevance

- It is controversial whether supination is stronger than pronation. Some studies report no difference, and others report supination torque is more than pronation torque.[45]
- Biceps brachii activity is highest in midsupination when the length of the muscle is shorter.[45]
- The supinator is considered the prime mover of supination by some authorities, as supination is the only movement it performs and forearm position is irrelevant. The biceps, however, is a far stronger supinator, as its mass is 5× that of the supinator, but the biceps performs optimally when elbow flexion and supination are combined.[45]

(Supinator and Biceps brachii)

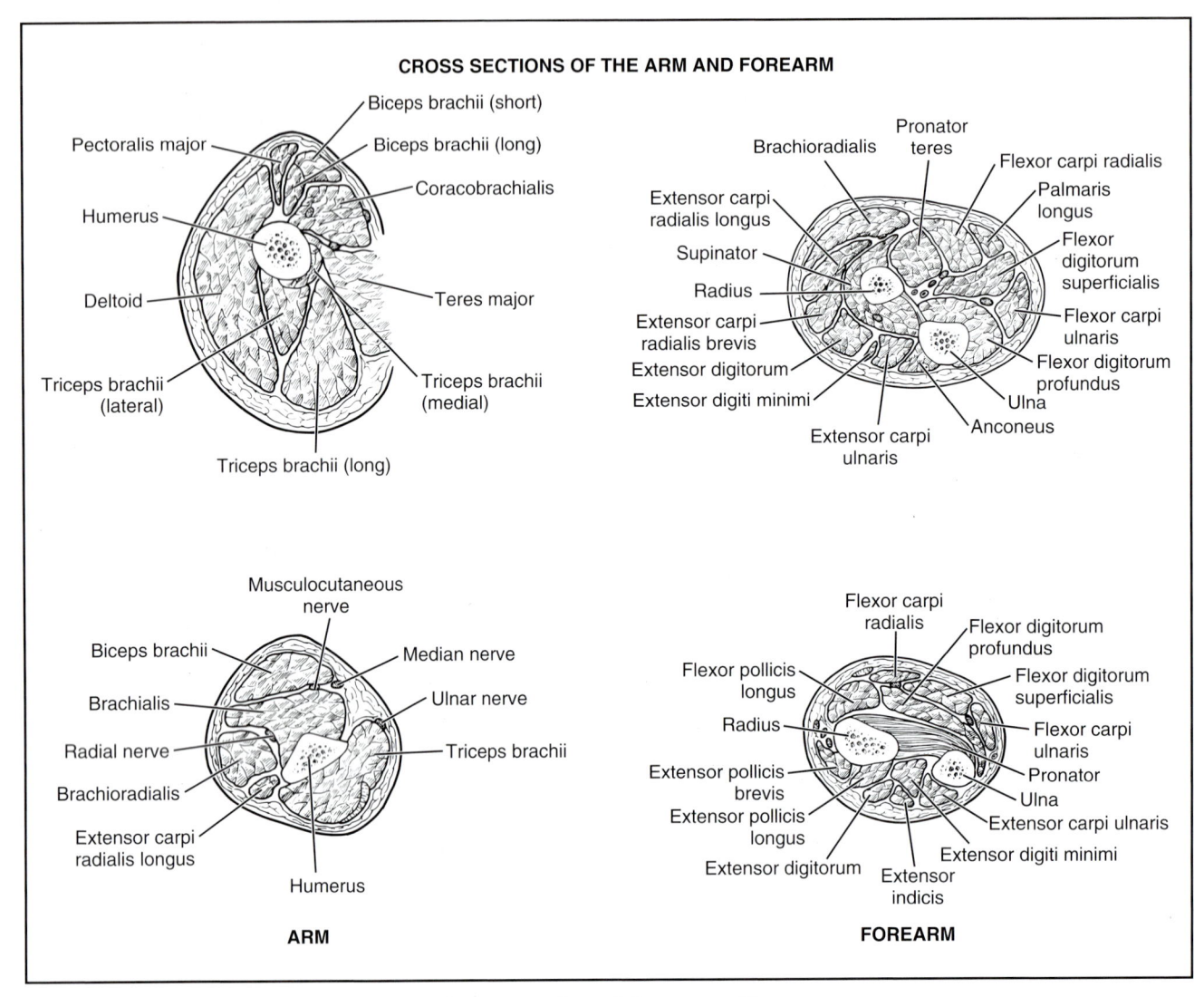

CROSS SECTIONS OF THE ARM AND FOREARM

ARM

FOREARM

PLATE 4 Cross sections of the arm and forearm.

Pronator teres

Pronator quadratus

PALMAR

FIGURE 5.129

C5
C6
C7
C8
T1

Median n.
To: Pronator teres
C6-C7
Pronator quadratus
C7-C8

FIGURE 5.130

Pronator
teres

Median
nerve

Radius

Ulna

Pronator
quadratus

Radius

Ulna

FIGURE 5.131 Arrow indicates level of cross section.

FOREARM PRONATION

(Pronator teres and Pronator quadratus)

Range of Motion

0°–80°

Table 5.17 FOREARM PRONATION

I.D.	Muscle	Origin	Insertion	Function
146	**Pronator teres**		Radius (midshaft, lateral surface)	Pronation of forearm with resisted pronation or rapid pronation Elbow flexion (accessory)[2,45]
	Humeral head	Humerus (shaft proximal to medial epicondyle) Common tendon of origin of flexor muscles Intermuscular septum Antebrachial fascia		
	Ulnar head	Ulna (coronoid process, medial) Joins humeral head in common tendon		
147	Pronator quadratus	Ulna (oblique ridge on distal quarter of anterior surface) Muscle aponeurosis	Radius (shaft, anterior surface distally; also area above ulnar notch)	Pronation of forearm
Other				
151	Flexor carpi radialis	See Table 5.18		*Pronation of forearm (weak assist)* Flexion of wrist Radial deviation (abduction) of wrist Extends fingers (tenodesis action) Flexion of elbow (weak assist)

Grade 5, Grade 4, and Grade 3

Position of Patient: Short sitting or may sit at a table. Arm at side with elbow flexed to 90° and forearm in supination.

Instructions to Clinician: Stand at side or in front of patient. Ask patient to turn palm down from supinated position. If sufficient range is present, proceed to apply resistance in test position. Support the elbow. Hand used for resistance applies resistance with hypothenar eminence over radius on the volar (flexor) surface of the forearm at the wrist (Fig. 5.132). Avoid pressure on the head of the radius and gripping the forearm for patient comfort.

Test: Patient attempts to pronates the forearm. Clinician resists motion at the wrist in the direction of supination for Grades 4 and 5.

Alternate Test: Grasp patient's hand as if to shake hands, cradling the elbow with the other hand and resisting pronation via the hand grip. This alternate test may be used if the patient has Grade 5 or 4 wrist and hand strength. This alternate test should not be used in the presence of wrist instability.

Instructions to Patient: "Turn your palm down. Hold it. Don't let me turn it up. Keep your wrist and fingers relaxed."

Grading

Grade 5: Holds test position against maximal resistance.

Grade 4: Holds test position against strong to moderate resistance.

Grade 3: Completes available range without resistance (Fig. 5.133, showing end range).

Grade 2: Complete partial range of motion.

FIGURE 5.132

FIGURE 5.133

(Pronator teres and Pronator quadratus)

Grade 1 and Grade 0

Instructions to Clinician: Stand to the side of the patient. Support the forearm just distal to the elbow. The fingers of the other hand are used to palpate the pronator teres over the upper third of the volar (flexor) surface of the forearm on a diagonal line from the medial condyle of the humerus to the lateral border of the radius (Fig. 5.134).

Test: Patient attempts to pronate the forearm.

Instructions to Patient: "Try to turn your palm down."

Grading

Grade 1: Visible or palpable contractile activity with no motion of the part.

Grade 0: No discernable palpable contractile activity.

FIGURE 5.134

Substitution

Patient may internally rotate the shoulder or abduct it during attempts at pronation (Fig. 5.135). When this occurs, the forearm rolls into pronation without the benefit of activity by the pronator muscles.

FIGURE 5.135

Clinical Relevance

- Nondominant arm elicits 81% to 95% of the force of the dominant arm in forearm rotation.[46]
- Pronation is strongest in the position of 45° of elbow flexion.[47]
- Men are 63% stronger in pronation and 68% stronger in supination than women, measuring as high as 12.6 to 14.8 nm.[48]
- In isokinetic studies, women's forearm strength is equal to 5.0 to 5.4 nm.[48]

Flexor
carpi
radialis

FIGURE 5.136

Flexor
carpi
ulnaris

PALMAR

FIGURE 5.137

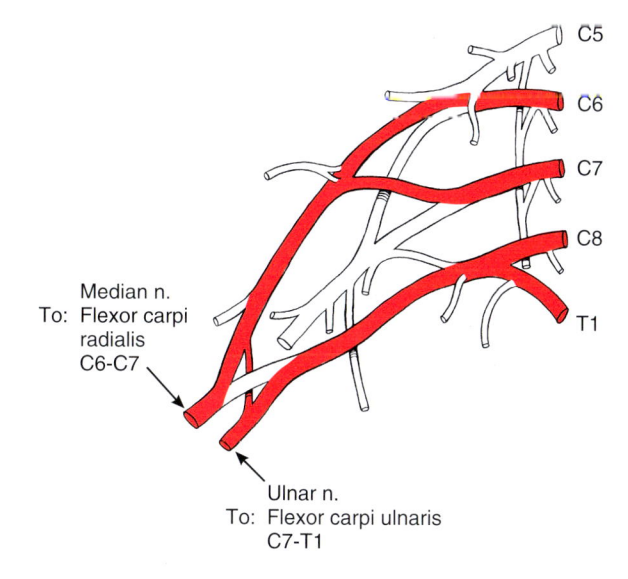

C5

C6

C7

C8

T1

Median n.
To: Flexor carpi
radialis
C6-C7

Ulnar n.
To: Flexor carpi ulnaris
C7-T1

FIGURE 5.138

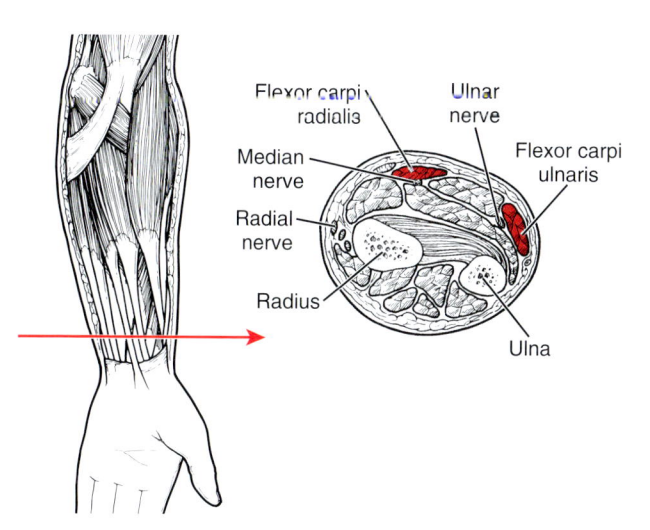

Flexor carpi
radialis

Ulnar
nerve

Flexor carpi
ulnaris

Median
nerve

Radial
nerve

Radius

Ulna

FIGURE 5.139 Arrow indicates level of cross section.

WRIST FLEXION

(Flexor carpi radialis and Flexor carpi ulnaris)

Table 5.18 **WRIST FLEXION**

I.D.	Muscle	Origin	Insertion	Function
151	**Flexor carpi radialis**	Humerus (medial epicondyle via common flexor tendon) Antebrachial fascia Intermuscular septum	2nd and 3rd metacarpals (base, palmar surface)	Flexion of wrist Radial deviation (abduction) of wrist Extends fingers (tenodesis action) Flexion of elbow (weak assist) Pronation of forearm (weak assist)
153	**Flexor carpi ulnaris** **Two heads**	Humeral head (medial epicondyle via common flexor tendon) Ulnar head (olecranon, medial margin; shaft, proximal two-thirds posterior via an aponeurosis) Intermuscular septum	Pisiform bone Hamate bone 5th metacarpal, base	Flexion of wrist Ulnar deviation (adduction) of wrist Flexion of elbow (assist)
Others				
156	Flexor digitorum superficialis	See Table 5.20		
157	Flexor digitorum profundus	See Table 5.20		
169	Flexor pollicis longus	See Table 5.24		

(Flexor carpi radialis and Flexor carpi ulnaris)

Grade 5 and Grade 4

Position of Patient (All Tests): Short sitting. Forearm is supinated (Fig. 5.140). Wrist is in neutral position or slightly extended.

Test: Patient flexes the wrist, keeping the digits and thumb relaxed.

Instructions to Clinician: Sit or stand in front of the patient and ask the patient to bend the wrist (Grade 3). If sufficient range is present, proceed to test strength by placing the hand in the test position. One hand supports the patient's forearm under the wrist (see Fig. 5.140), while the other hand applies resistance over the volar (palmar) surface of the hand (Fig. 5.141).

To Test Both Wrist Flexors: Apply resistance to the palm of the test hand using four fingers or hypothenar eminence (see Fig. 5.141). Resistance is given evenly across the hand in a straight-down direction into wrist extension.

To Test the Flexor Carpi Radialis: Place the patient's wrist in radial deviation and slight wrist extension. Resistance is applied with the index and long fingers over the first and second metacarpal (radial side of the hand) in the direction of extension and ulnar deviation (Fig. 5.142).

To Test the Flexor Carpi Ulnaris: Place the wrist in ulnar deviation and slight wrist extension. Resistance is applied over the fifth metacarpal (ulnar side of the hand) in the direction of extension and radial deviation (Fig. 5.143).

Instructions to Patient (All Tests): "Hold it. Don't let me pull it down. Keep your fingers relaxed."

Grading

Grade 5: Holds test position of wrist flexion against maximal resistance.

Grade 4: Holds test position of wrist flexion against strong to moderate resistance.

FIGURE 5.140

FIGURE 5.142

FIGURE 5.141

FIGURE 5.143

(Flexor carpi radialis and Flexor carpi ulnaris)

Grade 3:

Both Wrist Flexors: Patient flexes the wrist through full range without resistance and without radial or ulnar deviation.

Flexor Carpi Radialis: Patient flexes the wrist in radial deviation through full range without resistance. This is a small movement as compared with ulnar deviation described later (Fig. 5.144).

The illustration is shown from the extensor surface to better illustrate the small movement.

Flexor Carpi Ulnaris: Patient flexes the wrist in ulnar deviation through full range without resistance (Fig. 5.145).

FIGURE 5.144

FIGURE 5.145

Grade 2

Position of the Patient: Sitting with elbow supported on table. Forearm in mid position with hand resting on ulnar side (Fig. 5.146).

Instructions to Clinician: Support patient's forearm proximal to the wrist.

Test: Patient flexes wrist with the ulnar surface gliding across or not touching the table (see Fig. 5.146, end position). To test the two wrist flexors separately, hold the forearm so that the wrist does not lie on the table and ask the patient to perform the flexion motion while the wrist is in ulnar and then radial deviation.

Instructions to Patient: "Bend your wrist, keeping your fingers relaxed."

Grading

Grade 2: Completes available range of wrist flexion with gravity minimized.

FIGURE 5.146

(Flexor carpi radialis and Flexor carpi ulnaris)

Grade 1 and Grade 0

Position of the Patient: Supinated forearm supported on table.

Instructions to Clinician: Support the wrist in flexion; the index finger of the other hand is used to palpate the appropriate tendons.

Palpate the tendons of the flexor carpi radialis (Fig. 5.147) and the flexor carpi ulnaris (Fig. 5.148) in separate tests.

The flexor carpi radialis lies on the lateral palmar aspect of the wrist lateral to the palmaris longus.

The tendon of the flexor carpi ulnaris (see Fig. 5.147) lies on the medial palmar aspect of the wrist (at the base of the fifth metacarpal).

Test: Patient attempts to flex the wrist.

Instructions to Patient: "Try to bend your wrist. Relax. Bend it again." Patient should be asked to repeat the test so the clinician can feel the tendons during both relaxation and contraction.

Grading

Grade 1: One or both tendons may exhibit visible or palpable contractile activity, but the part does not move.

Grade 0: No discernable palpable contractile activity.

FIGURE 5.147

FIGURE 5.148

Clinical Relevance

Flexor carpi ulnaris contributes to adduction (ulnar deviation) most strongly in the supinated position as compared with the pronated and neutral positions.[49]

Suggested Exercises

• Wrist curls with resistance

(Extensor carpi radialis longus, Extensor carpi radialis brevis, and Extensor carpi ulnaris)

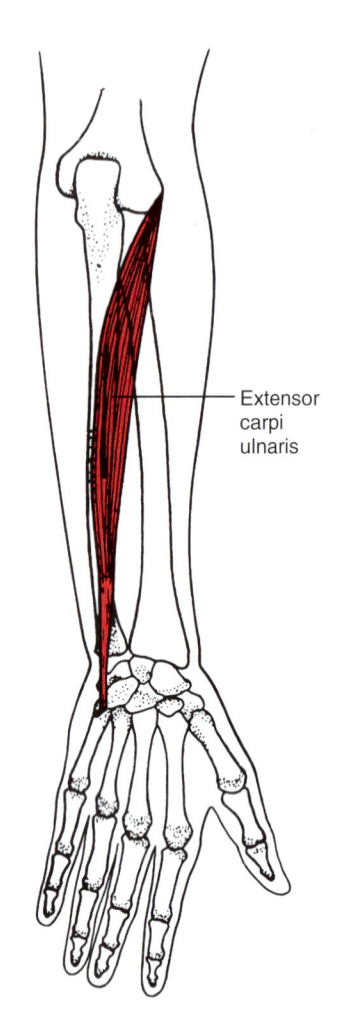

Extensor
carpi
ulnaris

FIGURE 5.149

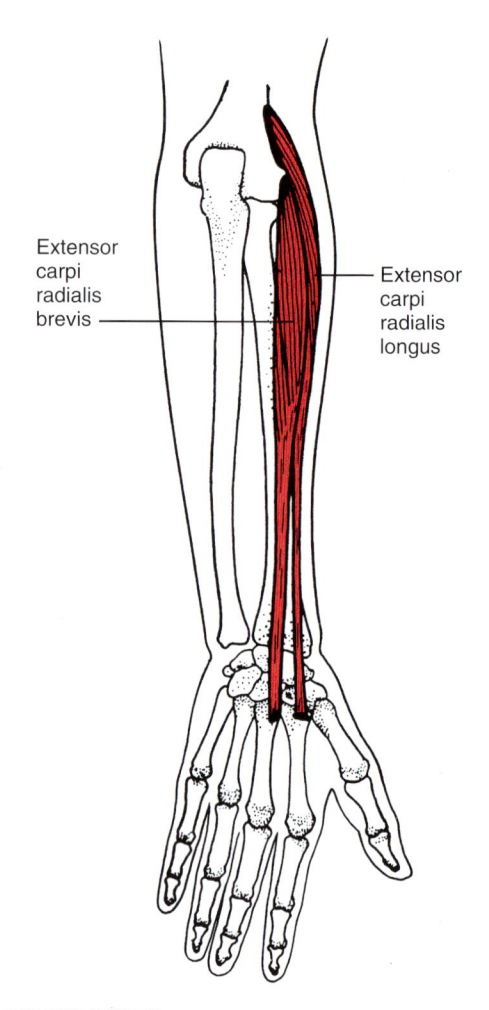

Extensor
carpi
radialis
brevis

Extensor
carpi
radialis
longus

DORSAL VIEWS

FIGURE 5.150

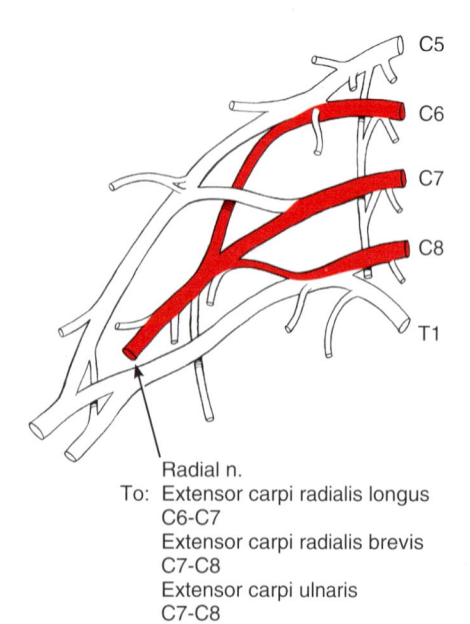

C5
C6
C7
C8
T1

Radial n.
To: Extensor carpi radialis longus
C6-C7
Extensor carpi radialis brevis
C7-C8
Extensor carpi ulnaris
C7-C8

FIGURE 5.151

Radius

Extensor carpi
radialis longus

Extensor carpi
radialis brevis

Radial
nerve

Ulna

Extensor
carpi
ulnaris

FIGURE 5.152 Arrow indicates level of cross section.

(Extensor carpi radialis longus, Extensor carpi radialis brevis, and Extensor carpi ulnaris)

Range of Motion

0°–70°

Table 5.19 WRIST EXTENSION

I.D.	Muscle	Origin	Insertion	Function
148	**Extensor carpi radialis longus**	Humerus (lateral supracondylar ridge, distal one-third) Common forearm extensor tendon Lateral intermuscular septum	2nd metacarpal bone (base on radial side of dorsal aspect)	Extension and radial deviation of wrist Synergist for finger flexion by stabilization of wrist Elbow flexion (accessory)
149	Extensor carpi radialis brevis	Humerus (lateral epicondyle via common forearm extensor tendon) Radial collateral ligament of elbow joint Aponeurosis of muscle	3rd metacarpal bone (base of dorsal surface on radial side) 2nd metacarpal (occasionally)	Extension of wrist Radial deviation of wrist (weak) Finger flexion synergist (by stabilizing the wrist)
150	Extensor carpi ulnaris	Humerus (lateral epicondyle via common extensor tendon) Ulna (posterior border by an aponeurosis)	5th metacarpal bone (tubercle on medial side of base)	Extension of wrist Ulnar deviation (adduction) of wrist
Others				
154	Extensor digitorum	See Table 5.20		
158	Extensor digiti minimi	See Table 5.20		
155	Extensor indicis	See Table 5.20		

The ability to extend the wrist is an essential function for most hand activity. A minimum of 25° of wrist extension is necessary for optimal grip strength.[50] Most activities of daily living (ADLs) (personal care, hygiene, writing, food preparation, etc.) require 40° of wrist extension.[51]

The radial wrist extensors are considerably stronger than the ulnar wrist extensor. The extensor carpi radialis brevis' muscle belly is 5× larger than the extensor carpi radialis longus.[52] Wrist extensor strength of the dominant side is approximately 10% stronger than the nondominant side, but only for right-handed persons.[53] Left-handed persons do not demonstrate a statistically different difference in grip strength.[54] There is a strong correlation between grip strength and wrist extension strength. Lateral epicondylitis (tennis elbow) most often affects the extensor carpi radialis brevis at its insertion on the lateral epicondyle, resulting in painful wrist extension.

Grade 5, Grade 4, and Grade 3

Position of the Patient: Short sitting. Elbow is flexed, forearm is fully pronated, and forearm is supported on the table.

Instructions to Clinician: Sit or stand at a diagonal in front of patient. Ask the patient to lift hand (Grade 3). If sufficient range is available, proceed to apply resistance by placing the patient's hand in the test position of full extension (Fig. 5.153). The hand used for resistance is placed over the dorsal (extensor) surface of the metacarpals.

To test all three muscles, the patient extends the wrist without deviation. Resistance is given with four fingers or

FIGURE 5.153

(Extensor carpi radialis longus, Extensor carpi radialis brevis, and Extensor carpi ulnaris)

Grade 5, Grade 4, and Grade 3 Continued

hypothenar eminence in a forward and downward direction over the second to fifth metacarpals for Grades 4 and 5 (Fig. 5.154).

To test the extensor carpi radialis longus and brevis (extension with radial deviation), position wrist in extension and radial deviation. Resistance is given on the dorsal (extensor) surface of the second and third metacarpals (radial side of hand) in the direction of flexion and ulnar deviation (Fig. 5.155).

To test the extensor carpi ulnaris (extension and ulnar deviation), position wrist in extension and ulnar deviation. Patient extends (lifts) the wrist, leading with the ulnar side of the hand. Resistance is given on the dorsal (extensor) surface of the fifth metacarpal (ulnar side of hand) in the direction of flexion and radial deviation (Fig. 5.156).

Test: For the combined test of the three wrist extensor muscles, the patient extends the wrist (lifts the hand) through the full available range. Do not permit extension of the fingers.

To test the two radial extensors, the patient extends the wrist, leading with the thumb side of the hand. The wrist may be prepositioned in some extension and radial deviation to direct the patient's motion.

To test the extensor carpi ulnaris, the patient extends the wrist, leading with the ulnar side of the hand. The clinician may preposition the wrist to direct the movement toward the ulna.

Instructions to Patient: "Hold it. Don't let me push it down."

For Grade 3: "Bring your hand up." (Add "to the side" when testing for radial or ulnar deviation.)

Grading

Grade 5: Holds test position against maximal resistance. Full extension is not required for the tests of radial and ulnar deviation.

Grade 4: Holds test position of wrist extension against strong to moderate resistance when all muscles are being tested. When testing the individual muscles, full wrist extension range of motion will not be achieved.

Grade 3: Completes full range of motion without resistance in the test for all three muscles. In the separate tests for the radial and ulnar extensors, the deviation required precludes full range of motion.

FIGURE 5.155

FIGURE 5.154

FIGURE 5.156

(Extensor carpi radialis longus, Extensor carpi radialis brevis, and Extensor carpi ulnaris)

Grade 2

Position of the Patient: Forearm supported on table in neutral position.

Instructions to Clinician: Support the patient's wrist. This elevates the hand from the table and removes friction (Fig. 5.157).

Test: Patient extends the wrist.

Instructions to Patient: "Bend your hand back."

Grading

Grade 2: Completes full range with gravity minimized.

FIGURE 5.157

WRIST EXTENSION

(Extensor carpi radialis longus, Extensor carpi radialis brevis, and Extensor carpi ulnaris)

Grade 1 and Grade 0

Position of the Patient: Hand and forearm supported on table with forearm fully pronated.

Instructions to Clinician: Support the patient's wrist in extension. The other hand is used for palpation. Use one finger to palpate one muscle in each test.

Extensor Carpi Radialis Longus: Palpate the tendon on the dorsum of the wrist in line with the second metacarpal (Fig. 5.158).

Extensor Carpi Radialis Brevis: Palpate the tendon on the dorsal surface of the wrist in line with the third metacarpal bone (Fig. 5.159).

Extensor Carpi Ulnaris: Palpate the tendon on the dorsal wrist surface proximal to the fifth metacarpal and just distal to the ulnar styloid process (Fig. 5.160).

Test: Patient attempts to extend the wrist.

Instructions to Patient: "Try to lift your hand."

Grading

Grade 1: For any given muscle, there is visible or palpable contractile activity, but no wrist motion ensues.

Grade 0: No discernable contractile activity.

Substitution

The most common substitution occurs when the finger extensors are allowed to participate. This can be avoided to a large extent by ensuring that the patient's fingers are relaxed and are not permitted to extend.

FIGURE 5.158

FIGURE 5.160

FIGURE 5.159

(Extensor carpi radialis longus, Extensor carpi radialis brevis, and Extensor carpi ulnaris)

Clinical Relevance

- Preferred position of the wrist when gripping is 35° of extension and 7° of ulnar deviation, where grip strength is the strongest. A minimum of 25° of wrist extension is necessary for optimal grip strength.[50]
- A patient with complete quadriplegia at C5-C6 will have only the radial wrist extensors remaining. Radial deviation during extension is therefore the prevailing extensor motion at the wrist.

Suggested Exercises for Wrist Extensors

- Wrist curls in pronated position
- Gripping/squeezing a ball or putty
- Wrist radial and ulnar deviation

INTRODUCTION TO MUSCLE TESTING OF THE HAND

(Extensor carpi radialis longus, Extensor carpi radialis brevis, and Extensor carpi ulnaris)

Evaluating the hand following a nerve injury is the primary reason single muscles or movements are tested. Because of the innervation pattern of the hand, grading of movements may be more appropriate than grading specific muscles. Because the hand muscles have multiple functions and can be active in combined movements, the clinician should incorporate knowledge of function, anatomy, and kinesiology to master strength testing of the hand. For example, the only muscles of the hand that can be purely isolated are the first dorsal interosseous (radial abduction of the index finger) and the flexor pollicis longus (flexion of the thumb interphalangeal [IP] joint).[55] Alternatively, grip strength is considered a gross, functional measure of hand strength. Asking the patient to make a fist and straighten out the fingers will provide a general idea of active range of motion of the digits and help to provide focus of the muscular exam.

When evaluating the muscles of the hand, care must be taken to use graduated and appropriate resistance, especially following surgical intervention. Because of the small muscle mass of the hand muscles, the clinician should only use one or two fingers to resist hand motions.

Clinical judgment is required when applying appropriate resistance in a safe fashion, especially in the surgically repaired hand. In the surgically repaired hand, the clinician may only want to assure the presence of a muscle contraction, as certain movements may be prohibited by the surgeon. Similarly, the amount of motion allowed or encouraged should be monitored in conjunction with the surgeon. Too much force or force too quickly applied may be harmful to the surgical repair or reconstruction. The clinician should have a thorough understanding of the type of surgery and any contraindications to movement before muscle testing the surgically repaired hand. Considerable practice in testing normal hands and comparing injured hands with their normal contralateral sides should provide some of the necessary judgment with which to approach the surgically repaired hand.

It is difficult to differentiate between Grades 5 and 4 in many of the small muscles of the hand, and differentiating between Grades 5 and 4 may not be clinically relevant. Therefore, Grades 5 and 4 have been combined for some muscles. It takes experience and skill to discern weakness in the actively contracting hand muscle. This text remains true to the principles of testing in the ranges of grades 5, 4, and 3 with respect to gravity. It is admitted, however, that the influence of gravity on the fingers is inconsequential, so gravity and antigravity positions are not considered in valid muscle tests of the hand.

Two common groupings of the hand muscles are the intrinsics, innervated mostly by the median and ulnar nerve, and the extrinsics, innervated primarily by the radial and median nerves. The extrinsics originate in the forearm and the intrinsics originate distal to the wrist. In general, each finger has six muscles controlling its movements, three extrinsic muscles (two long flexors and one long extensor) and three intrinsic muscles (dorsal and palmar interosseous and lumbrical muscles). The little finger and index finger each have an additional extrinsic extensor.[56]

The hand section of this chapter is organized by extrinsics, intrinsics, and the thumb (combined extrinsic and intrinsics).

EXTRINSIC MUSCLES

The extrinsic muscles of the hand originate above the wrist on the forearm and are made up of flexors and extensors. The tendons of the extrinsics are held in place at the wrist by the palmar carpal ligament and flexor retinaculum. The extrinsics are innervated by the radial, ulnar, and median nerves.

(Flexor digitorum superficialis and Flexor digitorum profundus)

Flexor
digitorum
superficialis

FIGURE 5.161

Flexor
digitorum
profundus

PALMAR

FIGURE 5.162

Median n.
To: Flexor digitorum
superficialis
C8-T1
Flexor digitorum
profundus
fingers 2, 3
C8-T1

C5
C6
C7
C8
T1

Ulnar n.
To: Flexor digitorum profundus
fingers 4, 5
C8-T1

FIGURE 5.163

Median
nerve

Flexor
digitorum
superficialis

Ulnar
nerve

Radius

Ulna

Flexor
digitorum
profundus

FIGURE 5.164 Arrow indicates level of cross section.

FINGER PIP AND DIP FLEXION

(Flexor digitorum superficialis and Flexor digitorum profundus)

Range of Motion

PIP joints: 0°–100°

DIP joints: 0°–90°

Table 5.20 **PIP AND DIP FINGER FLEXION**

I.D.	Muscle	Origin	Insertion	Function
156	**Flexor digitorum superficialis (2 heads)**	Humeroulnar head: humerus (medial epicondyle via common flexor tendon)	Four tendons arranged in 2 pairs Superficial pair: middle and ring fingers (sides of middle phalanges)	Flexion of PIP joints of digits 2–5 Flexion of MCP joints of digits 2–5 (assist) Flexion of wrist (accessory, especially in forceful grasp)
		Ulna (medial collateral ligament of elbow joint); coronoid process (medial side) Intermuscular septum *Radial head*: radius (oblique line on anterior shaft)	Deep pair: index and little fingers (sides of middle phalanges)	
157	**Flexor digitorum profundus**	Ulna (proximal three-quarters of anterior and medial shaft; medial coronoid process) Interosseous membrane (ulnar)	Four tendons to digits 2–5 (distal phalanges, at base of palmar surface)	Flexion of DIP joints of digits 2–5 Flexion of MCP and PIP joints of digits 2–5 (assist) Flexion of wrist (accessory)

DIP, Distal interphalangeal, *MCP*, metacarpophalangeal; *PIP*, proximal phalanges.

(Flexor digitorum superficialis and Flexor digitorum profundus)

The flexor digitorum superficialis (FDS) is innervated by the median nerve, while the flexor digitorum profundus (FDP) is innervated by the median and ulnar nerve. The FDP has two heads, flexing the middle and ring fingers together and the index and little fingers. If a tendon injury or nerve injury is the reason for testing, each digit should be tested separately. Otherwise, all digits can be tested together to assess the integrity and strength of the finger flexors.

COMBINED DIP AND PIP TESTS

Grade 5, Grade 4, and Grade 3

Position of the Patient: Forearm supinated, wrist in neutral. Fingers are relaxed.

Instructions to Clinician: Sit in front of the patient, with patient's forearm and hand supported on a table with wrist fully supinated. Ask patient to touch the pads of the fingers to the distal palm while keeping the metacarpals extended (flat on the table) (Fig. 5.165).

If sufficient range is present, proceed to apply resistance. Stabilization is provided by the hand position. With a finger of the hand providing resistance in the patient's palm under the digits, pull up to try to straighten the digits (Fig. 5.166).

Grading

Grade 5 and Grade 4: Holds against strong resistance.

Grade 3: Completes range of motion without resistance.

Grade 2, Grade 1, and Grade 0: Refer to isolated proximal interphalangeal (PIP) and distal interphalangeal (DIP) tests.

FIGURE 5.165

FIGURE 5.166

(Flexor digitorum superficialis)

Grade 5, Grade 4, and Grade 3

Position of the Patient: Forearm supinated, wrist in neutral. Finger to be tested is in slight flexion at the metacarpophalangeal (MCP) joint (Fig. 5.167).

Instructions to Clinician: Hold all fingers (except the one being tested) in extension at all joints (see Fig. 5.167) so as to block the action of the profundus action. Isolation of the index finger may not be complete. Ask the patient to bend the middle joint towards the proximal palm. If full range is present (Grade 3), apply appropriate resistance. Clinician resists the distal end of the middle phalanx of the test finger in the direction of extension (Fig. 5.168).

Test: Patient flexes the PIP joint without flexing the DIP joint. Do not allow motion of any joints of the other fingers. Repeat for other fingers, if indicated. Alternatively, you can test all fingers together (see Fig. 5.166, combined test above).

Flick the terminal end of the finger being tested with the thumb to make certain that the FDP is not active; that is, the DIP joint goes into extension. The distal phalanx should be relatively floppy.

Instructions to Patient: "Bend your index (then long, ring, and little) finger at the middle joint; hold it. Don't let me straighten it. Keep your other fingers relaxed."

Grading

Grade 5 and Grade 4: Holds against strong finger resistance.

Grade 3: Completes range of motion without resistance (see Fig. 5.167).

FIGURE 5.167

FIGURE 5.168

Grade 2, Grade 1, and Grade 0

Position of the Patient: Forearm is in midposition to eliminate the influence of gravity on finger flexion.

Instructions to Clinician: Same as for Grades 5, 4, and 3.
Palpate the FDS on the palmar surface of the wrist between the palmaris longus and the flexor carpi ulnaris (Fig. 5.169).

Test: Patient flexes the PIP joint.

Instructions to Patient: "Bend your middle finger." (Select other fingers individually.)

Grading

Grade 2: Completes range of motion.

Grade 1: Palpable or visible contractile activity, which may or may not be accompanied by a flicker of motion.

Grade 0: No discernable palpable contractile activity.

FIGURE 5.169

Substitutions

- The major substitution for this motion is offered by the flexor digitorum profundus, and this will occur if the DIP joint is allowed to flex.
- If the wrist is allowed to extend, tension increases in the long finger flexors, and may result in passive flexion of the IP joints. This is referred to as a "tenodesis" action.
- Relaxation of IP extension will result in passive IP flexion.

Clinical Relevance

Many people cannot isolate the little finger. When this is the case, test the little and ring fingers at the same time.

(Flexor digitorum profundus)

Grade 5, Grade 4, and Grade 3

Position of the Patient: Forearm in supination, wrist in neutral, and proximal PIP joint in extension.

Instructions to Clinician: Stabilize the middle phalanx in extension by grasping it on either side (Fig. 5.170). Ask the patient to bend the tip of the finger. If full range is present (Grade 3), apply appropriate resistance. Resistance is provided on the distal phalanx in the direction of extension (not illustrated).

Test: Test each finger individually if indicated. Patient flexes distal phalanx of each finger. Test all digits together by patient flexing all distal phalanxes together.

Instructions to Patient: "Bend the tip (or tips) of your finger. Hold it (them). Don't let me straighten it (them)."

Grading

Grade 5 and Grade 4: Able to hold flexed position against strong finger resistance.

Grade 3: Completes active range without resistance (see Fig. 5.170).

Grade 2, Grade 1, and Grade 0

Testing grades 2, 1, and 0 is the same as that used with higher grades except that the position of the forearm is in neutral to eliminate the influence of gravity.

Grades are assigned as for the PIP tests.

The tendon of the flexor digitorum profundus can be palpated on the palmar surface of the middle phalanx of each finger.

FIGURE 5.170

Substitutions

- The wrist must be kept in a neutral position and must not be allowed to extend to rule out the tenodesis effect of the wrist extensors.
- Don't be fooled if the patient extends the distal phalanges and then relaxes, which can give the impression of active finger flexion.
- In a power grip task, greater forces are applied on the distal phalanges of the long fingers compared with the middle and proximal ones, making the flexor digitorum profundus an important muscle to strengthen.[57]

(Extensor digitorum, Extensor indicis, and Extensor digiti minimi)

Extensor digitorum

FIGURE 5.171

Extensor digiti minimi

Extensor indicis

DORSAL

FIGURE 5.172

Radial nerve

Radius

Ulna

Extensor digitorum

Extensor indicis

Extensor digiti minimi

FIGURE 5.174 Arrow indicates level of cross section.

C5

C6

C7

C8

T1

Radial n.
To: Extensor digitorum
C7-C8
Extensor digiti minimi
C7-C8
Extensor indicis
C7-C8

FIGURE 5.173

FINGER MCP EXTENSION

(Extensor digitorum, Extensor indicis, and Extensor digiti minimi)

Range of Motion
0°–45°

Table 5.21 **MCP FINGER EXTENSION**

I.D.	Muscle	Origin	Insertion	Function
154	**Extensor digitorum**	Humerus (lateral epicondyle via common extensor tendon) Intermuscular septum Antebrachial fascia	Via four tendons to digits 2–5 (via the extensor expansion, to dorsum of middle and distal phalanges; one tendon to each finger)	Extension of MCP, PIP, and DIP joints, digits 2–5 Extensor digitorum can extend any and all joints over which it passes via the dorsal expansion Independent action of the extensor digitorum: Hyperextends MCP joint (proximal phalanges) by displacing dorsal expansion proximally Extends IP joints (middle and distal phalanges) when MCP joints are slightly flexed by intrinsics Wrist extension (accessory) Abduction of ring, index, and little fingers with extension but no such action on the middle finger
155	Extensor indicis	Ulna (posterior surface of shaft) Interosseous membrane	2nd digit (via tendon of extensor digitorum into extensor hood)	Extension of MCP joint of index finger Extension of IP joints (with intrinsics) Adduction of index finger (accessory) Wrist extension (accessory)
158	Extensor digiti minimi	Humerus (lateral epicondyle via common extensor tendon) Intermuscular septa	5th digit (extensor hood)	Extension of MCP, IP, and DIP joints of digit 5 (little finger) Wrist extension (accessory) Abduction of digit 5 (accessory)

DIP, Distal interphalangeal; *MCP*, metacarpophalangeal; *PIP*, proximal interphalangeal.

(Extensor digitorum, Extensor indicis, and Extensor digiti minimi)

Grade 5, Grade 4, and Grade 3

Position of the Patient: Forearm in pronation, wrist in neutral. MCP and IP joints are in relaxed flexion posture.

Instructions to Clinician: Sit at table or side of patient. Stabilize the wrist in neutral. Place the index finger of the resistance hand across the dorsum of all proximal phalanges just distal to the MCP joints to stabilize. Ask the patient to straighten the knuckles as far as possible. Demonstrate motion to patient and instruct to copy. If full range is present (Grade 3), apply appropriate resistance. Give resistance in the direction of flexion.

Test:

Extensor Digitorum: Patient extends MCP joints (all fingers simultaneously), allowing the IP joints to be in slight flexion (Fig. 5.175).

Extensor Indicis: Patient extends the MCP joint of the index finger.

Extensor Digiti Minimi: Patient extends the MCP joint of the 5th digit.

Instructions to Patient: "Straighten (lift) your knuckles as far as they will go."

FIGURE 5.175

Grading

Grade 5 and Grade 4: Able to hold position with appropriate level of resistance. (Extensor is not as strong as the flexor.)

Grade 3: Completes active range without resistance.

Grade 2, Grade 1, and Grade 0

Procedures: Test is the same as that for Grades 5, 4, and 3 except that the forearm is in the midposition.

The four tendons of the extensor digitorum, the tendon of the extensor indicis, and the tendon of the extensor digiti minimi are readily apparent on the dorsum of the hand, as they course in the direction of each finger.

Grading

Grade 2: Completes range.

Grade 1: Visible tendon activity but no joint motion.

Grade 0: No discernable palpable contractile activity.

Substitution

Flexion of the wrist will produce interphalangeal extension through a tenodesis action.

Clinical Relevance

- Metacarpophalangeal extension of the fingers is not a strong motion, and only slight resistance is required to "break" the end position.
- It is usual for the active range of motion to be considerably less than the available passive range. In this test, therefore, the "full available range" is not used, and the active range is accepted.
- Another way to check whether there is functional extensor strength in the fingers is to "flick" the proximal phalanx of each finger downward; if the finger rebounds, it is functional.

(Interossei and Lumbricals)

INTRINSIC MUSCLES

The intrinsic muscles are traditionally divided into five groups: thenar, hypothenar, palmar interossei, dorsal interossei, and lumbricals (Table 5.22). The primary function of the interossei is MCP flexion/stabilization with extension of the IP joints. This motion is assisted by the lumbricals, which can contract without adding flexion torque at the MCP joint.[56] Although efficient, the lumbricals are weak, with the smallest physiological cross-sectional area of all the intrinsic hand muscles. Without the interossei, the fingers are unstable and will collapse into the "claw" (i.e., intrinsic minus) position of hyperextension of the MCP joint and flexion of the IP joints when loaded.[56] The Mannerfelt sign is a sign of interosseous muscle weakness when the index PIP joint "collapses," resulting in hyperflexion, often greater than 90°. Another sign of weakness is the Thomas sign, when wrist flexion occurs to try to open the hand by means of increasing the pull on the extensor digitorum.[56]

The inability to adduct and abduct the fingers occurs with the loss of the interossei muscles. These actions are quite important to people who play musical instruments or operate keyboards, but for most people, this does not result in a severe deficit.[56]

Table 5.22 **GROUPS OF INTRINSIC HAND MUSCLES**

Groups	Function	Muscles
Thenar	Thumb is brought lateral to medial position across the palm in opposition to the 4 ulnar digits	Abductor pollicis brevis Flexor pollicis brevis Opponens pollicis
Hypothenar	Little finger is brought in opposition to the thumb	Opponens digiti minimi Adductor pollicis
Palmar interossei (3)	Adduct the 4 ulnar digits together toward the 3rd finger First palmar interossei: tip pinch	
Dorsal interossei	First dorsal interossei: key pinch[56] Flex the MCP joints and extend the IP joints; abducts the 4 ulnar digits away from the 3rd finger	Four interossei Abductor digiti minimi
Lumbricals	Extension of the IP joints in any position of the MCP joints	Two radial lumbricals Two ulnar lumbricals

IP, Interphalangeal; *MCP*, metacarpophalangeal.

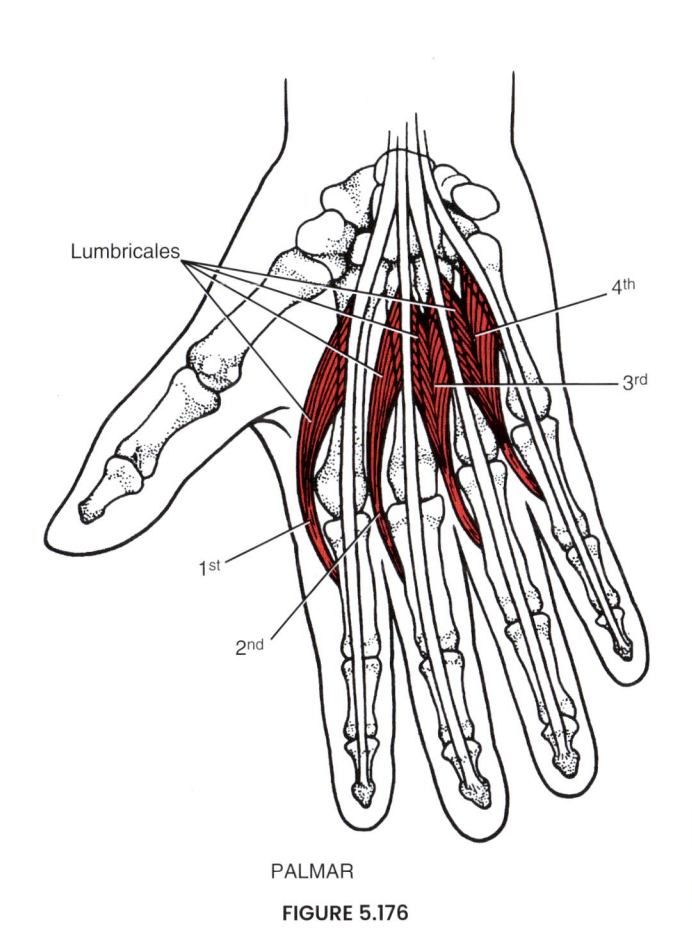

Lumbricales

4th

3rd

1st

2nd

PALMAR

FIGURE 5.176

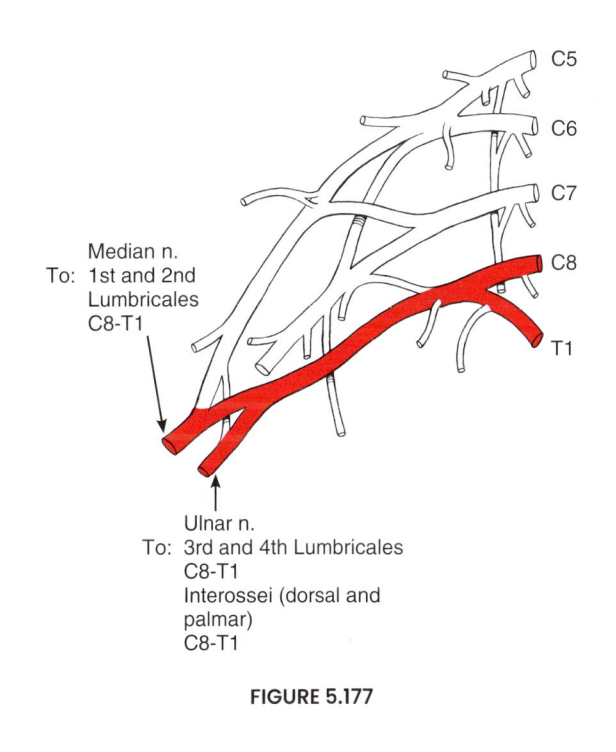

C5

C6

C7

C8

T1

Median n.
To: 1st and 2nd
Lumbricales
C8-T1

Ulnar n.
To: 3rd and 4th Lumbricales
C8-T1
Interossei (dorsal and
palmar)
C8-T1

FIGURE 5.177

Range of Motion
MCP joints: 0°–90°

(Interossei and Lumbricals)

Table 5.23 MCP FLEXION AND ABDUCTION AND ADDUCTION OF THE FINGERS

I.D.	Muscle	Origin	Insertion	Function
164	Dorsal interossei (four bipennate muscles) 1st dorsal interosseus (often named *abductor indicis*)	Metacarpal bones (each muscle arises by two heads from adjacent sides of metacarpals between which each lies)	All: dorsal expansion Proximal phalanges (bases)	Abduction of fingers away from an axis drawn through the center of the long (middle) finger Flexion of fingers at MCP joints (assist) Extension of fingers at IP joints (assist) Thumb adduction (assist)
		1st dorsal: between thumb and index finger	1st dorsal: index finger (radial side)	
		2nd dorsal: between index and long finger	2nd dorsal: long finger (radial side)	
		3rd dorsal: between long and ring fingers	3rd dorsal: long finger (ulnar side)	
		4th dorsal: between ring and little fingers	4th dorsal: ring finger (ulnar side)	
165	Palmar interossei three muscles (a 4th muscle often is described)	Metacarpal bones 2, 4, and 5 (muscles lie on palmar surfaces of metacarpals rather than between them) No palmar interosseous on long finger All muscles lie on aspect of metacarpal facing the long finger	All: Dorsal expansion Proximal phalanges	Adduction of fingers (index, ring, and little) toward an axis drawn through the center of the long finger Flexion of MCP joints (assist) Extension of IP joints (assist) Opposition of digit 5 (3rd interosseous)
		1st palmar: 2nd metacarpal (ulnar side)	1st palmar: index finger (ulnar side)	
		2nd palmar: 4th metacarpal (radial side)	2nd palmar: ring finger (radial side)	
		3rd palmar: 5th metacarpal (radial side)	3rd palmar: little finger (radial side)	
159	Abductor digiti minimi	Pisiform bone Tendon of flexor carpi ulnaris Pisohamate ligament	5th digit (base of proximal phalanx, ulnar side) Dorsal expansion of extensor digiti minimi	Abduction of 5th digit away from ring finger Flexion of proximal phalanx of 5th digit at the MCP joint Opposition of 5th digit (assist)
163	Lumbricals (4 in number)	Tendons of flexor digitorum profundus:	Extensor digitorum expansion Each muscle runs distally to the *radial* side of its corresponding digit, attaches to the dorsal digital expansion	Flexion of MCP joints (proximal phalanges) of digits 2–5 and simultaneous extension of the PIP and DIP joints

Continued

Table 5.23 MCP FLEXION AND ABDUCTION AND ADDUCTION OF THE FINGERS—cont'd

I.D.	Muscle	Origin	Insertion	Function
	1st lumbrical	Index finger (radial side, palmar surface)	1st lumbrical to index finger	
	2nd lumbrical	Middle finger (radial side, palmar surface)	2nd lumbrical to long finger	
	3rd lumbrical	Middle and ring fingers (double heads from adjacent sides of tendons)	3rd lumbrical to ring finger	
	4th lumbrical	Ring and little fingers (adjacent sides of tendons)	4th lumbrical to little finger	Opposition of digit 5 (4th lumbrical) Flexion of MCP joints (proximal phalanges) of digits 2–5 and simultaneous extension of the PIP and DIP joints
Others				
156	Flexor digitorum superficialis	See Table 5.20		
157	Flexor digitorum profundus	See Table 5.20		
160	Flexor digiti minimi brevis			
161	Opponens digiti minimi			
154	Extensor digitorum (no action on long finger)	See Table 5.21		
158	Extensor digiti minimi (little finger)	See Table 5.21		

DIP, Distal phalanges; *IP*, interphalangeal; *MCP*, metacarpophalangeal; *PIP*, proximal phalanges.

The lumbricals are the smallest muscles of all the intrinsic hand muscles and thus are weak compared with the interossei muscles. It is impossible to separate the interossei from the lumbricals because of their synergistic action through the extensor hood mechanism.[56] The lumbricals have a rich composition of muscle spindles, making them important for sensory input and in fast, alternating movements, for example, in typing and playing musical instruments.[56]

The test for the interossei and lumbricals is often called the lumbrical test, but it is the interossei that are being graded for their strength in stabilizing the MCP joints in flexion and therefore is more accurately referred to as the intrinsic plus test (or rooftop)[55] (Fig. 5.178). This position demands the interosseous muscles (and to some extent, the lumbricals) to move adjacent joints in opposite directions, creating a competition between movement at the MCP and IP joints.

FIGURE 5.178

FINGER MCP FLEXION

(Interossei and Lumbricals)

Grade 5, Grade 4, and Grade 3

Position of the Patient: Short sitting or elbow flexed and resting on table with hand pointed up. Forearm in neutral. Hand relaxed.

Instructions to Clinician: Sit in front or to the side of the patient. Demonstrate the intrinsic plus position (see Fig. 5.178) to patient and insist on practice to get the motions performed correctly and simultaneously. While stabilizing the metacarpals (dorsum of hand on the table) to maintain flexion of the MCP joints, ask the patient to lift the fingers so that IP joints are straight. This action tests the lumbricals of each finger. If this position can be achieved (Grade 3), apply appropriate resistance over each digit, one finger at a time, distal to the PIP joint (pushing down) (Fig. 5.179).

To test the MCP flexion part of the lumbrical function, the patient should be in the intrinsic plus position in a fully pronated position. Stabilize the metacarpals. Give resistance on the palmar PIP in the direction of extension (Fig. 5.180).

Test: Patient simultaneously flexes the MCP joints and extends the IP joints (intrinsic plus position). Fingers may be tested separately if indicated (see Fig. 5.179). Do not allow fingers to curl; they must remain extended.

Instructions to Patient: MCP joint portion: "Lift your fingers up. Hold them. Don't let me move your fingers."

IP portion: "Hold your fingers straight. Don't let me bend them."

Grading (Both Movements Are Graded Together)

Grade 5 and Grade 4: Patient holds position against strong resistance. Resistance can be given to fingers individually because of the variant strength of the different interossei and lumbricals and because the interossei and lumbricals have different innervations.

Grade 3: Patient completes both motions correctly and simultaneously without resistance.

FIGURE 5.179

FIGURE 5.180

Grade 2, Grade 1, and Grade 0

Position of the Patient: Forearm and wrist in mid position to remove influence of gravity. MCP joints are fully extended; all IP joints are flexed.

Instructions to Clinician: Stabilize metacarpals.

Test: Patient attempts to flex MCP joints through full available range while extending IP joints (Fig. 5.181).

Instructions to Patient: "Try to straighten your fingers while keeping your knuckles bent." Demonstrate motion to patient and allow practice.

FIGURE 5.181

Grading

Grade 2: Completes full range of motion in gravity-minimized position.

Grade 1: Except in the hand that is markedly atrophied, the palmar interossei and lumbricals cannot be palpated. A grade of 1 is given for minimal motion.

Grade 0: A grade of 0 is given in the absence of any discernable palpable contraction.

Substitution

The long finger flexors may substitute for the lumbricals. To avoid this pattern, make sure that the patient's interphalangeal joints fully extend.

Clinical Relevance

- In the normal hand, the metacarpophalangeal (MCP) and interphalangeal (IP) joints extend at the same time and also flex at the same time. When attempting to flex the MCP joints and extend the IP joints simultaneously, it is increasingly difficult to maintain full IP extension at or near end range of MCP joint flexion. The converse is also true: full MCP joint flexion is not possible if full IP joint extension is maintained.
- In most cases of early nerve palsy, weakness of the index and middle fingers is apparent when they are tested in the intrinsic plus position.[55]

(Dorsal interossei)

FIGURE 5.182

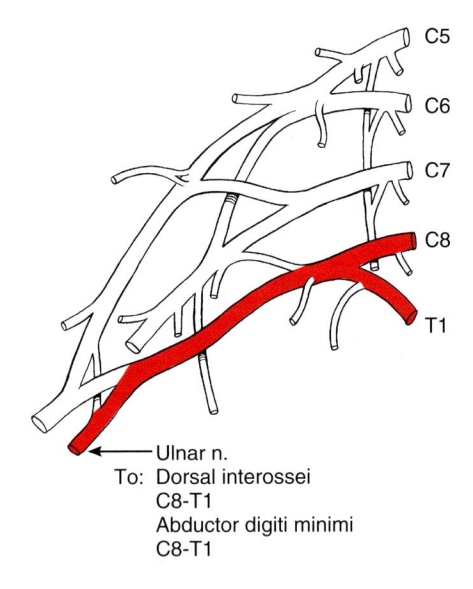

Ulnar n.
To: Dorsal interossei
C8-T1
Abductor digiti minimi
C8-T1

FIGURE 5.183

Range of Motion
0°–20°

Grade 5 and Grade 4

Position of the Patient: Forearm pronated, wrist in neutral. Fingers start in extension and adduction. MCP joints in neutral and avoid hyperextension.

Instructions to Clinician: Sit at table or side of patient. Support the wrist in neutral. Ask the patient to spread the fingers. If full range is present (Grade 3), apply appropriate resistance. The fingers of the other hand are used to give resistance on the distal phalanx, the radial side of the finger, and the ulnar side of the adjacent finger (i.e., they are squeezed together). The direction of resistance will cause any pair of fingers to approximate (Fig. 5.184).

Test: Abduction of fingers (individual tests):

Dorsal Interossei:
Abduction of ring finger toward little finger
Abduction of middle finger toward ring finger
Abduction of middle finger toward index finger
Abduction of index finger toward thumb

   The long (middle) finger (digit 3, finger 2) will move one way when tested with the index finger and the opposite way when tested with the ring finger (see Fig. 5.182, which shows a dorsal interosseous on either side). When

FIGURE 5.184

Grade 5 and Grade 4 Coninued

testing the little finger with the ring finger, the abductor digiti minimi is being tested along with the fourth dorsal interosseous.

Abductor Digiti Minimi: Patient abducts fifth digit away from ring finger.

Instructions to Patient: "Hold your fingers apart. Don't let me push them together."

Grading

Neither the dorsal interossei nor the abductor digiti minimi will tolerate much resistance.

Grade 5 and Grade 4: Patient holds test position against strong finger resistance. Fig. 5.185 illustrates the test for second and fourth dorsal interossei. Alternatively, provide resistance for a Grade 5 test by flicking each finger toward adduction; if the finger tested rebounds, the grade is 5.

Grade 3: Patient can abduct any given finger. Remember that the long finger has two dorsal interossei and therefore must be tested as it moves away from the midline in both directions (Fig. 5.186).

Grade 2, Grade 1, and Grade 0

Procedures and Grading: Same as for higher grades in this test. A Grade 2 should be assigned if the patient can complete only a partial range of abduction for any given finger. The only dorsal interosseous that is readily palpable is the first at the base of the proximal phalanx (Fig. 5.187).

The abductor digiti minimi is palpable on the ulnar border of the hand.

FIGURE 5.185

FIGURE 5.186

FIGURE 5.187

FINGER ADDUCTION

(Palmar interossei)

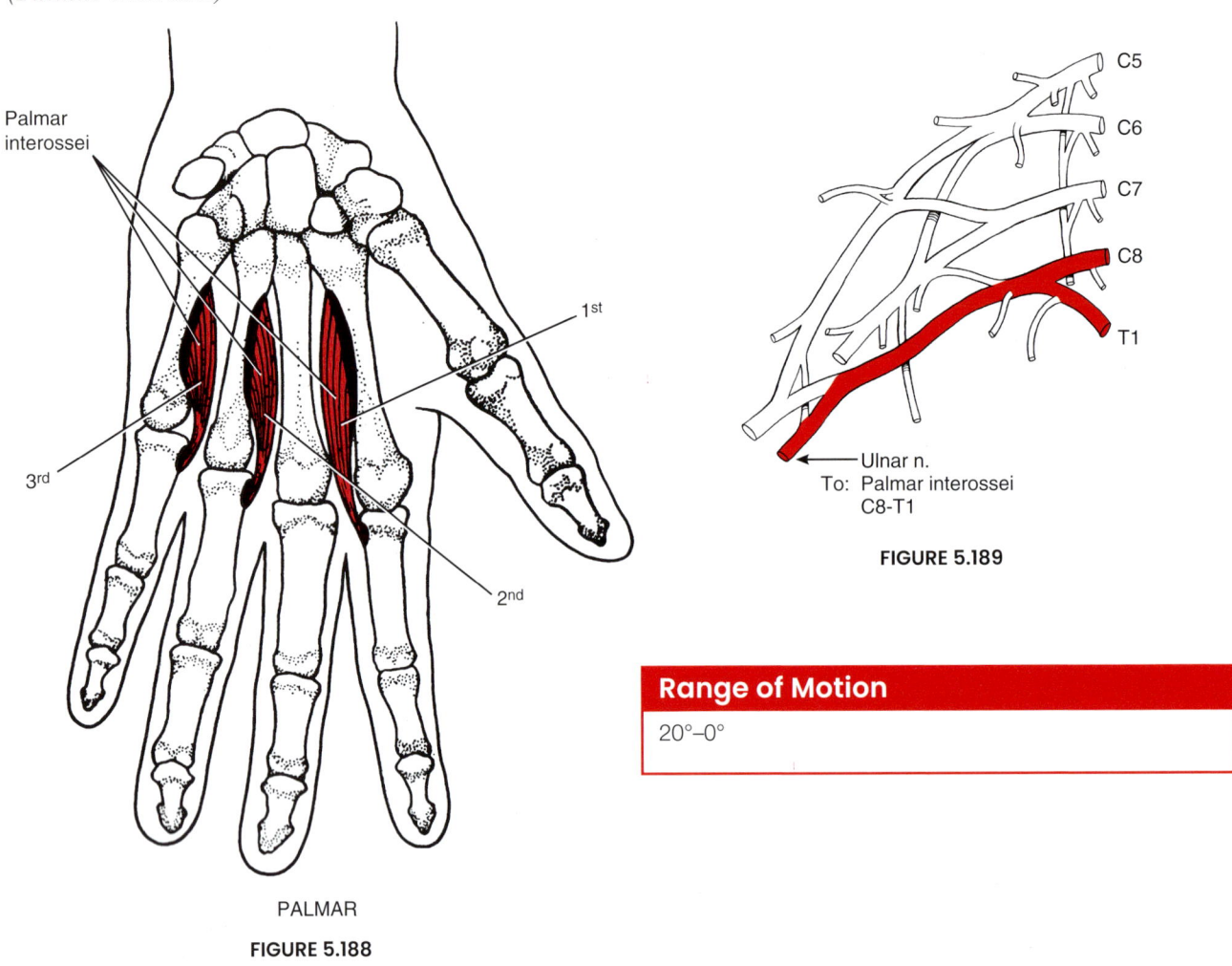

Palmar interossei

3rd

1st

2nd

C5
C6
C7
C8
T1

Ulnar n.
To: Palmar interossei
C8-T1

FIGURE 5.189

Range of Motion

20°–0°

PALMAR

FIGURE 5.188

Grade 5 and Grade 4

Position of the Patient: Forearm pronated (palm down), wrist in neutral, and fingers extended and adducted. MCP joints are neutral; avoid flexion.

Instructions to Clinician: Sit at table or to side of patient. Ask the patient to hold the fingers together. If the patient is able (Grade 3) and resistance is appropriate, grasp the middle phalanx on each of two adjoining fingers (Fig. 5.190) and try to pull the finger in the direction of abduction for each finger tested. The clinician is trying to "pull" the fingers apart. Each finger should be resisted separately.

Test: Adduction of fingers (individual tests):
Adduction of little finger toward ring finger
Adduction of ring finger toward long finger
Adduction of index finger toward long finger
Adduction of thumb toward index finger

Occasionally, there is a fourth palmar interosseous (not illustrated in Fig. 5.188) that some consider a separate muscle from the adductor pollicis. In any event, the two muscles cannot be clinically separated.

Because the middle finger (also called the long finger, digit 3, or finger 2) has no palmar interosseous, it is not tested in adduction.

FIGURE 5.190

(Palmar interossei)

Grade 5 and Grade 4 Coninued

Instructions to Patient: "Hold your fingers together. Don't let me spread them apart."

Grading

Grade 5 and Grade 4: Patient holds test position against strong finger resistance. Distinguishing between Grades 5 and 4 is difficult and, clinically, perhaps not important. The grade awarded will depend on the amount of the clinician's experience with normal hands.

Grade 3: Patient can adduct fingers toward middle finger (Fig. 5.191).

FIGURE 5.191

Grade 2, Grade 1, and Grade 0

Procedures: Same as for Grades 5, 4, and 3.

For Grade 2, the patient can adduct each of the fingers tested through a partial range of motion. The test for Grade 2 is begun with the fingers abducted.

Palpation of the palmar interossei is rarely feasible. By placing the clinician's finger against the side of a finger to be tested, the clinician may detect a slight outward motion for a muscle less than Grade 2.

Substitution

Caution must be used to ensure that finger flexion does not occur because the long finger flexors can contribute to adduction.

Clinical Relevance

- The fingers can be assessed quickly by grasping the distal phalanx and flicking the finger in the direction of abduction. If the finger rebounds or snaps back, that interosseous is functional.
- A quick test for ulnar nerve integrity is to place a piece of paper between each finger and instruct the patient to not let the clinician pull the paper out from between the fingers (Fig. 5.192).

FIGURE 5.192

(Palmar interossei)

THUMB MUSCLES

The thumb muscles are made up of three extrinsics and four intrinsics. Three of these muscles, the abductor pollicis brevis (APB), opponens pollicis (OP), and flexor pollicis brevis (FPB), form the fleshy mass at the radial border of the thumb. There are eight motions of the thumb (Plate 5), which are possible because of the medial and lateral rotation at its carpometacarpal (CMC) joint.[58] To fully understand the muscles of the thumb, the complex motions of the thumb must be understood. The thumb musculature dynamically allows for precision pinching and power gripping. Thumb stability is actively maintained by muscles rather than articular constraints.

The thenar intrinsics that medially rotate and oppose the thumb (APB, OP, and FPB) can be quickly assessed by asking the patient to touch the tip of the thumb to each of the pads of the fingers so that the thumb nail is parallel to the fingertips. It is important to palpate the thenar muscles to note an active contraction.

It is difficult to differentiate between Grade 5 and 4 in many of the small muscles of the hand and may not be clinically relevant. Therefore, Grades 5 and 4 have been combined for some muscles. It takes experience and skill to discern weakness in the actively contracting hand muscle.

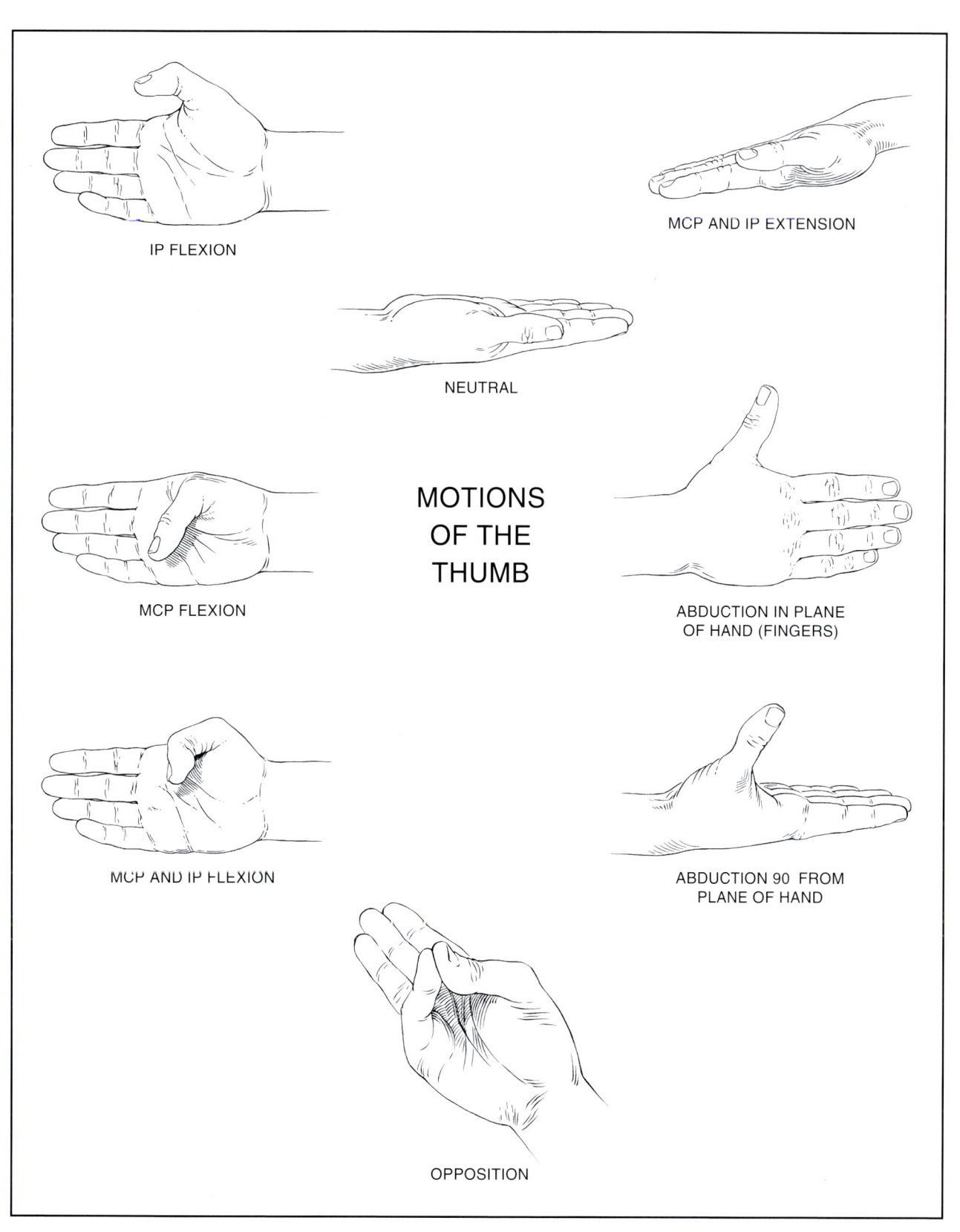

IP FLEXION

MCP AND IP EXTENSION

NEUTRAL

MOTIONS
OF THE
THUMB

MCP FLEXION

ABDUCTION IN PLANE
OF HAND (FINGERS)

MCP AND IP FLEXION

ABDUCTION 90 FROM
PLANE OF HAND

OPPOSITION

PLATE 5 Motions of the thumb.

(Flexor pollicis brevis and Flexor pollicis longus)

Flexor pollicis brevis

Flexor pollicis longus

PALMAR

FIGURE 5.193

FIGURE 5.194

Median n.
To: Flexor pollicis longus
C8-T1
Flexor pollicis brevis
(superficial head)
C8-T1

Ulnar n.
To: Flexor pollicis brevis (deep head)
C8-T1

C5
C6
C7
C8
T1

FIGURE 5.195

Median nerve

Flexor pollicis longus

FIGURE 5.196 Arrow indicates level of cross section.

Range of Motion

MCP flexion: 0°–50°

IP flexion: 0°–80°

Table 5.24 THUMB MCP AND IP FLEXION

I.D.	Muscle	Origin	Insertion	Function
MCP Flexion				
170	Flexor pollicis brevis Superficial head (often blended with opponens pollicis)	Flexor retinaculum (distal) Trapezoid bone (tubercle, distal)	Thumb (base of proximal phalanx, radial side)	Flexion of the MCP and CMC joints of the thumb Opposition of thumb (assist)
	Deep head	Trapezium bone Capitate bone Palmar ligaments of distal carpal bones		
IP Flexion				
169	Flexor pollicis longus	Radius (anterior surface of middle half) and adjacent interosseous membrane Ulna (coronoid process, lateral border [variable]) Humerus (medial epicondyle [variable])	Thumb (base of distal phalanx, palmar surface)	Flexion of IP joint of thumb Flexion of the MCP and CMC joints of thumb (accessory) Flexion of wrist (accessory)

CMC, Carpometacarpal; *IP*, interphalangeal; *MCP*, metacarpophalangeal.

(Flexor pollicis brevis)

The FPB is an intrinsic muscle of the thumb. The innervation of the two heads can be variable, innervated by the median nerve, the ulnar nerve, or both.[59] The FPB and longus are implicated in texting motions.

Grade 5 to Grade 0

Position of the Patient: Forearm in supination, wrist in neutral. CMC joint is at 0°; IP joint is at 0°. Thumb in adduction, lying relaxed and adjacent to the second metacarpal.

Instructions to Clinician: Sit at table or to side of patient. Demonstrate thumb flexion and have patient practice the motion. Stabilize the first metacarpal firmly to avoid any wrist or CMC motion. Ask the patient to bend the thumb toward the palm, keeping the IP straight. If the motion can be accomplished (Grade 3), apply appropriate resistance with one-finger resistance to MCP flexion on the proximal phalanx in the direction of extension (Fig. 5.197).

Test: Patient flexes the MCP joint of the thumb, keeping the IP joints straight (see Fig. 5.197).

Instructions to Patient: "Don't bend the tip of the finger. Hold it. Don't let me pull it back."

Grading

Grade 5 and Grade 4: Can hold position against strong thumb resistance. Distinguishing between Grades 5 and 4 is difficult and clinically, perhaps not important. The grade awarded will depend on the amount of the clinician's experience with normal hands.

Grade 3: Completes full range of motion.

Grade 2: Cannot complete full range of motion.

Grade 1: Palpate the muscle by initially locating the tendon of the flexor pollicis longus in the thenar eminence (Fig. 5.198). Then, palpate the muscle belly of the FPB on the ulnar side of the longus tendon in the thenar eminence.

Grade 0: No discernable palpable activity.

Substitution by Flexor Pollicis Longus

- The long thumb flexor can substitute but only after flexion of the IP joint begins. To avoid this substitution, do not allow flexion of the distal joint of the thumb.
- Work-related thumb pain in physical therapists is related to decreased stability and strength of the thumb.[60] This instability may result in the inability to maintain thumb extension during mobilization techniques, a frequent complaint of clinicians.[61]

FIGURE 5.197

FIGURE 5.198

Grade 5 to Grade 0

Position of the Patient: Forearm supinated with wrist in neutral and MCP joint of thumb in extension.

Instructions to Clinician: Sit at table or side of patient. Stabilize the MCP joint of the thumb firmly in extension by grasping the patient's thumb across that joint. Ask the patient to bend the tip of the thumb. If sufficient range is present (Grade 3), apply resistance with the tip of your finger against the palmar surface of the distal phalanx of the thumb in the direction of extension (Fig. 5.199).

Test: Patient flexes the IP joint of the thumb.

Instructions to Patient: "Bend the end of your thumb. Hold it. Don't let me straighten it."

FIGURE 5.199

Grading

Grade 5 and Grade 4: Patient tolerates maximal finger resistance from clinician for Grade 5. This muscle is very strong, and a Grade 4 muscle will also tolerate strong resistance.

Grade 3: Completes full range of motion with minimal resistance because gravity is minimized.

Grade 2: Holds test position.

Grade 1 and Grade 0: Palpate the tendon of the flexor pollicis longus on the palmar surface of the proximal phalanx of the thumb. Palpable activity is graded 1; no discernable palpable activity is graded 0.

Substitution

Do not allow the distal phalanx of the thumb to extend at the beginning of the test. If the distal phalanx is extended and then relaxes, the clinician may think active flexion has occurred.

THUMB MCP AND IP EXTENSION

(Extensor pollicis brevis and Extensor pollicis longus)

Extensor pollicis brevis

Extensor pollicis longus

DORSAL

FIGURE 5.200

FIGURE 5.201

Radial n.
To: Extensor pollicis brevis
C7-C8
Extensor pollicis longus
C7-C8

FIGURE 5.202

Radius
Radial nerve
Extensor pollicis brevis
Extensor pollicis longus
Ulna

FIGURE 5.203 Arrow indicates level of cross section.

(Extensor pollicis brevis and Extensor pollicis longus)

Range of Motion

MCP extension: 50°–0°

IP extension: 80°–0°

Table 5.25 **THUMB MCP AND IP EXTENSION**

I.D.	Muscle	Origin	Insertion	Function
MCP Extension				
168	Extensor pollicis brevis (radiomedial wall of "anatomical snuffbox")	Radius (posterior surface) Adjacent interosseous membrane	Thumb (proximal phalanx, base, dorsolateral surface)	Extension of MCP joint of thumb Extension and abduction of 1st CMC joint of thumb Radial deviation of wrist (accessory)
IP Extension				
167	Extensor pollicis longus (ulnar wall of "anatomical snuffbox")	Ulna (shaft, middle one-third on posterior-lateral surface) Adjacent interosseous membrane	Thumb (base of distal phalanx)	Extension of the thumb at all joints: Distal phalanx (alone) MCP and CMC joints (along with extensor pollicis brevis and abductor pollicis longus) Radial deviation of wrist (accessory)

CMC, Carpometacarpal; *IP*, interphalangeal; *MCP*, metacarpophalangeal.

THUMB MCP AND IP EXTENSION

(Extensor pollicis brevis and Extensor pollicis longus)

The extensor pollicis brevis (EPB) is a muscle with common variations that often blends with the extensor pollicis longus (EPL); therefore, it is not possible to separate the brevis from the longus by clinical tests, and the test for the longus prevails. The EPL and EPB with the abductor pollicis longus form the borders of the anatomical snuff box. The snuff box is most visible with thumb extension.

Grade 5, Grade 4, and Grade 3

Position of the Patient: Forearm in midposition, wrist in neutral with ulnar side of hand resting on the table. Thumb relaxed in a flexion posture.

Instructions to Clinician: Sit or stand near the patient. Use the table to support the hand. Ask patient to lift just the thumb. If full range is present (Grade 3), apply the appropriate resistance over the dorsal surface of the distal phalanx of the thumb in the direction of flexion (Fig. 5.204).

Test: Patient lifts the thumb from the table, extending the IP joint of the thumb.

Instructions to Patient: "Hold it. Don't let me push it down."

Grading

Grade 5 and Grade 4: This is not a strong muscle, so resistance must be applied accordingly. The distinction between Grades 5 and 4 is based on comparison with the contralateral normal hand and, barring that, extensive experience in testing the hand.

Grade 3: Completes full range of motion without resistance.

FIGURE 5.204

Grade 2, Grade 1, and Grade 0

Position of the Patient: Forearm in pronation with wrist in neutral and thumb in relaxed flexion posture to start.

Instructions to Clinician: Stabilize the wrist over its dorsal surface. Stabilize the fingers by gently placing the other hand across the fingers just below the MCP joints (Fig. 5.205).

Test: Patient extends distal joint of the thumb (see Fig. 5.205).

Instructions to Patient: "Straighten the end of your thumb."

Grading

Grade 2: Thumb completes range of motion.

Grade 1: Palpate the tendon of the EPL on the ulnar side of the "anatomical snuffbox" or, alternatively, on the dorsal surface of the proximal phalanx (Fig. 5.206).

Grade 0: No discernable palpable contractile activity.

Substitution

The muscles of the thenar eminence (abductor pollicis brevis [APB], flexor pollicis brevis [FPB], and adductor pollicis [AP]) can extend the interphalangeal joint by flexing the carpometacarpal joint (an extensor tenodesis).

FIGURE 5.205

FIGURE 5.206

Clinical Relevance

- A quick way to assess the functional status of the long thumb extensor is to flick the distal phalanx into flexion; if the finger rebounds or snaps back, it is a useful muscle.
- The trapeziometacarpal (TMC) joint is the most common site of symptomatic osteoarthritis in the hand, with radiographic prevalence of 7% for men and 15% for women over age 30 years,[62] reaching 90% in both men and women 80 years of age.[63]
- TMC arthritis leads to a loss of abduction-adduction in the TMC joint and at the MCP joint and often reduces pronation-supination.[64]
- TMC pain affects the ability to open jars (grasp) and turn keys (pinch).
- Resisted thumb extension that reproduced the patients' pain had a sensitivity of 0.94 and specificity of 0.95 for TMC arthritis. A positive test of either adduction or extension movements yielded a sensitivity of 1.00 and specificity of 0.91 for TMC arthritis.[63]
- The dorsal radial ligament is the prime opposer of TMC translation and is also mechanically robust, anatomically thick, and well innervated.[65]

THUMB ABDUCTION

(Abductor pollicis longus and Abductor pollicis brevis)

Abductor pollicis brevis

Abductor pollicis longus

PALMAR

FIGURE 5.208

Median n.
To: Abductor pollicis brevis C8-T1

Radial n.
To: Abductor pollicis longus C7-C8

FIGURE 5.209

DORSAL

FIGURE 5.207

Range of Motion
0°–70°

Table 5.26 THUMB ABDUCTION

I.D.	Muscle	Origin	Insertion	Function
166	Abductor pollicis longus (radiolateral wall of "anatomical snuffbox")	Ulna (posterior surface laterally) Radius (shaft, middle one-third of posterior aspect) Interosseous membrane	Thumb: 1st metacarpal (radial side of base) Trapezium bone	Abduction of thumb at CMC joint Extension of thumb at IP joint (in concert with thumb extensors) Radial deviation of wrist (assist)
171	Abductor pollicis brevis	Flexor retinaculum Scaphoid bone (tubercle) Trapezium bone (tubercle) Tendon of abductor pollicis longus	Medial fibers: Thumb (base of proximal phalanx, radial side) Lateral fibers: Extensor expansion of thumb	Abduction of thumb CMC and MCP joints (in a plane 90° from the palm) Opposition of thumb (assist) Extension of IP joint (assist)
Others				
152	Palmaris longus (if present)			
168	Extensor pollicis brevis	See Table 5.25		

CMC, Carpometacarpal; *IP,* interphalangeal; *MCP,* metacarpophalangeal.

The palmaris longus can abduct the thumb, if present.[66]

ABDUCTOR POLLICIS LONGUS

Grade 5 to Grade 0

Position of the Patient: Forearm supinated and wrist in neutral; thumb relaxed in adduction.

Instructions to Clinician: Sit or stand near the patient. Demonstrate the movement. Then, stabilize the metacarpals of the four fingers and the wrist. Ask the patient to lift the thumb straight up to 90° from the palm. If full range of motion is present (Grade 3), then apply appropriate resistance on the distal end of the first metacarpal in the direction of adduction (Fig. 5.210).

Test: Patient abducts the thumb away from the hand in a plane parallel to the finger metacarpals.

Instructions to Patient: "Lift your thumb straight up."

Grading

Grade 5 and Grade 4: Can hold against strong resistance. Distinguishing Grades 5 and 4 may be difficult.

Grade 3: Completes full range of motion without resistance.

Grade 2: Completes partial range of motion.

Grade 1: Palpate tendon of the abductor pollicis longus at the base of the first metacarpal on the radial side of the EPB (Fig. 5.211). It is the most lateral tendon at the wrist.

Grade 0: No discernable palpable contractile activity.

Substitution

The extensor pollicis brevis can substitute for the abductor pollicis longus. If the line of pull is toward the dorsal surface of the forearm (extensor pollicis brevis), substitution is occurring.

Clinical Relevance

- If the abductor pollicis longus is stronger than the brevis, the thumb will deviate toward the radial side of the hand.
- If the abductor pollicis brevis is stronger, deviation will be toward the ulnar side.
- De Quervain tenosynovitis, affecting the abductor pollicis longus and extensor pollicis brevis tendons, is indicated by the Finkelstein test. To perform this test, ask the patient to close the fingers around the thumb so the thumb is tucked into the palm. Then, ask the patient to ulnarly deviate the wrist. If pain is on the thumb side of the wrist, the test is positive. The condition has been linked to texting more than 50 messages/day.[67,68] Can also be referred to as "Gamer thumb."

FIGURE 5.210

FIGURE 5.211

THUMB ABDUCTION

(Abductor pollicis longus and Abductor pollicis brevis)

ABDUCTOR POLLICIS BREVIS

Grade 5, Grade 4, and Grade 3

Position of the Patient: Dorsum of hand is on table with forearm in supination, wrist in neutral, and thumb relaxed in adduction.

Instructions to Clinician: Sit or stand near the patient. Demonstrate the movement. Ask the patient to lift the thumb to point towards the ceiling. If full range is present (Grade 3), apply appropriate resistance with index finger to the lateral aspect of the proximal phalanx of the thumb in the direction of adduction (Fig. 5.212).

Test: Patient abducts the thumb in a plane perpendicular to the palm. Observe wrinkling of the skin over the thenar eminence.

Instructions to Patient: "Lift your thumb vertically until it points to the ceiling." Demonstrate motion to the patient.

Grading

Grade 5: Holds motion with maximal finger resistance.

Grade 4: Tolerates moderate resistance.

Grade 3: Completes full range of motion without resistance.

Grade 2, Grade 1, and Grade 0

Position of the Patient: Forearm in midposition, wrist in neutral, and thumb relaxed in adduction.

Instructions to Clinician: Stabilize wrist in neutral.

Test: Patient abducts thumb in a plane perpendicular to the palm.

Instructions to Patient: "Try to lift your thumb so it points at the ceiling."

Grading

Grade 2: Completes partial range of motion.

Grade 1: Palpate the belly of the APB in the center of the thenar eminence, medial to the OP (Fig. 5.213).

Grade 0: No discernable palpable contractile activity.

Substitution

If the plane of motion is not perpendicular but toward the radial side of the hand, the substitution may be by the abductor pollicis longus.

FIGURE 5.212

FIGURE 5.213

To: Adductor pollicis
C8-T1

Ulnar n.

FIGURE 5.215

<table>
<tr><td style="background:red;color:white">**Range of Motion**</td></tr>
<tr><td>70°–0°</td></tr>
</table>

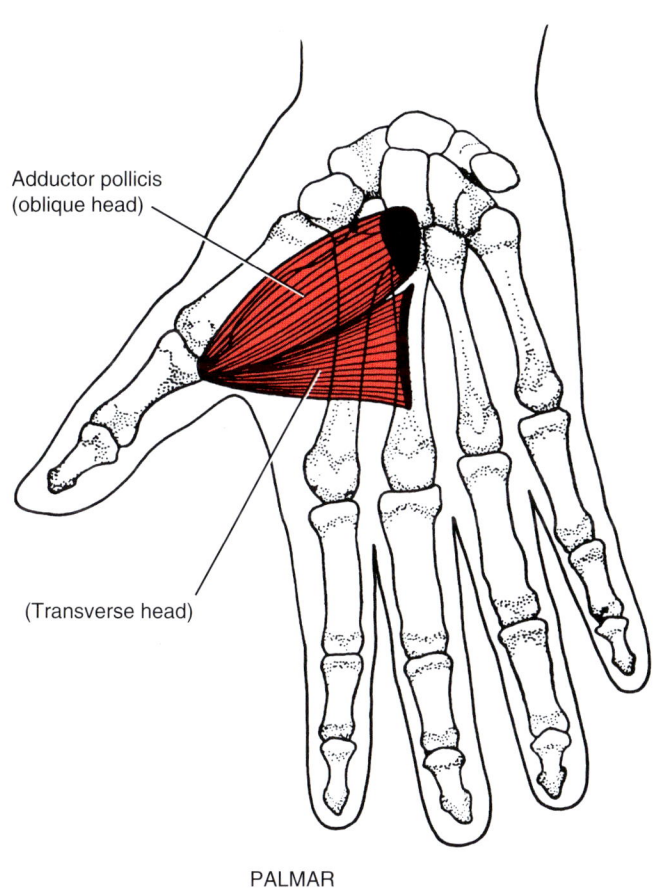

Adductor pollicis
(oblique head)

(Transverse head)

PALMAR

FIGURE 5.214

Table 5.27 THUMB ADDUCTION

I.D.	Muscle	Origin	Insertion	Function
173	Adductor pollicis		Thumb (proximal phalanx, ulnar side of base)	Adduction of CMC joint of thumb (approximates the thumb to the palm) Adduction and flexion of MCP joint (assist)
	Oblique head	Capitate bone 2nd and 3rd metacarpals (bases) Palmar ligaments of carpal bones Sheath of tendon of flexor carpi radialis		
	Transverse head	3rd metacarpal bone (palmar surface of distal two-thirds)		

CMC, Carpometacarpal; *MCP*, metacarpophalangeal.

THUMB ADDUCTION

(Adductor pollicis)

Grade 5, Grade 4, and Grade 3

Position of the Patient: Forearm in pronation, wrist in neutral, and thumb relaxed and hanging down in abduction.

Instructions to Clinician: Sit or stand near the patient. Demonstrate the movement. Stabilize the metacarpals of the four fingers by grasping the patient's hand around the ulnar side. If full range is present (Grade 3), apply appropriate resistance on the medial side of the proximal phalanx of the thumb in the direction of abduction (Fig. 5.216). Do not allow ulnar deviation. Alternatively, place a sheet of paper between the thumb and the index finger (adduction) and ask the patient to hold it while the clinician tries to pull the paper away. This is strong movement, and the patient should be able to hold a paper without difficulty.

Test: Patient adducts the thumb by bringing the first metacarpal up to the second metacarpal.

Instructions to Patient: "Bring your thumb up to your index finger." OR "Hold the paper. Don't let me pull it out."

Grading

Grade 5 and Grade 4: Holds test position against strong resistance. Patient can resist rigidly (Grade 5), or the muscle yields (Grade 4).

Grade 3: Completes full range of motion without resistance.

FIGURE 5.216

(Adductor pollicis)

Grade 2 and Grade 1

Position of the Patient: Forearm in midposition, wrist in neutral resting on table, and thumb in abduction.

Instructions to Clinician: Stabilize wrist on the table and use a hand to stabilize the finger metacarpals (Fig. 5.217).

Test: Patient moves thumb horizontally in adduction. The end position is shown in Fig. 5.217.

Instructions to Patient: "Return your thumb to its place next to your index finger." Demonstrate motion to patient.

Grading

Grade 2: Completes full range of motion.

Grade 1: Palpate the adductor pollicis on the palmar side of the web space of the thumb by grasping the web between the index finger and thumb (Fig. 5.218). The adductor lies between the first dorsal interosseous and the first metacarpal bone. This muscle is difficult to palpate, and the clinician may have to ask the patient to perform a palmar pinch to assist in its location.

FIGURE 5.217

FIGURE 5.218

THUMB ADDUCTION

(Adductor pollicis)

Substitutions

- A positive Froment's sign indicates the lack of strength of the adductor pollicis when the motor branch of the ulnar nerve is affected. The patient will use the flexor pollicis longus for pinch grip, which will result in obvious bending of the interphalangeal joint of the thumb (Fig. 5.219).
- The extensor pollicis longus may attempt to substitute for the adductor pollicis, in which case the carpometacarpal joint will extend (not shown).

FIGURE 5.219

Clinical Relevance

- Resisted thumb adduction that reproduces the patient's pain had a sensitivity of 0.94 and specificity of 0.93 for trapeziometacarpal (TMC) arthritis. A positive test of either thumb adduction or thumb extension yielded a sensitivity of 1.00 and specificity of 0.91 for TMC arthritis.[63]
- The tip pinch (index finger to thumb) is the functional task that is most compromised in people with MCP osteoarthritis.[69]

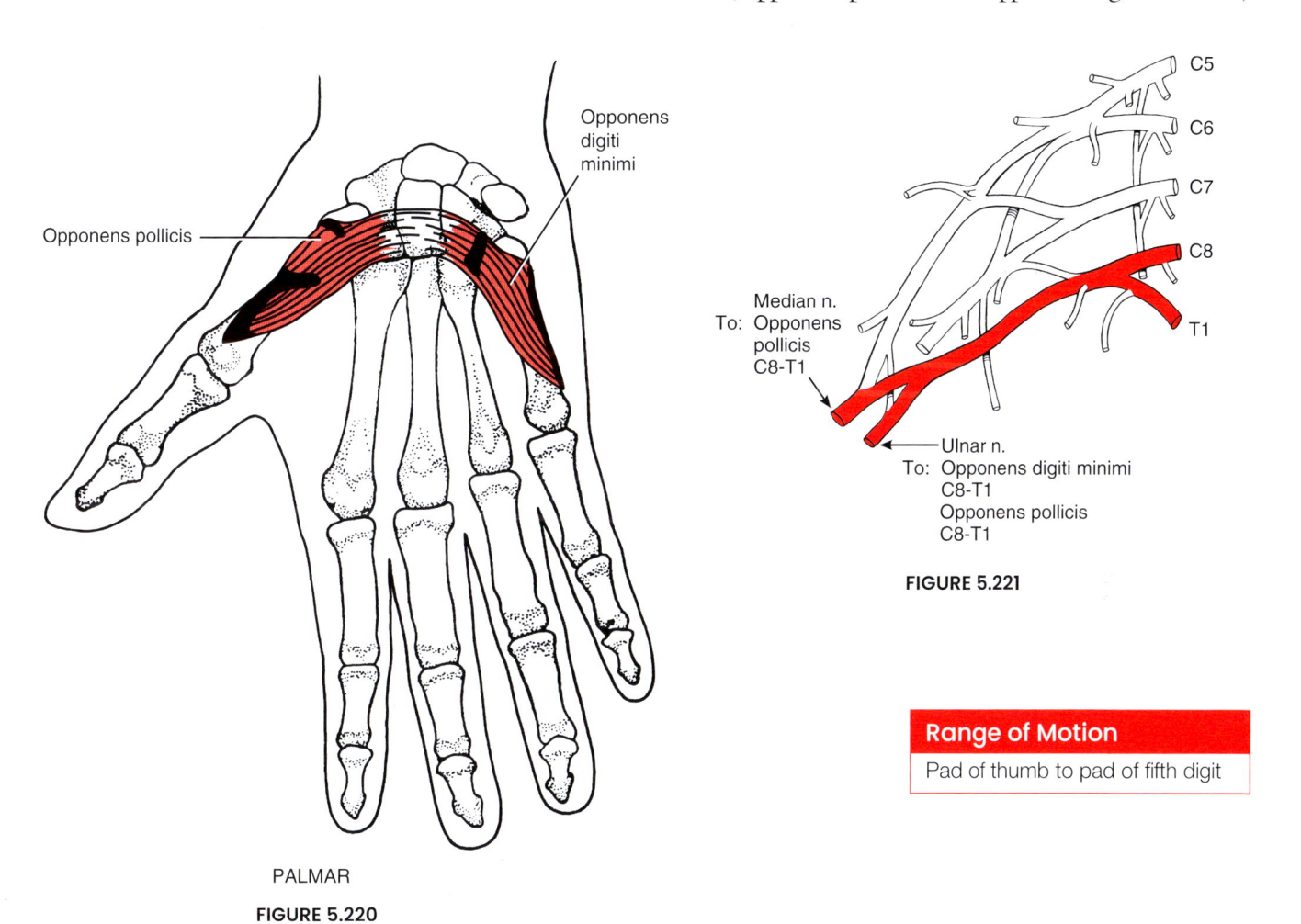

Opponens digiti minimi

Opponens pollicis

PALMAR

FIGURE 5.220

C5
C6
C7
C8
T1

Median n.
To: Opponens pollicis C8-T1

Ulnar n.
To: Opponens digiti minimi
C8-T1
Opponens pollicis
C8-T1

FIGURE 5.221

Range of Motion

Pad of thumb to pad of fifth digit

Table 5.28 OPPOSITION (THUMB TO LITTLE FINGER)[A]

I.D.	Muscle	Origin	Insertion	Function
172	Opponens pollicis	Trapezium bone (tubercle) Flexor retinaculum	1st metacarpal (entire length of lateral border and adjoining lateral half of palmar surface)	Flexion of CMC joint medially across the palm Medial rotation of CMC joint
161	Opponens digiti minimi	Hamate (hook) Flexor retinaculum	5th metacarpal (whole length of ulnar margin and adjacent palmar surface)	
Others				
171	Abductor pollicis brevis	See Table 5.26		
170	Flexor pollicis brevis	See Table 5.24		

[a]This motion is a combination of abduction, flexion, and medial rotation of the thumb. The two muscles in thumb-to-fifth-digit opposition (opponens pollicis and opponens digiti minimi) should be graded separately.
CMC, Carpometacarpal.

OPPOSITION (THUMB TO LITTLE FINGER)

(Opponens pollicis and Opponens digiti minimi)

Grade 5 to Grade 0

Position of the Patient: Forearm is supinated and supported on table, wrist in neutral, and thumb in adduction with MCP and IP flexion.

Instructions to Clinician: Sit or stand near patient. Ask patient to bring the thumb and little finger together (Grade 3) (Fig. 5.222). The table provides stabilization of the hand. Both thumb and fifth digits should be observed individually. If full range is present in each movement (Grade 3), apply appropriate finger resistance at CMP joint of thumb and digit to test both actions simultaneously Fig. 5.223).

Opponens Pollicis: Apply resistance for the OP at the head of the 1st metacarpal in the direction of lateral rotation, extension, and adduction (Fig. 5.224).

Opponens Digiti Minimi: Give resistance for the opponens digiti minimi on the palmar surface of the 5th metacarpal in the direction of medial rotation (flattening the palm) (Fig. 5.225).

Test: Patient approximates the pad of the thumb and pad of fifth digit (see Fig. 5.222). Such apposition must be pad to pad and not tip to tip. Opposition also can be evaluated by asking the patient to hold an object between the thumb and little finger (in opposition), which the clinician tries to pull it away.

FIGURE 5.222

FIGURE 5.224

FIGURE 5.223

FIGURE 5.225

Grade 5 to Grade 0 Continued

Instructions to Patient: "Bring your thumb to your little finger and touch the two pads, forming the letter 'O' with your thumb and little finger." Demonstrate motion to the patient and require practice.

Grading

Grade 5: Holds against maximal thumb resistance.

Grade 4: Holds against moderate resistance.

Grade 3: Moves thumb and fifth digit through full range of opposition without resistance.

Grade 2: Moves through range of opposition. (The two opponens muscles are evaluated separately.)

Grade 1: Palpate the OP along the radial shaft of the 1st metacarpal (Fig. 5.226). It lies lateral to the APB. During Grades 5 and 4 contractions, the clinician will have difficulty in palpating the OP because of nearby muscles. In Grade 3 muscles and below, the weaker contractions do not obscure palpation.

Palpate the opponens digiti minimi on the hypothenar eminence on the radial side of the fifth metacarpal (Fig. 5.227). The clinician should be careful not to cover the muscle with the finger or thumb used for palpation lest any contractile activity be missed.

Grade 0: No discernable palpable contractile activity.

FIGURE 5.227

FIGURE 5.226

OPPOSITION (THUMB TO LITTLE FINGER)

(Opponens pollicis and Opponens digiti minimi)

Substitutions

- The flexor pollicis longus and the flexor pollicis brevis can draw the thumb across the palm toward the little finger. If such motion occurs in the plane of the palm, it is not opposition; contact will be at the tips, not the pads, of the digits.
- The abductor pollicis brevis may substitute, but the rotation component of the motion will not be present.

Clinical Relevance

The muscles involved in opening a 66-mm-diameter jar lid are the flexor pollicis longus, flexor pollicis brevis, abductor pollicis brevis, adductor pollicis, and opponens pollicis.[70]

Pinch strength, especially key pinch is less in patients with early thumb CMC arthritis.[71]

Grip strength is an efficient way to measure the composite strength of the hand and wrist, but grip strength is also related to general health and age. For example, grip strength peaks at 20 to 40 years of age and declines thereafter with advancing age.[72,73] In the older adult, grip strength has been shown to be a reliable predictor of mortality.[74,75]

Position of the Patient: Seated erect with shoulders level and neutrally rotated. The elbow is flexed to 90°, forearm in neutral and wrist between 0° and 30° of extension (Fig. 5.228A).[72]

Instructions to Clinician: Both hands are tested, one at a time. Record which hand is dominant, as it will be most often stronger. Stand in front of the patient to be able to see the dial. Place the dynamometer in the patient's hand with the dial facing away from patient (see Fig. 5.228B). Adjust the position of the dynamometer handle so that the patient's fingers can comfortably grasp and squeeze it. Most often, this is in the second position. Repeat three times. Alternate hands with each trial.

Instructions to Patient: "When I say go, squeeze as hard as you can in a smooth manner. Do not jerk the tool while you are gripping. Stop immediately if you experience any unusual pain or discomfort." (See Fig. 5.228).

Scoring

Three trials are recorded for each hand, averaging the three scores for the final score. Scores are compared with the appropriate age and sex categories for accurate interpretation (see Tables 5.29 and 5.30).

FIGURE 5.228 A and B

GRIP STRENGTH

Clinical Relevance

- The position of the patient (sitting vs supine with extended or flexed elbow) did not affect grip strength results.[76]
- Grip strength of 9 kg (20 pounds) is commonly considered functional and is necessary to perform most daily activities.[73]
- Grip strength of 25 kg for women and 42 kg for men (maximum) is associated with all-cause mortality.[77]
- Grip strength is correlated significantly with upper limb function in older adults and in people with certain disorders but not in young, healthy patients.[78,79]
- Grip strength is affected by certain disorders that impair results, such as carpal tunnel syndrome, lateral epicondylitis, dementia, arthritis, and stroke.
- The interossei can be tested by hand grip using a hand-grip dynamometer. Use the smallest distance between handle positions because the intrinsics are most active in this position.[80]
- The average decrease in grip strength after an ulnar nerve block is 38%.[81]

Table 5.29 MEAN REFERENCE DATA FOR HAND GRIP STRENGTH (KG)[82]

Age (years)	MEN			WOMEN		
	Right	Left	BMI	Right	Left	BMI
20–29	47 (9.5)	45 (8.8)	26.4 (5.1)	30 (7)	28 (6.1)	25.1 (5.8)
30–39	47 (9.7)	47 (9.8)	28.3 (5.2)	31 (6.4)	29 (6)	27.3 (6.8)
40–49	47 (9.5)	45 (9.3)	28.4 (4.6)	29 (5.7)	28 (5.7)	27.7 (7.7)
50–59	45 (8.4)	43 (8.3)	28.7 (4.3)	28 (6.3)	26 (5.7)	29.1 (6.4)
60–69	40 (8.3)	38 (8)	28.6 (4.4)	24 (5.3)	23 (5)	28.1 (5.1)
70+	33 (7.8)	32 (7.5)	27.2 (3.9)	20 (5.8)	19 (5.5)	27 (4.7)

Date collected using the position described in Fig. 5.224A and B.
BMI, Body mass index.

Table 5.30 GRIP STRENGTH VALUES FOR AGES 4–14 (KG)[83]

Age (years)	BOYS			GIRLS		
	Dominant	Nondominant	BMI	Dominant	Nondominant	BMI
4	5.7 (2)	5.3 (2)	15.42	5.1 (2)	4.7 (2)	15.42
6	10.2 (3)	9.4 (3)	16	9.0 (3)	8.3 (3)	16
8	15.9 (4)	14.6 (3)	16.5	14.4 (3)	13.1 (3)	17.75
10	19.6 (2)	18.1 (3)	17.6	19.1 (4)	17.2 (4)	18.5
12	24.7 (5)	22.9 (5)	19	24.2 (5)	22.3 (4)	18.75
14	36.0 (7)	33.5 (7)	19.6	29.1 (5)	26.6 (5)	19.3

BMI, Body mass index.

Supplemental Video Resources

Visit Elsevier eBooks+ (eBooks.Health.Elsevier.com) to access supplemental videos about the following tests:

- Scapular Abduction and Upward Rotation
- Scapular Adduction
- Scapular Depression and Adduction
- Scapular Depression
- Introduction to Shoulder Muscle Testing
- Shoulder Extension
- Shoulder Abduction
- Shoulder Horizontal Abduction
- Shoulder Horizontal Adduction
- Elbow Flexion
- Elbow Extension
- Forearm Supination
- Forearm Pronation
- Wrist Flexion
- Wrist Extension
- Finger MCP Flexion
- PIP Tests
- DIP Tests
- Finger MCP Extension
- Finger Abduction
- Finger Adduction
- Thumb MCP and IP Flexion
- Thumb MCP and IP Flexion Tests
- Thumb MCP and IP Extension
- Thumb MCP Extension Tests
- Thumb IP Extension Tests
- Abductor Pollicis Longus Test
- Adductor Pollicis Brevis Test
- Thumb Adduction
- Opposition (Thumb to Little Finger)

1. Standring S, ed. *Gray's Anatomy: The Anatomical Basis for Clinical Practice.* 41st ed. New York: Elsevier; 2016.
2. Neumann DA. *Kinesiology of the Musculoskeletal System.* 3rd ed. St. Louis, MO: Elsevier; 2017.
3. Scibek JS, Carcia CR. Assessment of scapulohumeral rhythm for scapular plane shoulder elevation using a modified digital inclinometer. *World J Orthop.* 2012;3(6): 87–94.
4. Sagano M, Magee D, Katayose M. The effect of glenohumeral rotation on scapular upward rotation in different positions of scapular-plane elevation. *J Sport Rehab.* 2006;15:144–155.
5. Ekstrom RA, Donatelli RA, Soderberg GL. Surface electromyographic analysis of exercises for the trapezius and serratus anterior muscles. *J Orthop Sports Phys Ther.* 2003;33:247–258.
6. Ekstrom RA, Soderberg GL, Donatelli RA. Normalization procedures using maximum voluntary isometric contractions for the serratus anterior and trapezius muscles during surface EMG analysis. *J Electromyogr Kinesiol.* 2005;15(4):418–428.
7. Neumann D.A., Camargo P.R. Kinesiologic considerations for targeting activation of scapulothoracic muscles - part 1: serratus anterior. Braz J Phys Ther. 2019;23(6):459–466. https://doi.org/10.1016/j.bjpt.2019.01.008. Epub 2019 Feb 2. PMID: 30737019; PMCID: PMC6849091.
8. Escamilla RF, Yamashiro K, Paulos L, et al. Shoulder muscle activity and function in common shoulder rehabilitation exercises. *Sports Med.* 2009;39(8):663–685.
9. Cricchio M, Frazer C. Scapulothoracic and scapulohumeral exercises: a narrative review of electromyographic studies. *J Hand Ther.* 2011;24(4):322–333.
10. Schory A, Bidinger E, Wolf J, et al. A systematic review of the exercises that produce optimal muscle ratios of the scapular stabilizers in normal shoulders. *Int J Sports Phys Ther.* 2016;11(3):321–336.
11. Smith J, Padgett DJ, Kaufman KR, et al. Rhomboid muscle electromyography activity during 3 different manual muscle tests. *Arch Phys Med Rehabil.* 2004;85:987–992.
12. Camargo PR, Neumann DA. Kinesiologic considerations for targeting activation of scapulothoracic muscles – part 2: trapezius. *Braz J Phys Ther.* 2019,23(6).467–475.
13. Perry J. Muscle control of the shoulder. In: Rowe CR, ed. *The Shoulder.* New York: Churchill-Livingstone; 1988:17–34.
14. Arlotta M, LoVasco G, McLean L. Selective recruitment of the lower fibers of the trapezius muscle. *J Electromyogr Kinesiol.* 2011;21(3):403–410.
15. Kendall FP, McCreary EK, Provance PG, et al. *Muscles: Testing and Function with Posture and Pain.* 5th ed. Baltimore, MD: Lippincott, Williams & Wilkins; 2005:297–305.
16. De Freias V, Vitti M, Furlani J. Electromyographic study of levator scapulae and rhomboideus major muscles in movements of the shoulder and arm. *Electromyogr Clin Neurophysiol.* 1980;20:205–216.
17. Signorile JF, Zink AJ, Szwed SP. A comparative electromyographical investigation of muscle utilization patterns using various hand positions during the lat pull-down. *J Strength Cond Res.* 2002;16(4):539–546.
18. Lehman GJ, Buchan DD, Lundy A, et al. Variations in muscle activation levels during traditional latissimus dorsi weight training exercises: an experimental study. *Dyn Med.* 2004;3(1):4.
19. Park SY, Yoo WG. Comparison of exercises inducing maximum voluntary isometric contraction for the latissimus dorsi using surface electromyography. *J Electromyogr Kinesiol.* 2013;23(5):1106–1110.
20. Travell JG, Simons DG. Myofascial pain and dysfunction. In: *The Trigger Point Manual.* Baltimore MD: Williams & Wilkins; 1983:433.
21. Ackland DC, Pak P, Richardson M, et al. Moment arms of the muscles crossing the anatomical shoulder. *J Anat.* 2008;213(4):383–390.
22. Freeman S, Karpowicz A, Gray J, et al. Quantifying muscle patterns and spine load during various forms of the push-up. *Med Sci Sports Exerc.* 2006;38(3):570–577.
23. Lauver JD, Cayot TE, Scheuermann BW. Influence of bench angle on upper extremity muscular activation during bench press exercise. *Eur J Sport Sci.* 2016;16(3):309–316.
24. Trebs AA, Brandenburg JP, Pitney WA. An electromyography analysis of 3 muscles surrounding the shoulder joint during the performance of a chest press exercise at several angles. *J Strength Cond Res.* 2010;24(7):1925–1930.
25. Boettcher CE, Ginn KA, Cathers I. Standard maximum isometric voluntary contraction tests for normalizing shoulder muscle. *J Orthop Res.* 2008;26(12):1591–1597.
26. Reinold MM, Wilk KE, Fleisig GS, et al. Electromyographic analysis of the rotator cuff and deltoid musculature during common shoulder external rotation exercises. *J Orthop Sports Phys Ther.* 2004;34:385–394.
27. Ferreira MI, Büll ML, Vitti M. Electromyographic validation of basic exercises for physical conditioning programmes. I. Analysis of the deltoid muscle (anterior portion) and pectoralis major muscle (clavicular portion) in rowing exercises with middle grip. *Electromyogr Clin Neurophysiol.* 1995;35(4):239–245.
28. Gregori JH, Bureau NJ, Billuart F, et al. Coaptation/elevation role of the middle deltoid muscle fibers: a static biomechanical pilot study using shoulder MRI. *Surg Radiol Anat.* 2014;36(10):1001–1007.
29. Ackmann T, Schneider KN, Schorn D, et al. Comparison of efficacy of supraspinatus tendon tears diagnostic tests: a prospective study on the "full-can," the "empty-can," and the "Whipple" tests. *Musculoskelet Surg.* 2021;105(2):149–153. https://doi.org/10.1007/s12306-019-00631-0. Epub 2019 Nov 5. PMID: 31691179.
30. Anauate Nicolao F, Yazigi Junior JA, Matsunaga FT, et al. Comparing shoulder maneuvers to magnetic resonance imaging and arthroscopic findings in patients with supraspinatus tears. *World J Orthop.* 2022;13(1):102–111. https://doi.org/10.5312/wjo.v13.i1.102. PMID: 35096540; PMCID: PMC8771410.
31. Marcolin G, Petrone N, Moro T, et al. Selective activation of shoulder, trunk, and arm muscles: a comparative analysis of different push-up variants. *J Athl Train.* 2015;50(11):1126–1132.
32. Decker MJ, Tokish JM, Ellis HB, et al. Subscapularis muscle activity during selected rehabilitation exercises. *Am J Sports Med.* 2003;31(1):126–134.
33. Hughes PC, Green RA, Taylor NF. Isolation of infraspinatus in clinical test positions. *J Sci Med Sport.* 2014;17(3):256–260.
34. McKay MJ, Baldwin JN, Ferreira P, et al. 1000 Norms Project Consortium. Normative reference values for strength and flexibility of 1,000 children and adults. *Neurology.* 2017;88(1):36–43.
35. Lädermann A, Collin P, Zbinden O, et al. Diagnostic accuracy of clinical tests for subscapular-

is tears: a systematic review and meta-analysis. *Orthop J Sports Med*. 2021;9(9):23259671211042011. https://doi.org/10.1177/23259671211042011. PMID: 35146034; PMCID: PMC8822023.

36. Tokish JM, Decker MJ, Ellis HB, et al. The belly-press test for the physical examination of the subscapularis muscle: electromyographic validation in comparison to the lift-off test. *J Shoulder Elbow Surg*. 2003;12:427–430.

37. Kadaba MP, Cole A, Wootten ME, et al. Intramuscular wire electromyography of the subscapularis. *J Orthop Res*. 1992;10(3):394–397.

38. Date S, Kurumadani H, Nakashima Y, et al. Brachialis muscle activity can be measured with surface electromyography: a comparative study with surface and fine-wire electrodes. *Front Physiol*. 2021;12:2021. https://doi.org/10.3389/fphys.2021.809422.

39. Kleiber T, Kunz L, Disselhorst-Klug C. Muscular coordination of biceps brachii and brachioradialis in elbow flexion with respect to hand position. *Front Physiol*. 2015;6:215.

40. Basmajian JV, Travill J. Electromyography of the pronator muscles in the forearm. *Anat Rec*. 1961;139:45–49.

41. Klein CS, Marsh GD, Petrella RJ, et al. Muscle fiber number in the biceps brachii muscle of young and old men. *Muscle Nerve*. 2003;28(1):62–68.

42. Oliveira LF, Matta TT, Alves DS, et al. Effect of the shoulder position on the biceps brachii in different dumbbell curls. *J Sports Sci Med*. 2009;8(1):24–29.

43. Snarr RL, Esco MR. Electromyographic comparison of traditional and suspension push-ups. *J Hum Kinet*. 2013;39:75–83.

44. Youdas JW, Budach BD, Ellerbusch JV, et al. Comparison of muscle-activation patterns during the conventional push-up and perfect· pushup exercises. *J Strength Cond Res*. 2010;24(12):3352–3362.

45. Gordon KD, Pardo RD, Johnson JA, et al. Electromyographic activity and strength during maximum isometric pronation and supination efforts in healthy adults. *J Orthop Res*. 2004;22(1):208–213.

46. Matsuoka J, Berger R, Berglund LJ, et al. An analysis of symmetry of torque strength of the forearm under resisted forearm rotation in normal subjects. *J Hand Surg*. 2006;31:801–805.

47. O'Sullivan LW, Gallwey TJ. Upper-limb surface electromyography at maximum supination and pronation torques: the effect of elbow and forearm angle. *J Electromyogr Kinesiol*. 2002;12:275–285.

48. Wong CK, Moskovitz N. New assessment of forearm strength: reliability and validity. *Am J Occup Ther*. 2010;64:809–813.

49. Narita A, Sagae M, Suzuki K, et al. Strict actions of the human wrist flexors: a study with an electrical neuromuscular stimulation method. *J Electromyogr Kinesiol*. 2015;25(4):689–696.

50. Lee JA, Sechachalam S. The effect of wrist position on grip endurance and grip strength. *J Hand Surg Am*. 2016;41(10):e367–e373. https://doi.org/10.1016/j.jhsa.2016.07.100. Epub 2016 Aug 25. PMID: 27569783.

51. Gates DH, Walters LS, Cowley J, et al. Range of motion requirements for upper-limb activities of daily living. *Am J Occup Ther*. 2016;70(1):7001350010p1–7001350010p10. https://doi.org/10.5014/ajot.2016.015487. PMID: 26709433; PMCID: PMC4690598.

52. Kerver AL, Carati L, Eilers PH, et al. An anatomical study of the ECRL and ECRB: feasibility of developing a preoperative test for evaluating the strength of the individual wrist extensors. *J Plast Reconstr Aesthet Surg*. 2013;66(4):543–550.

53. Richards RR, Gordon R, Beaton D. Measurement of wrist, metacarpophalangeal joint, and thumb extension strength in a normal population. *J Hand Surg Am*. 1993;18(2):253–261.

54. Armstrong C, Oldham JA. A comparison of dominant hand strengths. *J Hand Surg Br*. 199;24(4):421–425.

55. Brandsma JW, Schreuders TA. Sensible manual muscle strength testing to evaluate and monitor strength of the intrinsic muscles of the hand: a commentary. *J Hand Ther*. 2001;14(4):273–278.

56. Schreuders TA, Brandsma JW, Stam HJ. The intrinsic muscles of the hand. Function, assessment and principles for therapeutic intervention. *Phys Med Rehab Kuror*. 2007;17:20–27. Accessed at: https://www.academia.edu/15339468/The_Intrinsic_Muscles_of_the_Hand March 7. 2023.

57. Goislard de Monsabert B, Rossi J, Berton E, et al. Quantification of hand and forearm muscle forces during a maximal power grip task. *Med Sci Sports Exerc*. 2012;44(10):1906–1916.

58. Ladd AL, Crisco JJ, Hagert E, et al. The 2014 ABJS Nicolas Andry Award: the puzzle of the thumb: mobility, stability, and demands in opposition. *Clin Orthop Relat Res*. 2014;472(12):3605–3622. https://doi.org/10.1007/s11999-014-3901-6. Epub 2014 Aug 30. PMID: 25171934; PMCID: PMC4397810.

59. Gupta S, Michelsen-Jost H. Anatomy and function of the thenar muscles. *Hand Clin*. 2012;28:1–7.

60. Snodgrass SJ, Rivett DA, Chiarelli P, et al. Factors related to thumb pain in physiotherapists. *Aust J Physiother*. 2003;49(4):243–250.

61. Wajon A, Ada L, Refshauge K. Work-related thumb pain in physiotherapists is associated with thumb alignment during performance of PA pressures. *Man Ther*. 2007;12(1):12–16.

62. Haara MM, Heliövaara M, Kröger H, et al. Osteoarthritis in the carpometacarpal joint of the thumb. Prevalence and associations with disability and mortality. *J Bone Joint Surg Am*. 2004;86-A(7):1452–1457.

63. Gelberman RH, Boone S, Osei DA, et al. Trapeziometacarpal arthritis: a prospective clinical evaluation of the thumb adduction and extension provocative tests. *J Hand Surg Am*. 2015;40(7):1285–1291.

64. Hamann N, Heidemann J, Heinrich K, et al. Effect of carpometacarpal joint osteoarthritis, sex, and handedness on thumb in vivo kinematics. *J Hand Surg Am*. 2014;39(11):2161–2167.

65. Lin JD, Karl JW, Strauch RJ. Trapeziometacarpal joint stability: the evolving importance of the dorsal ligaments. *Clin Orthop Relat Res*. 2014;472(4):1138–1145.

66. Gangata H, Ndou R, Louw G. The contribution of the palmaris longus muscle to the strength of thumb abduction. *Clin Anat*. 2010;23(4):431–436.

67. Ashurst JV, Turco DA, Lieb BE. Tenosynovitis caused by texting: an emerging disease. *J Am Osteopath Assoc*. 2010;110(5):294–296.

68. Ali M, Asim M, Danish SH, et al. Frequency of De Quervain's tenosynovitis and its association with SMS texting. *Muscles Ligaments Tendons J*. 2014;4(1):74–78.

69. Cantero-Téllez R, Martín-Valero R, Cuesta-Vargas A. Effect of muscle strength and pain on hand function in patients with trapeziometacarpal osteoarthritis. A cross-sectional study. *Reumatol Clin*. 2015;11(6):340–344.

70. Kuo LC, Chang JH, Lin CF, et al. Jar-opening challenges. Part 2: estimating the force-generating capacity of thumb muscles in healthy young adults during jar-opening tasks. *Proc Inst Mech Eng H.* 2009;223(5):577–588.

71. McQuillan TJ, Kenney D, Crisco JJ, et al. Weaker functional pinch strength is associated with early thumb carpometacarpal osteoarthritis. *Clin Orthop Relat Res.* 2016;474(2):557–561.

72. Fess EE. *Grip Strength.* 2nd ed. Chicago: American Society of Hand Therapists; 1992.

73. Bohannon RW, Bear-Lehman J, Desrosiers J, et al. Average grip strength: a meta-analysis of data obtained with a Jamar dynamometer from individuals 75 years or more of age. *J Geriatr Phys Ther.* 2007;30:28–30.

74. López-Bueno R, Andersen LL, Koyanagi A, et al. Thresholds of handgrip strength for all-cause, cancer, and cardiovascular mortality: a systematic review with dose-response meta-analysis. *Ageing Res Rev.* 2022;82:101778. https://doi.org/10.1016/j.arr.2022.101778. Epub 2022 Nov 1. PMID: 36332759.

75. Leong DP, Teo KK, Rangarajan S, et al. Prognostic value of grip strength: findings from the Prospective Urban Rural Epidemiology (PURE) study. *Lancet.* 2015;386(9990):266–273. https://doi.org/10.1016/S0140-6736(14)62000-6. Epub 2015 May 13. PMID: 25982160 .

76. Vargas-Pinilla OC, Rodríguez-Grande EI. Reproducibility and agreement between three positions for handgrip assessment. *Sci Rep.* 2021;11:12906. https://doi.org/10.1038/s41598-021-92296-8.

77. López-Bueno R, Andersen LL, Calatayud J, et al. Associations of handgrip strength with all-cause and cancer mortality in older adults: a prospective cohort study in 28 countries. *Age Ageing.* 2022;51(5):afac117. https://doi.org/10.1093/ageing/afac117. PMID: 35639798; PMCID: PMC9351371.

78. Kallman DA, Plato CC, Tobin JD. The role of muscle loss in the age-related decline of grip strength: cross-sectional and longitudinal perspectives. *J Gerontol.* 1990;45:M82–M88.

79. Hinson M, Gench BE. The curvilinear relationship of grip strength to age. *Occup Ther J Res.* 1989;9:53–60.

80. Janda DH, Geiringer SR, Hankin FM, et al. Objective evaluation of grip strength. *J Occup Med.* 1987;29(7):569–571.

81. Kozin SH, Porter S, Clark P, et al. The contribution of the intrinsic muscles to grip and pinch strength. *J Hand Surg Am.* 1999;24(1):64–72.

82. Massy-Westropp NM, Gill TK, Taylor AW, et al. Hand grip strength: age and gender stratified normative data in a population-based study. *BMC Res Notes.* 2011;4:127.

83. Ploegmakers JJ, Hepping AM, Geetzen JH, et al. Grip strength is strongly associated with height, weight and gender in childhood a cross sectional of 2241 children and adolescents providing reference values. *J Physiotherapy.* 2013;59(4):255–261.

Testing the Muscles of the Lower Extremity

Hip Flexion

Hip Flexion, Abduction, and External Rotation with Knee Flexion

Hip Extension

  Hip Extension Test to Isolate Gluteus Maximus

  Hip Extension Tests Modified for Hip Flexion Tightness

  Supine Hip Extension Test

Hip External Rotation

Hip Internal Rotation

Hip Abduction and Pelvic Stabilization

Hip Abduction from Flexed Position

Hip Adduction

Knee Flexion

  Hamstring Muscles in Aggregate

  Medial Hamstring Test (Semitendinosus and Semimembranosus)

Lateral Hamstring Test (Biceps Femoris)

Knee Extension

Ankle Plantar Flexion

  Gastrocnemius and Soleus Combined Test

Foot Dorsiflexion and Inversion

Foot Inversion

Foot Eversion with Plantar Flexion

Hallux and Toe Metatarsophalangeal (MP) Flexion

  Hallux MP Flexion

  Toe MP Flexion

Hallux and Toe DIP and PIP Flexion

Hallux and Toe MP and IP Extension

FIGURE 6.1

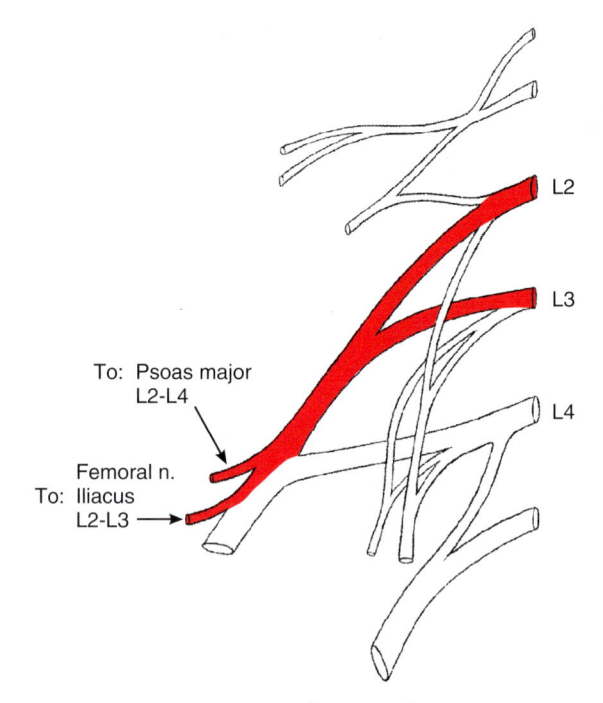

FIGURE 6.2 Innervation is L2-3 (primarily). From Mahan, M. A., Sanders, L. E., Guan, J., et al. (2017). Anatomy of psoas muscle innervation: Cadaveric study. *Clinical Anatomy. 30*(4):479–486.

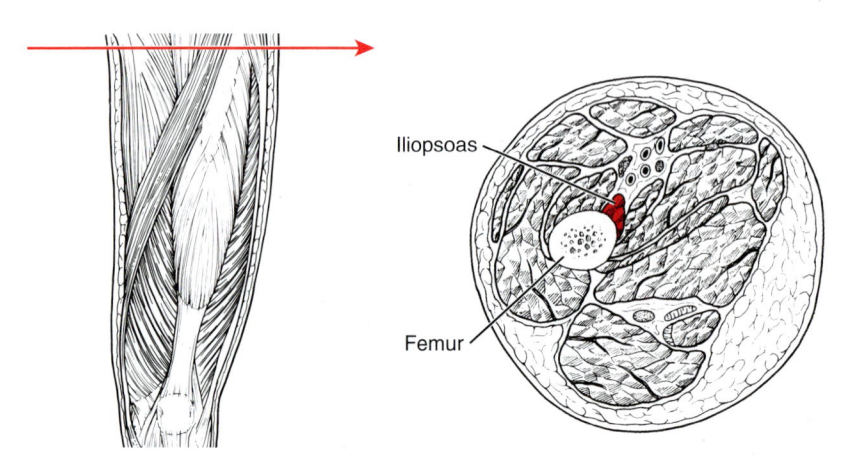

FIGURE 6.3 Arrow indicates level of cross section.

(Psoas major and Iliacus)

Range of Motion
0°–120°

Table 6.1 **HIP FLEXION**

I.D.	Muscle	Origin	Insertion	Function
176	**Iliacus**	Ilium (superior 1/3 of iliac fossa) Iliac crest (inner lip) Anterior sacroiliac and iliolumbar ligaments Sacrum (upper lateral surface)	Femur (lesser trochanter via insertion on tendon of the psoas major) Femoral shaft below lesser trochanter	Hip flexion up to 110° Internal rotation Abduct femur in external rotation Flexes pelvis on femur
174	**Psoas major**	L1-L5 vertebrae (transverse processes) T12-L5 vertebral bodies (sides) and their intervertebral discs	Femur (lesser trochanter)	Hip flexion with origin fixed Trunk flexion (sit-up) with insertion fixed (These two functions occur in conjunction with the iliacus) Hip external (lateral) rotation Flexion of lumbar spine (muscles on both sides) Lateral bending of lumbar spine to same side (muscle on one side)
177	Pectineus			Accessory in hip flexion
195	Sartorius			Hip flexion (combined with external rotation and abduction)
196	Rectus femoris			Hip flexion
185	Tensor fasciae latae			Hip flexion Hip abduction
Others				
180	Adductor brevis			Hip flexion
178	Gracilis			Hip flexion
184	Gluteus minimus (anterior fibers)			Hip flexion
175	Psoas minor	T12-L1 vertebral bodies (sides) and the intervertebral disc between them	Pecten pubis (i.e., pectineal line) Ilium (iliopectineal eminence and linea terminalis of the inner surface of the pelvis) Iliac fascia	Controversial

The iliopsoas muscle is a compound muscle consisting of the iliacus and the psoas major, which join in a common tendon of insertion on the lesser trochanter of the femur (Table 6.1). The psoas minor is a normal anatomical variant and is present in approximately 60% of people.[1] It cannot be tested clinically.

The function of the psoas is to connect the upper body to the lower body, the appendicular to the axial skeleton. The psoas major muscle has a biomechanical and postural function during moving and static states. It contributes to postural stability while standing erect and, when sitting, flexes the torso from a supine position. The iliopsoas and rectus femoris are also necessary for initiation and some continuation of leg swing during gait, contributing an estimated 10% of the net metabolic cost of walking.[2] Hip flexion strength was not found to be a significant predictor of or contributor to walking speed.[3] The function of the iliopsoas may be more important in transfer activities and stair climbing as well as in uphill running.[4]

HIP FLEXION

(Psoas major and Iliacus)

Grade 5, Grade 4, and Grade 3

Position of Patient: Short sitting with thighs fully supported on table and legs hanging over the edge. Patient may use arms to provide trunk stability by grasping table edge or with hands on table at each side (Fig. 6.4).

Instructions to Clinician: Stand next to leg to be tested. Ask patient to lift the thigh off the table. If adequate range is present (thigh clears the table), proceed to apply maximum resistance at midrange (Grade 5) over distal thigh just proximal to the knee joint, being careful not to grasp the thigh (see Fig. 6.4).

Test: Patient flexes hip to end of range, clearing the table and maintaining neutral rotation. Patient then brings the hip to midrange and holds that position against clinician's resistance, which is given in a downward direction toward the floor.

Instructions to Patient: "Sit tall and hold your thigh up. Don't let me push it down."

Grading

Grade 5: Patient holds test position against maximal resistance.

Grade 4: Patient holds test position against strong to moderate resistance. There may be some "give" with maximum resistance, making the grade a 4.

Grade 3: Patient completes test range and holds the position without added resistance (Fig. 6.5).

FIGURE 6.4

FIGURE 6.5

Clinical Relevance

The position of the pelvis influences the action of the hip flexors. An anterior or posterior pelvic tilt influences the length tension of the hip flexors, thereby making them appear stronger or weaker. To eliminate the influence of the pelvis, the pelvis and spine should be in neutral as in Fig. 6.4.

Grade 2

Position of Patient: Side lying with leg to be tested uppermost and supported by clinician (Fig. 6.6). Trunk and pelvis in neutral alignment. Lowermost leg may be flexed for stability. A powder board under the upper leg may be used instead of clinician supporting the leg.

Instructions to Clinician: Stand behind patient. Cradle test leg in one arm with hand support under the slightly flexed knee or use a powder board with patient's hip in slight extension and knee in slight flexion. Opposite hand stabilizes the hip and maintains trunk alignment (see Fig. 6.6).

Test Patient flexes hip with supported leg. Knee is permitted to flex to prevent hamstring tension.

Instruction to Patient: "Bring your knee up toward your chest."

Grading

Grade 2: Patient completes the range of motion in side-lying position without assistance.

Grade 1 and Grade 0

Position of Patient: Supine.

Instructions to Clinician: Stand at side of leg to be tested. Test leg is supported under calf with hand behind knee. Free hand palpates the muscle just distal to the inguinal ligament on the medial side of the sartorius (Fig. 6.7).

Test: Patient attempts to flex hip.

Instructions to Patient: "Try to bring your knee up to your nose."

Grading

Grade 1: Palpable contraction but no visible movement.

Grade 0: No discernable palpable contraction of muscle.

FIGURE 6.6

FIGURE 6.7

(Psoas major and Iliacus)

Substitutions

- Use of the sartorius will result in external rotation and abduction of the hip. The sartorius contraction will be seen because it is superficial and can be palpated along its entire length (Fig. 6.8).
- If the tensor fasciae latae substitutes for the hip flexors, internal rotation and abduction of the hip will result. The tensor may be seen and palpated at its origin on the anterior superior iliac spine.
- Patient may try to flex trunk as effort is made to flex hip or lean back to enhance length tension or the hip flexors.

FIGURE 6.8

Clinical Relevance

- The hip flexors are rather small muscles (see Fig. 6.3) and therefore do not provide a lot of force, especially compared with the quadriceps or gluteus maximus. Therefore, a negative break test is rarely achieved if using a straight-arm technique. Consequently, Fig. 6.4 shows the clinician with a bent arm while providing resistance. Experience is necessary to appreciate what constitutes a normal level of resistance.
- The hip flexors are prone to shortening as a consequence of prolonged sitting. Power generation is often reduced when a muscle is not at its optimal length. To increase the power generation ability of chronically shortened hip flexors, a contact-relax technique may be effective.
- Weak hip flexors during gait may be apparent by the substitution of hip external rotation or circumduction of the leg to advance the leg.
- Abdominal muscles serve as proximal stabilizers for the hip flexors, improving the efficiency of the hip flexors. If the abdominal muscles are weak and therefore not providing adequate stabilization during hip flexion contraction, the pelvis may rotate anteriorly.[4,5,5a]
- Hip flexor weakness may predict progression of mobility disability in older adults.[6]
- Hip flexor weakness may be improved through hip flexion resistance training through its full range.[7]
- Iliopsoas weakness, in a supine position, may be the earliest clinical sign of spinal stenosis but should be differentiated from ipsilateral hip joint degeneration.[8]

Suggested Strength Exercises for Iliopsoas

- Straight leg raise (SLR)
- Marching (high knees)
- Standing SLR
- V-sit up (flexing knees with semireclined trunk)

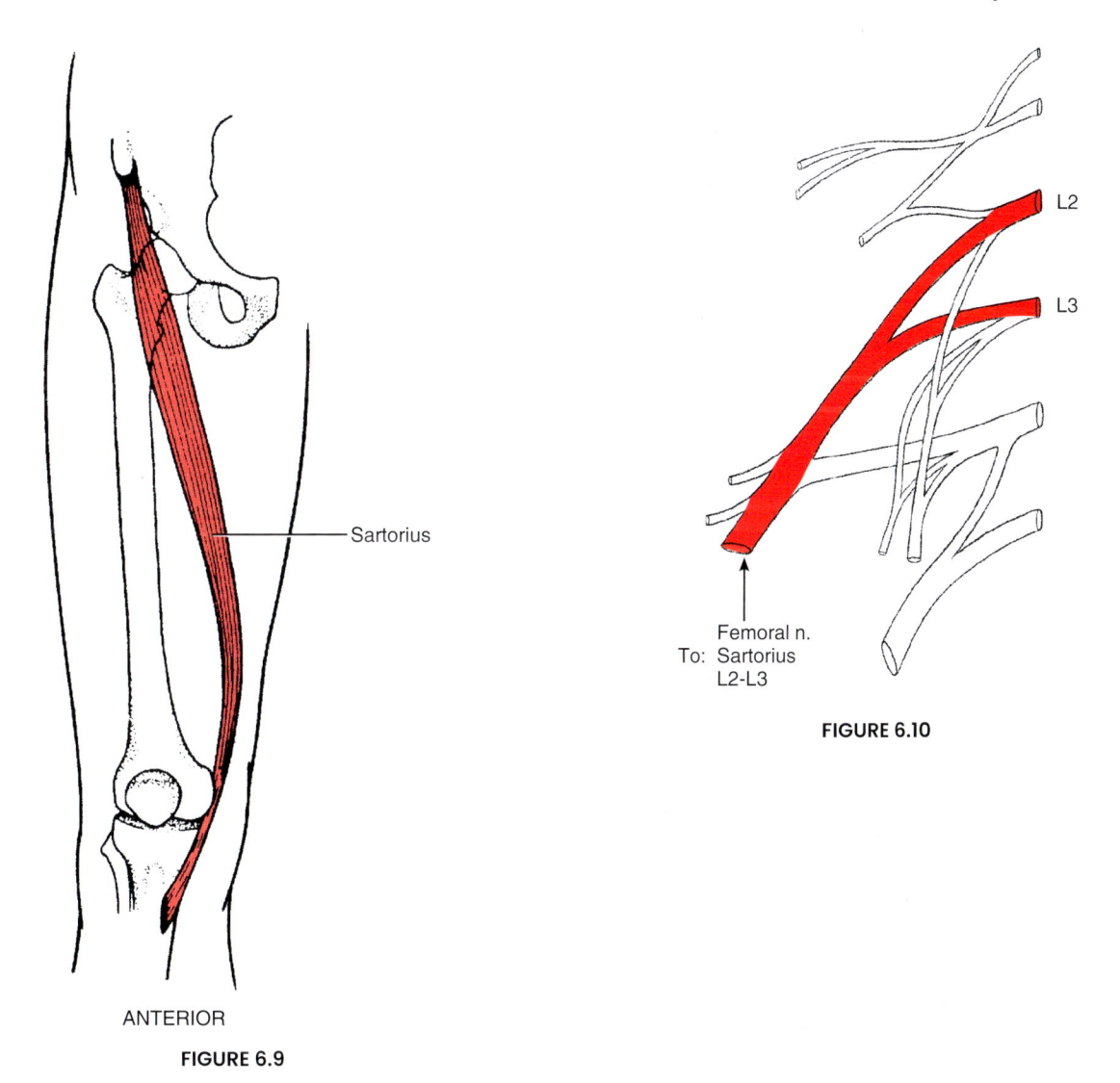

Sartorius

ANTERIOR

FIGURE 6.9

L2

L3

Femoral n.
To: Sartorius
L2-L3

FIGURE 6.10

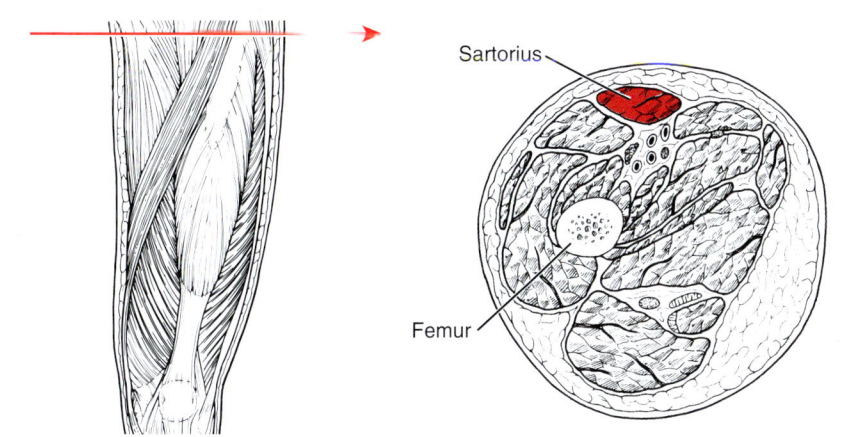

Sartorius

Femur

FIGURE 6.11 Arrow indicates level of cross section.

HIP FLEXION, ABDUCTION, AND EXTERNAL ROTATION WITH KNEE FLEXION

(Sartorius)

Table 6.2 HIP FLEXION, ABDUCTION, AND EXTERNAL ROTATION

I.D.	Muscle	Origin	Insertion	Function
195	Sartorius	Ilium (ASIS) Iliac notch below ASIS	Tibia (shaft, proximal medial surface) Capsule of knee joint (via slip) Aponeurosis	Hip external rotation, abduction, and flexion Knee flexion Knee internal rotation Assists in "tailor sitting"
Others				
	Hip and knee flexors			
	Hip external rotators			

ASIS, Anterior superior iliac spine.

The sartorius is the longest muscle in the body, crossing the thigh from the anterior superior iliac spine (ASIS) to the medial surface of the knee. The sartorius is considered a two-joint muscle. The word sartorius comes from the Latin word sartor, meaning tailor. The sartorius facilitates the movement of crossing one leg over the other one, as in a "tailor sit" (cross-legged sitting).

Grade 5, Grade 4, and Grade 3

Position of Patient: Short sitting with thighs supported on table and legs hanging over side. Arms may be used for support.

Instructions to Clinician: Stand lateral to the leg to be tested. Ask patient to flex, abduct, and externally rotate the hip, with the knee flexed. If adequate range is present, place one hand on the lateral side of the knee, the other hand over the medial-anterior surface of the distal leg (Fig. 6.12). Apply appropriate resistance with both hands, resisting hip flexion and abduction (in a down and inward direction) with the proximal hand and hip external rotation and knee flexion (up and outward) with the hand at the distal leg.

Test: Patient flexes, abducts, and externally rotates the hip while maintaining knee flexion (see Fig. 6.12).

Instructions to Patient: Clinician may demonstrate the required motion passively and then ask patient to repeat the motion, or clinician may place the leg in the desired test position.

"Hold it! Don't let me move your leg or straighten your knee."

Alternate instruction: "Slide your heel up the shin of your other leg."

Grading

Grade 5: Holds test position against maximal resistance; leg does not "give."

Grade 4: Tolerates moderate to strong resistance while maintaining position.

Grade 3: Completes movement and holds test position without resistance (Fig. 6.13).

FIGURE 6.12

FIGURE 6.13

HIP FLEXION, ABDUCTION, AND EXTERNAL ROTATION WITH KNEE FLEXION

(Sartorius)

Grade 2

Position of Patient: Supine. Heel of leg to be tested is placed on contralateral shin (Fig. 6.14).

Instructions to Clinician: Stand at side of leg to be tested. Support leg as necessary to maintain alignment.

Test: Patient slides test heel upward along shin to knee.

Instruction to Patient: "Slide your heel up to your knee."

Grading

Grade 2: Completes desired movement.

FIGURE 6.14

Clinical Relevance

- The clinician is reminded that failure of the patient to complete the full range of motion in the Grade 3 test is not an automatic Grade 2. The patient should be tested in the supine position to ascertain whether the correct grade is 2 or less.
- The abdominal muscles must generate a posterior pelvic tilt of sufficient force to neutralize the strong anterior pelvic tilt potential of the hip flexors.[5]
- In the presence of weakness, patients will attempt to substitute using the knee flexors, external rotators, and tensor fascia lata, but the movement would deviate out of the expected plane.

Grade 1 and Grade 0

Position of Patient: Supine.

Instructions to Clinician: Stand on side to be tested. Cradle test leg under calf with hand supporting leg behind knee. Opposite hand palpates sartorius on medial side of thigh where the muscle crosses the femur (Fig. 6.15). Clinician may prefer to palpate near the muscle origin just below the ASIS.

Test: Patient attempts to slide heel up shin toward knee.

Instruction to Patient: "Try to slide your heel up to your knee."

Grading

Grade 1: Clinician can detect slight contraction of muscle; no visible movement.

Grade 0: No discernable palpable contraction.

FIGURE 6.15

Substitution

Substitution by the iliopsoas or the rectus femoris results in pure hip flexion without abduction and external rotation.

Suggested Strength Exercises for the Sartorius Muscle

- Multidirectional lunge (forward, side, lateral)
- High-box step-ups
- Closed-stance squats
- Leg lifts with hip externally rotated

HIP EXTENSION

(Gluteus maximus)

Gluteus
maximus

Biceps femoris
(long head)

Semitendinosus

POSTERIOR

FIGURE 6.16

Semimembranosus

FIGURE 6.17

Inferior gluteal n.
To: Gluteus maximus
L5-S2

L4

L5

S1

S2

S3

S4

Sciatic

Tibial

Sciatic nerve, tibial part
To: Semimembranosus
L5-S2
Semitendinosus
L5-S2
Biceps femoris (long head)
L5-S2

FIGURE 6.18

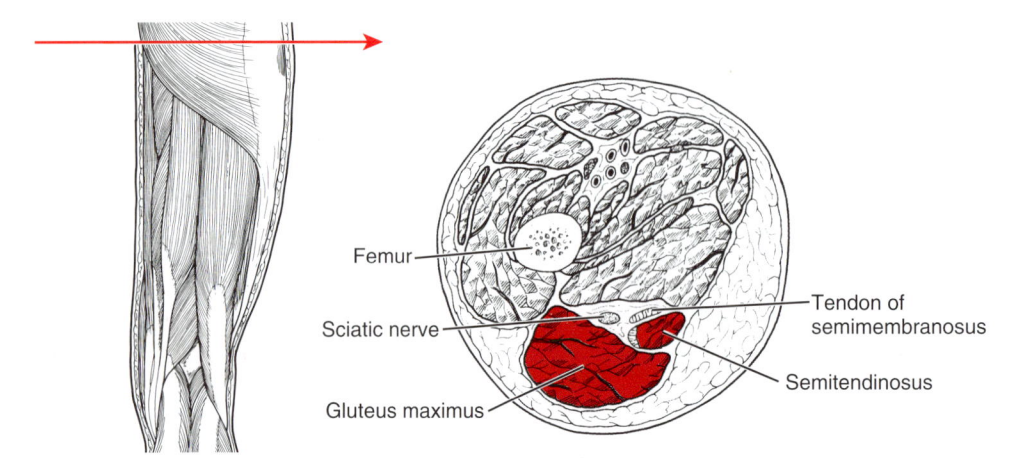

Femur

Sciatic nerve

Gluteus maximus

Tendon of
semimembranosus

Semitendinosus

FIGURE 6.19 Arrow indicates level of cross section.

Range of Motion
0°–20°
Some authors say as low as 0°–5°.

Table 6.3 HIP EXTENSION

I.D.	Muscle	Origin	Insertion	Function
182	Gluteus maximus	Ilium (posterior gluteal line) Iliac crest (posterior medial)	Femur (gluteal tuberosity)	Extends the thigh from a flexed position to in line with the body and raising the trunk from a flexed position)
		Sacrum (dorsal surface of lower part) Coccyx (side) Sacrotuberous ligament Aponeurosis over gluteus medius	Iliotibial tract of fascia lata	Hip external (lateral) rotation Posteriorly rotates pelvis
193	Semitendinosus	Ischial tuberosity (upper area, inferomedial impression via tendon shared with biceps femoris) Aponeurosis (between the two muscles)	Tibia (proximal medial shaft) Pes anserinus	Knee flexion Hip extension by assisting with raising the trunk from a flexed position Hip internal rotation (accessory)
194	Semimembranosus	Ischial tuberosity (superolateral impression)	Tibia (medial condyle, posterior aspect) Oblique popliteal ligament of knee joint Aponeurosis over distal muscle (variable)	Knee flexion Hip extension by assisting with raising the trunk from a flexed position Hip internal rotation (accessory)
192	Biceps femoris (long head)	Ischial tuberosity (inferomedial impression via tendon shared with semitendinosus) Sacrotuberous ligament	Fibula (head) Tibia (lateral condyle) Aponeurosis	Hip extension by assisting with raising the trunk from a flexed position and (weak) external rotation
181	Adductor magnus (posterior)		When the femur is flexed, this muscle can be a powerful extensor. In earlier anatomy texts, this muscle was classified as a fourth hamstring	
Others				
183	Gluteus medius (posterior)			

The gluteus maximus is the largest muscle in the body, accounting for 16% of the total cross-sectional area of the lower extremity.[9] Eighty percent of the gluteus maximus inserts into the iliotibial band. It has at least six regions within the muscle that respond to different movements. The action of the gluteus maximus is most effective in near full extension. Its pennate structure and long muscle length suggest it produces both high levels of force at low speeds through small ranges of motion and low levels of force at high speeds through large ranges of motion. It is a mix of slow and fast twitch fibers. It is often used to accelerate the body upward and forward from a position of hip flexion ranging from 40° to 60° (as in sprinting, squatting, and climbing a steep hill).[10]

The muscle test that will elicit the greatest force in the gluteus maximus is shown in Fig. 6.20, with the hip and knee extended. However, this muscle test position (Fig. 6.20) also implicates the hamstrings because of the effort required to keep the knee extended to resist the clinician's force at the ankle. The muscle test performed with the knee flexed (see Fig. 6.25) provides for isolation of the gluteus maximus, but a maximum contraction cannot be elicited in most patients in this position.

(Gluteus maximus)

Grade 5, Grade 4, and Grade 3 (Aggregate of All Hip Extensor Muscles)

Position of Patient: Prone. Arms may be at the side of the body or abducted to hold sides of table. (Note: If there is a hip flexion contracture, immediately go to the test described for hip extension modified for hip flexion tightness [see page 250].)

Instructions to Clinician: Stand at level of pelvis on side of leg to be tested. (Note: Fig. 6.20 shows clinician on opposite side to avoid obscuring activity.) Ask patient to lift the leg off the table as high as possible while keeping the knee straight. If sufficient range is achieved, place the hand providing resistance on the posterior leg just above the ankle. The opposite hand may be used to stabilize or maintain pelvis alignment in the area of the posterior superior spine of the ilium (see Fig. 6.20). This can be a demanding test on the clinician because of the size of the muscle and the length of the lever arm.

Alternate Position: The hand that gives resistance is placed on the posterior thigh just above the knee (Fig. 6.21). This alternate position is a less demanding test. Optimal resistance cannot be applied because of the shorter lever arm, and thus, the highest grade a patient can attain is a Grade 4.

This test is not recommended unless absolutely necessary (e.g., unstable, painful knee, above-knee amputee).

Test: Patient extends hip through entire available range of motion. Resistance is given straight downward toward the floor.

Instructions to Patient: "Lift your leg off the table as high as you can without bending your knee. Hold it!" (see Fig. 6.20).

Grading

Grade 5: Patient holds test position against maximal resistance.

Grade 4: Patient holds test position against strong to moderate resistance.

Grade 3: Completes range and holds the position without resistance (Fig. 6.22).

FIGURE 6.22

FIGURE 6.20

FIGURE 6.21

Clinical Relevance

Excessive knee flexion should be avoided when applying maximum force to avoid biasing the hamstrings. Testing the gluteus maximus with knee in full (but not locked) extension is the ideal position to elicit a maximum contraction.

Knowledge of the patient's hip joint range is imperative before manual tests of hip strength are conducted. If tightness in the hip flexor muscles exists, test results will be inaccurate in the hip-extended test positions. The alternate test position shown in Fig. 6.28 must be used to elicit the muscle's maximum effort in the presence of hip flexor tightness. This position will decrease the influence of the flexion contracture and will allow the patient to move against gravity through the available range. The supine hip extensor test can also be used (see page 252) and may be the most demanding of the hip extensor manual tests.

Grade 2

Position of Patient: Side lying with test leg uppermost. Knee straight. Lowermost leg is flexed for stability.

Instructions to Clinician: Stand behind patient at thigh level. Clinician supports test leg just below the knee, cradling the leg (Fig. 6.23). Opposite hand is placed over the pelvic crest to maintain pelvic and hip alignment.

Test: Patient extends hip through full range of motion.

Instructions to Patient: "Bring your leg back toward me. Keep your knee straight."

Grading

Grade 2: Completes available range of motion in side-lying position.

FIGURE 6.23

Clinical Relevance

- Because of the strength of the gluteus maximus, it is imperative that the clinician achieve an optimal position to use a straight-arm technique to apply as much force as the muscle can bear. Shorter clinicians may need to step up on a stool or lower the table to apply adequate resistance.
- The clinician should be aware that the gluteus maximus is one of the most powerful muscles in the body, and most clinicians will not be able to "break" a Grade 5 hip extension. Care should be taken not to overestimate a Grade 4 muscle.

Grade 1 and Grade 0

Position of Patient: Prone.

Instructions to Clinician: Stand at level of pelvis on side to be tested. Palpate the gluteus maximus with deep finger pressure over the center of the buttock, including the upper and lower fibers (Fig. 6.24). Asking patient to externally rotate the leg with the knee flexed may assist clinician to feel the contraction.

Test: Patient attempts to extend hip in prone position or tries to squeeze buttocks together.

Instructions to Patient: "Try to lift your leg from the table." OR "Squeeze your buttocks together."

Grading

Grade 1: Palpable contraction of gluteus maximus but no visible joint movement. Contraction of gluteus maximus will result in narrowing of the gluteal crease.

Grade 0: No discernable palpable contraction.

FIGURE 6.24

Substitutions

Rotation of pelvis. Having the patient turn his or her head to the opposite side will help prevent trunk rotation.

Flexion of the knee to substitute hamstrings for gluteus maximus. The gluteus maximus (page 248) and hamstring (page 275) isolation tests may be a better indicator of specific muscle action.

HIP EXTENSION

(Gluteus maximus)

HIP EXTENSION TEST TO ISOLATE GLUTEUS MAXIMUS

Grade 5, Grade 4, and Grade 3

Position of Patient: Prone with knee flexed to 90° and hip abducted and externally rotated. The abducted and externally rotated hip positions are difficult to visualize in Figs. 6.25 and 6.26. (Note: In the presence of a hip flexion contracture, do not use this test, but refer to the test for hip extension modified for hip flexion tightness [see page 250].)

Instructions to Clinician: Stand at the level of the pelvis on the side to be tested. (Note: Clinician in the illustration is shown on the wrong side to avoid obscuring test positions.) Ask patient to lift the thigh off the table as high as possible while bending the knee. If sufficient range is achieved, place the hand for resistance over the posterior thigh just above the knee. The opposite hand may stabilize or maintain the alignment of the pelvis (see Fig. 6.25).

For the Grade 3 test, the knee may be supported in flexion (by cradling at the ankle) if needed because of hamstring weakness.

Test: Patient extends the abducted and externally rotated hip through available extension range, maintaining knee flexion. Resistance is given in a straight downward direction (toward floor).

Instructions to Patient: "Lift your foot to the ceiling." OR "Lift your leg, keeping your knee bent."

Grading

Grade 5: Holds test position against maximal resistance.

Grade 4: Holds test position against strong to moderate resistance.

Grade 3: Completes available range of motion and holds test position but without resistance (see Fig. 6.26).

FIGURE 6.25

FIGURE 6.26

Grade 2

Position of Patient: Side lying with test leg uppermost. Knee is flexed and supported by clinician. Lowermost hip and knee should be flexed for stability (Fig. 6.27). Clinician provides stabilization and alignment through the uppermost hip by assuring that the pelvis and hip are in line with the shoulder.

Instructions to Clinician: Stand at the level of the pelvis behind patient. Clinician cradles uppermost leg with forearm. Other hand stabilizes pelvis in neutral alignment at the iliac crest.

Test: Patient extends hip with supported knee flexed.

Instruction to Patient: "Move your leg back toward me."

Grading

Grade 2: Completes available range of motion in side-lying position.

Grade 1 and Grade 0

This test is identical to the Grades 1 and 0 tests for aggregate hip extension (see Fig. 6.24). Patient is prone and attempts to extend the hip or squeeze the buttocks together while clinician palpates the gluteus maximus.

Clinical Relevance

- Hip extension range is less when the knee is flexed because of tension in the rectus femoris; therefore, a diminished hip extension range may be observed in tests that isolate the gluteus maximus.
- Often, cramping of the hamstrings will occur when the patient performs this test. The authors have found that decreasing knee flexion to 70° or applying resistance in the middle of the muscle belly during the test will decrease the likelihood of a cramp.
- Hip extension torque increases with hip flexion (increase of 41% with 15° hip flexion and 112% with 45° hip flexion [average of 1.9 Nm per degree of flexion]).[11]

FIGURE 6.27

HIP EXTENSION

(Gluteus maximus)

HIP EXTENSION TESTS MODIFIED FOR HIP FLEXION TIGHTNESS

Grade 5, Grade 4, and Grade 3

Position of Patient: Patient leans over the table with hips flexed so that the ASIS is "hooked" on the end of table (Fig. 6.28). The arms are used to "hug" the table for support. The knee of the non-test leg should be flexed to allow the test leg to rest on the floor at the start of the test.

Instructions to Clinician: Stand at side of leg to be tested. (Note: Fig. 6.28 shows clinician on the opposite side to avoid obscuring test positions.) Ask patient to lift his leg toward the ceiling. If sufficient range is achieved, place the hand used to provide resistance over the posterior thigh just above the knee. The opposite hand stabilizes the pelvis laterally to maintain hip and pelvis posture (see Fig. 6.28). Clinician's stabilizing hand may need to be placed over the hip to prevent the pelvis from rising (not shown).

Test: Patient extends hip through available range, but hip extension range is less when the knee is flexed. Keeping the knee in extension will test both the gluteus maximus and hamstrings; with the knee flexed, the gluteus maximus will be evaluated in isolation. Resistance is applied downward (toward floor).

Instruction to Patient: "Lift your foot off the floor as high as you can."

Grading

Grade 5: Holds test position against maximal resistance.

Grade 4: Holds test position against strong to moderate resistance.

Grade 3: Completes available range and holds test position without resistance.

Grade 2, Grade 1, and Grade 0

Do not test the patient with hip flexion contractures who has less than Grade 3 hip extensors in the standing position. Position patient side lying on the table. Conduct the test as described for the aggregate of extensor muscles (see page 249) or for the isolated gluteus maximus (see page 248).

Clinical Relevance

The modified hip extensor test is the preferred test for people who are not able or are unwilling to lie prone. This test may elicit a greater effort than the alternate supine hip extensor test.

FIGURE 6.28

CROSS SECTIONS OF THE THIGH

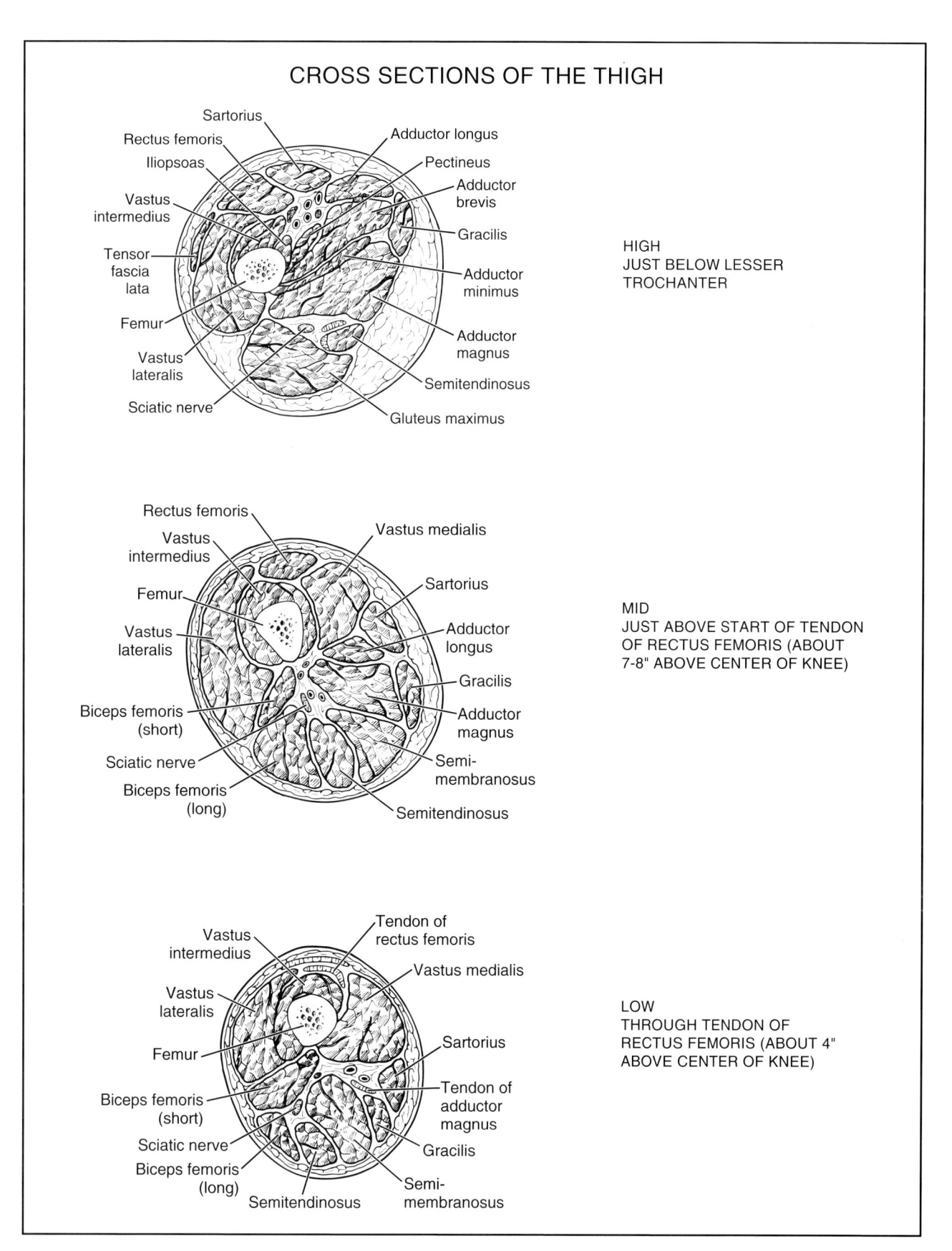

HIGH
JUST BELOW LESSER
TROCHANTER

MID
JUST ABOVE START OF TENDON
OF RECTUS FEMORIS (ABOUT
7-8" ABOVE CENTER OF KNEE)

LOW
THROUGH TENDON OF
RECTUS FEMORIS (ABOUT 4"
ABOVE CENTER OF KNEE)

PLATE 6

HIP EXTENSION

(Gluteus maximus)

SUPINE HIP EXTENSION TEST

An alternate test for the hip extensors (gluteus maximus and hamstrings) is the supine hip extension test. This supine test may be used to eliminate change of patient position or for those who cannot lie prone. Grades 5, 4, 3, and 2 have been validated in this position (*n* = 44 subjects) by measuring maximum hip extension torques recorded via a strain gauge dynamometer.[12]

Grade 5, Grade 4, Grade 3, and Grade 2

Position of Patient: Supine with heels off end of table. Arms folded across chest or abdomen. (Do not allow patient to push into table with upper extremities.)

Instructions to Clinician: Stand at end of table. Lift patient's leg to at least 65° of flexion. Determine patient's hip range by measuring from the heel to the table (Fig. 6.29). Approximately 35 inches from heel to table (approximately 65° of flexion) is necessary to perform this test and is the distance the leg should be lifted during the test. In a squat position (knees and hips bent and elbows straight), cup both hands under the heel and ask patient to push into clinician's hands, keeping the knee straight and hip locked (Fig. 6.30). Try to raise the leg to the height measured initially. Clinician will need excellent body mechanics to be able to resist this typically very strong muscle (Fig. 6.31). (Note: Ideally, the table should be lower than the one shown in these figures to allow for optimal clinician advantage and body mechanics.)

Test: Patient presses heel into clinician's cupped hands, attempting to maintain full extension of the leg as clinician raises the leg approximately 35 inches from the table. No instructions are given for the opposite leg except to relax.

Instructions to Patient: "Don't let me lift your leg from the table. Keep your hip locked tight (don't let it bend)."

FIGURE 6.29

FIGURE 6.30

FIGURE 6.31

Grade 5, Grade 4, Grade 3, and Grade 2 Continued

Grading

Grade 5: Hip locks in neutral (full extension) throughout this test. Pelvis and back elevate as one locked unit as clinician raises the leg (see Fig. 6.31). The opposite leg will rise involuntarily, illustrating a locked pelvis.

Grade 4: Hip flexes before pelvis and back elevate and lock as the leg is raised by clinician. Hip flexion should not exceed 30° before locking occurs (Fig. 6.32). The other leg will rise involuntarily but will have some hip flexion because the pelvis is not fully locked.

Grade 3: Full flexion of the hip to the end of the straight leg raising range (65° of hip flexion) with little or no elevation of the pelvis, demonstrated by the other leg remaining on the table. Clinician feels strong resistance throughout the test (Fig. 6.33).

Grade 2: Hip flexes fully with only minimal resistance felt (clinician should check to ensure that the resistance felt exceeds the weight of the leg; see Fig. 6.33).

There is no Grade 1.

Grade 0: Hip flexes fully with no active resistance felt by clinician as leg is raised. Clinician perceives that resistance is due to leg weight only.

Clinical Relevance

- To optimize the clinician's body mechanics and ability to generate sufficient force to resist this strong muscle action, the clinician should start in a squat position to enable elbows to be straight, necessitating the patient to be positioned on a low table or mat table.
- The supine hip extensor test was found to have higher hamstring activation than the unilateral bridge test.[13]
- When the trunk is held relatively stationary, contraction of the hip extensors and abdominal muscles function as a force couple to posteriorly tilt the pelvis.[5]
- Weight-bearing exercises with a greater base of stability (squats and lunges) may be implemented for more novice subjects, progressing to single-leg squats and step-up exercises.[14]

FIGURE 6.32

Suggested Strength Exercises for the Gluteus Maximus

Exercises are over 40% MVIC.[10] Exercises producing the greatest gluteus maximus EMG amplitude will be those performed in standing and place the gluteus maximus in a shortened position (pull-throughs, glute bridges, hip thrusts, horizontal back extensions).
- Sideways lunge
- Plank with bent knee hip extension
- Lateral step-up
- Transverse lunge
- Skater squat
- Quadruped with contralateral arm/leg lift (lifted knee bent or straight)
- Single-leg bridge (all knee angles and ankle angles)
- Barbell hip thrust
- Unilateral mini-squat
- Retro step-up
- Single-leg wall squat
- Single-leg squat with knee straight
- Single-leg deadlift
- Forward and lateral step down and up • Roman chair back extension

EMG, Electromyography; *MVIC,* maximum voluntary isometric contraction.

FIGURE 6.33

(Gluteus maximus [posterior])[5]

Obturator
externus

FIGURE 6.34

L3

L4

Inferior gluteal n.
To: Gluteus maximus
L5-S2

Obturator n.
To: Obturator
externus
L3-L4

L5

S1

S2

n. to
To: Piriformis
S1-S2

S3

S4

Sciatic

n. to Quadratus femoris
To: Quadratus femoris
L5-S1
Gemellus inferior
L5-S1

n. to Obturator internus
To: Obturator internus
L5-S1
Gemellus superior
L5-S1

FIGURE 6.36

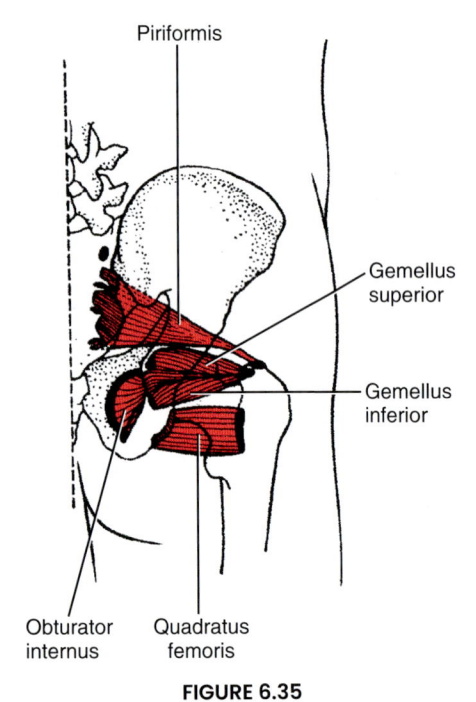

Piriformis

Gemellus
superior

Gemellus
inferior

Obturator
internus

Quadratus
femoris

FIGURE 6.35

Range of Motion
0°–35°[15]

Table 6.4 HIP EXTERNAL ROTATION[5a]

I.D.	Muscle	Origin	Insertion	Function
182	Gluteus maximus Posterior fibers	Ilium (posterior gluteal line and crest) Sacrum (dorsal and lower aspects) Coccyx (side) Sacrotuberous ligament Aponeurosis over gluteus medius	Femur (gluteal tuberosity) Iliotibial tract of fascia lata	Hip external (lateral) rotation Hip abduction with hip flexed (weak assist)
186	Piriformis	Sacrum (anterior surface) Ilium (gluteal surface near posterior inferior iliac spine) Sacrotuberous ligament Capsule of sacroiliac joint	Femur (greater trochanter, medial side)	Hip external (lateral) rotation Abducts the flexed hip (assist) (muscle probably too small to do much of this)
189	Gemellus superior (may be absent)	Ischium (spine, dorsal surface)	Femur (greater trochanter, medial surface) Blends with tendon of obturator internus	Hip external (lateral) rotation Hip abduction with hip flexed (accessory)
190	Gemellus inferior	Ischial tuberosity (upper part)	Femur (greater trochanter, medial surface) Blends with tendon of obturator internus	
187	Obturator internus	Pubis (inferior ramus) Ischium (ramus) Obturator fascia Obturator foramen (margin) Obturator membrane Upper brim of greater sciatic foramen	Femur (greater trochanter, medial) Tendon fuses with gemelli	Hip external (lateral) rotation Abduction of flexed hip (assist)
191	Quadratus femoris (may be absent)	Ischial tuberosity (external aspect)	Femur (quadrate tubercle on trochanteric crest)	Hip external (lateral) rotation
Others				
188	Obturator externus	Obturator membrane (external surface) Ischium (ramus) Pubis (inferior ramus) Pelvis (lesser pelvic cavity, inner surface)	Femur (trochanteric fossa)	Hip external (lateral) rotation Hip adduction (assist)
195	Sartorius			
192	Biceps femoris (long head)			
183	Gluteus medius (posterior)			
184	Gluteus minimus			

(Gluteus maximus [posterior])[5]

The gluteus maximus is potentially the most powerful external rotator of the hip, depending on its line of force.[16] The deep rotators are primarily responsible for stabilizing the hip. This stabilization can be visualized during an athletic cutting action when abruptly changing direction.[5]

Grade 5, Grade 4, Grade 3, and Grade 2

Position of Patient: Short sitting with thighs fully supported on table and legs hanging over the edge. (Trunk may be supported by placing hands flat or fisted at sides of chair or table [Fig. 6.37].)

Instructions to Clinician: Sit on a low stool or kneel beside leg to be tested. Ask patient to turn the leg in toward the other leg. If sufficient range is present, position leg in midposition between internal and external rotation. Place the hand providing resistance on the medial aspect of the ankle just above the malleolus (Fig. 6.38). The other hand, which will offer a stabilizing counterpressure, is contoured over the lateral aspect of the distal thigh just above the knee. The two forces are applied in counterdirections for this rotary motion (see Fig. 6.38).

Test: Patient externally rotates the hip.

Instructions to Patient: "Don't let me turn your leg out. Hold it!"

Grading

Grade 5: Holds test position in midrange against maximal resistance.

Grade 4: Holds test position in midrange against strong to moderate resistance.

Grade 3: Able to complete full range of motion with mild to no resistance (this is a gravity-eliminated position, so if patient is able to exert mild resistance, grade the effort a 3) (Fig. 6.39).

Grade 2: Completes full range of motion without resistance (this is a gravity-minimized position). Care needs to be taken to ensure that gravity is not the predominant force.

FIGURE 6.38

FIGURE 6.37

FIGURE 6.39

Grade 2 Alternate Test (If Patient Cannot Sit)

Position of Patient: Supine. Test leg is in internal rotation.

Instructions to Clinician: Stand at side of leg to be tested. Clinician may need to support the leg in internal rotation because gravity tends to pull the leg into external rotation.

Test: Patient externally rotates hip in available range of motion (Fig. 6.40). One hand may be used to maintain pelvic alignment at lateral hip.

Instruction to Patient: "Roll your leg out."

Grading

Grade 2: Completes external rotation range of motion. As the hip rolls past the midline, minimal resistance can be offered to offset the assistance of gravity.

Grade 1 and Grade 0

Position of Patient: Supine with test leg placed in internal rotation.

Instructions to Clinician: Stand at side of leg to be tested.

Test: Patient attempts to externally rotate hip.

Instruction to Patient: "Try to roll your leg out."

Grading

Grade 1 and Grade 0: The external rotator muscles, except for the gluteus maximus, are not palpable. If there is any discernable movement (contractile activity), a grade of 1 should be given; otherwise, a grade of 0 is assigned on the principle that whenever uncertainty exists, the lesser grade should be awarded.

Clinical Relevance

- There is wide variation in the amount of hip external rotation range that can be considered normal. It is imperative, therefore, that a patient's accurate range (in each test position) be known before manual muscle testing takes place. Muscles that are lengthened often test weak, which is why testing in the midposition between external rotation and internal rotation is recommended.[17]
- There is greater range of rotation at the hip when the hip is flexed than when it is extended, probably secondary to laxity of hip joint structures. Therefore, the sitting muscle test elicits a greater contraction than in prone.[18]
- In short-sitting tests, the patient should not be allowed to use the following motions, lest they add visual distortion and confound the test results:
  a. Lift the contralateral buttock off the table or lean in any direction to lift the pelvis;
  b. Increase flexion of the test knee;
  c. Abduct the test hip.
- The surgical posterior approach to hip arthroplasty cuts through at least part of the hip's posterior capsule, potentially disrupting several of the deep external rotator muscles. Insufficient repair of these external rotator muscle tendons can be a cause of hip dislocations.

Suggested Strength Exercises for Hip External Rotation

- Clamshell exercise against resistance
- Lateral step-up
- Seated external rotation against band or pulley

FIGURE 6.40

HIP INTERNAL ROTATION

(Gluteus minimus and medius; Tensor fasciae latae)

LATERAL

FIGURE 6.41

To: Superior gluteal n.
Gluteus medius
L4-S1
Gluteus minimus
L4-S1
Tensor fasciae latae
L4-S1

Gluteus minimus

FIGURE 6.42

Range of Motion
0°–40°[15]

Table 6.5 HIP INTERNAL ROTATION

I.D.	Muscle	Origin	Insertion	Function
184	Gluteus minimus (anterior fibers)	Ilium (outer surface between anterior and inferior gluteal lines) Greater sciatic notch	Femur (greater trochanter, anterior aspect) Fibrous capsule of hip joint	Hip abduction Hip internal (medial) rotation
185	Tensor fasciae latae	Iliac crest (outer lip) Fascia lata (deep) Anterior superior iliac spine (lateral surface)	Iliotibial tract (between its two layers ending 1/3 down femur)	Hip flexion Hip internal (medial) rotation
183	Gluteus medius (anterior fibers)	Ilium (outer surface between crest and posterior gluteal line) Gluteal fascia	Femur (greater trochanter, lateral surface)	Internal with hip flexion[17]
Others	Gluteus maximus (anterior fibers)			Internal rotator with hip flexed to 90°
193	Semitendinosus			
194	Semimembranosus			
180	Adductor brevis			
179	Adductor longus (position dependent)			

Unlike the external rotators, no one muscle stands out as the primary mover in internal rotation. Maximal-effort activity of the internal rotators increases as the hip approaches 90° of hip flexion.

Muscular imbalance, such as relative increased internal rotation and weakness of the abductors, external rotators, and hip extensors, often plays a role in biomechanical alignment at the knee.[5] Therefore, it is critical to consider the role of hip strength when knee pain or dysfunction is present.

Grade 5, Grade 4, Grade 3, and Grade 2

Position of Patient: Short sitting with thighs fully supported on table and legs hanging over the edge. (Trunk may be supported by placing hands flat or fisted at sides.)

Instructions to Clinician: Sit or kneel in front of patient. Ask patient to move the leg out, away from the other leg while maintaining hip stabilization. If sufficient range is present, position the leg in midposition between internal and external rotation. Place the hand providing resistance on the lateral surface of the ankle just above the malleolus (Fig. 6.43). The other hand, which offers counterpressure, is contoured over the medial surface of the distal thigh just above the knee. Stabilization is provided in a medially directed force at the knee, counteracting the lateral resistance provided at the ankle. Give resistance in a medially directed force at the ankle.

Test: The leg should be placed in midrange of hip rotation for best results (see Fig. 6.41).[17]

Instructions to Patient: "Don't let me turn your leg in. Hold it!"

Grading

Grade 5: Holds test position against maximal resistance.

Grade 4: Holds test position against strong to moderate resistance.

Grade 3: Able to complete full range of motion with mild to no resistance (this is a gravity-eliminated position, so if patient is able to exert mild resistance, grade the effort a 3) (Fig. 6.44).

Grade 2: Able to complete full range of motion but cannot tolerate resistance (this is a gravity-minimized position). Care needs to be taken to ensure that gravity is not the predominant force.

FIGURE 6.43

FIGURE 6.44

HIP INTERNAL ROTATION

(Gluteus minimus and medius; Tensor fasciae latae)

Alternate Grade 2 for Patient Who Cannot Sit

Position of Patient: Supine. Test leg in partial external rotation.

Instructions to Clinician: Stand next to test leg. Palpate the gluteus medius proximal to the greater trochanter and the tensor fasciae latae (Fig. 6.45) over the anterolateral hip below the ASIS.

Test: Patient internally rotates hip through available range.

Instruction to Patient: "Roll your leg in toward the other one."

Grading

Grade 2: Holds test position. As the hip rolls inward past the midline, minimal resistance can be offered to offset the assistance of gravity.

FIGURE 6.45

Grade 1 and Grade 0

Position of Patient: Patient supine with test leg placed in external rotation.

Instructions to Clinician: Stand next to test leg. One hand is used to palpate the gluteus medius (over the posterolateral surface of the hip above the greater trochanter). The other hand is used to palpate the tensor fasciae latae (on the anterolateral surface of the hip below the ASIS).

Test: Patient attempts to internally rotate hip.

Instruction to Patient: "Try to roll your leg in."

Grading

Grade 1: Palpable contractile activity in either or both muscles.

Grade 0: No discernable contractile activity.

Clinical Relevance

- The patient should not be allowed to extend the knee or adduct and extend the hip during performance of the test. These motions contaminate the test by offering visual distortion to the clinician.
- There is greater range of rotation at the hip when the hip is flexed than when it is extended, probably secondary to laxity of hip joint structures.
- In short-sitting tests, the patient should not be allowed to use the following motions, lest they add visual distortion and confound the test results:
  a. Lift the contralateral buttock off the table or lean in any direction to lift the pelvis;
  b. Increase flexion of the test knee;
  c. Adduct the test hip.

Suggested Strength Exercises for Hip Internal Rotation[19]

- Prone isometric with knee in 90° of flexion (can use opposite leg for resistance)
- Reverse clams

LATERAL

FIGURE 6.46

Superior gluteal n.
To: Gluteus medius
L4-S1
Gluteus minimus
L4-S1

L4

L5

S1

FIGURE 6.47

Range of Motion

0°–45°

Table 6.6 **HIP ABDUCTION**

I.D.	Muscle	Origin	Insertion	Function
183	Gluteus medius	Ilium (outer surface between crest and anterior and posterior gluteal lines) Fascia (over upper part)	Femur (greater trochanter, lateral aspect)	Pelvic stabilizer Hip abduction (in all positions) Hip internal rotation (anterior fibers) Hip external (lateral) rotation (posterior fibers) Hip flexion (anterior fibers) Hip extension (posterior fibers) as accessory functions
184	Gluteus minimus	Ilium (outer surface between anterior and inferior gluteal lines) Greater sciatic notch	Femur (greater trochanter, anterolateral ridge) Anterior and superior capsule of hip joint	Hip abduction Hip internal (medial) rotation
185	Tensor fasciae latae			
Others				
182	Gluteus maximus (upper fibers)			
195	Sartorius			
186	Piriformis			
196	Rectus femoris			

HIP ABDUCTION AND PELVIC STABILIZATION

(Gluteus medius and Gluteus minimus)

The gluteus medius is functionally divided into three parts: (1) anterior, (2) middle, and (3) posterior, each with separate branches from the superior gluteal nerve. Consequently, the three parts have different actions of rotation with abduction, dependent on the degree of hip flexion. The test described on page 262 captures all three parts during hip abduction. Functionally, the gluteus medius generates an exceptional amount of force, given its size.[10]

The greatest percentage of maximum voluntary contraction (MVC) in the gluteus medius was recorded during single-leg stance when the subject was simultaneously abducting the opposite leg, thus solidifying its primary as pelvic stabilizer during the single-leg support phase of gait.[20,21,5] Because of this stabilizing function, the gluteus medius generates the most force in a slightly abducted position rather than the maximally abducted position previously thought. In fact, the maximally abducted position, when the gluteus medius is at its shortest, is where the least force is generated.[5]

Grade 5, Grade 4, and Grade 3

Position of Patient: Side lying with test leg uppermost. Start test with the hip slightly extended beyond the midline and the pelvis rotated slightly forward (Fig. 6.48). Lowermost leg is flexed for stability.

Instructions to Clinician: Stand behind patient. Ask patient to lift the leg slightly past the width of the pelvis, giving verbal and tactile clues as necessary to keep the pelvis from rotating and the hip from flexing. If sufficient range is achieved, place hand used to give resistance at the ankle (Fig. 6.49). Applying resistance at the ankle creates a longer lever arm, thus requiring more patient effort to resist the movement. If patient cannot hold the leg against resistance at the ankle, then apply resistance at the lateral knee (Fig. 6.50). Clinician is reminded always to use the same lever in a given test sequence and in subsequent comparison tests.

FIGURE 6.49

FIGURE 6.48

FIGURE 6.50

(Gluteus medius and Gluteus minimus)

Test: Patient abducts hip without flexing the hip or rotating it in either direction. Resistance is given in a straight downward direction.

Instructions to Patient: "Lift your leg up and back. Hold it! Don't let me push it down."

Grading

Grade 5: Holds test position against maximal resistance at the ankle.

Grade 4: Holds test position against strong to moderate resistance at the ankle (the leg cannot hold the position) or with maximum resistance given at the knee.

Grade 3: Completes range of motion and holds test position without resistance (Fig. 6.51). Hip should not flex into frontal plane or rotate.

Grade 2

Position of Patient: Supine.

Instructions to Clinician: Stand on side of leg being tested. One hand supports and lifts the leg by holding it under the ankle or heel to raise leg just enough to decrease friction of the heel on the table surface. This hand offers no resistance, nor should it be used to offer assistance to the movement. On some smooth surfaces, such support may not be necessary (Fig. 6.52). (Note: Figs. 6.52 and 6.53 show clinician on opposite side of patient to avoid obscuring test positions.) The other hand palpates the gluteus medius just proximal to the greater trochanter of the femur (see Fig. 6.53).

Test: Patient abducts hip through available range.

Instructions to Patient: "Move your leg out to the side. Keep your kneecap pointing to the ceiling."

Grading

Grade 2: Completes range of motion supine with no resistance and minimal to zero friction.

FIGURE 6.52

FIGURE 6.51

FIGURE 6.53

HIP ABDUCTION AND PELVIC STABILIZATION

(Gluteus medius and Gluteus minimus)

Grade 1 and Grade 0

Position of Patient: Supine.

Instructions to Clinician: Stand at the side of the leg being tested at level of thigh. One hand supports the leg under the ankle just above the malleoli or at the heel. The hand should provide neither resistance nor assistance to movement (see Fig. 6.52). Palpate the gluteus medius on the lateral aspect of the hip just above the greater trochanter. The weight of the opposite leg stabilizes the pelvis. It is not necessary, therefore, to use a hand to manually stabilize the contralateral leg.

Test: Patient attempts to abduct hip.

Instruction to Patient: "Try to move your leg out to the side."

Grading

Grade 1: Palpable contraction of gluteus medius but no movement of the part.

Grade 0: No discernable contractile activity.

Substitutions

- Hip-hike substitution: If testing in the supine position, the patient may "hip hike" by approximating pelvis to thorax using the lateral trunk muscles, which moves the leg through partial abduction range (Fig. 6.54). This movement may be detected by observing the lateral trunk and hip (move clothing aside) and palpating the gluteus medius above the trochanter.
- External rotation and flexion (sartorius) substitution: The patient may try to externally rotate during the motion of abduction (Fig. 6.55). This could allow the oblique action of the hip flexors to substitute for the gluteus medius.
- Tensor fasciae latae substitution: If the test is allowed to begin with active hip flexion or with the hip positioned in flexion, there is an opportunity for the tensor fasciae latae to abduct the hip.

FIGURE 6.54

FIGURE 6.55

Clinical Relevance

- The force required to stabilize the body is about 2× the body weight, the majority of which is produced by the hip abductors.[5] The clinician should not be able to "break" a Grade 5 muscle (resistance applied at the knee), and most clinicians will not be able to "break" a Grade 4 muscle with a minimum of 100 pounds of push force required for a valid test.

- A patient should be able to stand on one leg, keeping the pelvis level with a muscle grade of 4 or 5. The inability to do so results in a gluteus medius limp, whereby the pelvis drops on the opposite side of the weakness. In gait, a pelvic drop would occur in every step. If weakness is bilateral, you will see the equivalent of a "waddling" gait where the pelvis drops on each side, with each step. A waddling gait is a sign of marked gluteus medius weakness.

- When a hip flexion contracture of 30° or more is present, the gluteus medius is compromised as an abductor, as its anterior fibers are now in the plane of flexion instead of abduction.

- Hip abductor and lateral rotator weakness can lead to knee valgus, hip adduction, and hip internal rotation, positions that can put undue stress on lower extremity joints.

- Hip compression forces can be three times the body weight while walking and five to six times body weight while running or ascending or descending stairs.[22,22a]

- Gluteus medius strength is associated with stair ascend/descend and five-chair rise test performance. In the presence of gluteus medius weakness, patients will display a gluteus medius limp during stair ascent. A gluteus medius limp is particularly prevalent in inactive older adults and those with hip osteoarthritis or arthroplasties.

- Strengthening the hip abductors in the presence of knee osteoarthritis reduces symptoms.[23]

- Tears or degenerative changes of the attachment of the gluteus medius and minimus may be a source of pain, often attributed to trochanteric bursitis.[5]

- Gluteus medius and minimus atrophy is greater in people with fall-related hip/pelvic fractures (odds ratio = 2.15).[24]

- The weight of the leg alone results in greater external peak torque during side-lying hip abduction than during most other hip abductor exercises.[25]

- The clamshell exercise may be most appropriate for early rehabilitation (motor control and recruitment) but is not sufficient for strengthening, particularly for the anterior and middle segments.[26]

Suggested Hip Abduction Strengthening Exercises (>40% MVIC)[10,27,28]

Lateral and forward step-up
- Quadruped with contralateral arm and leg lift
- Standing hip abduction (all three portions and gluteus minimus)
  - Open chain and isometric
- Supine single-leg bridge (middle portion and gluteus minimus)
- Wall squat (anterior portion)
- Side bridge to neutral spine position
- Standing erect pelvic drop with knee straight (all three portions)
- Single-leg deadlift
- Single-leg squat
- Side bridge with hip abduction
- Side-lying hip abduction with internal rotation (middle portion)

MVIC, Maximum voluntary isometric contraction.

HIP ABDUCTION FROM FLEXED POSITION

(Tensor fasciae latae)

Tensor
fascia lata

LATERAL

FIGURE 6.56

Superior gluteal n.
To: Tensor fasciae latae
L4-S1

L4

L5

S1

FIGURE 6.57

Tensor
fascia lata

Femur

FIGURE 6.58 Arrow indicates level of cross section.

Range of Motion

No specific range of motion can
be assigned solely to the tensor.

Table 6.7 **HIP ABDUCTION FROM FLEXION**

I.D.	Muscle	Origin	Insertion	Function
185	**Tensor fasciae latae**	Iliac crest (outer lip) Fasciae latae (deep) Anterior superior iliac spine (lateral surface)	Iliotibial tract (between its two layers, ending 1/3 of the way down)	Hip flexion Hip internal (medial) rotation
Others				
183	Gluteus medius			
184	Gluteus minimus			

(Tensor fasciae latae)

The tensor fascia latae (TFL) is the smallest of the three primary hip abductors, accounting for about 11% of the total abductor muscle cross-sectional area. The TFL lies inferior to the iliotibial band, originating at the anterior iliac crest and becoming fused with the fibers of the iliotibial band distally, generally below the greater trochanter. While the abductor function of the TFL has little consensus, it is generally thought the TFL helps to stabilize the opposite hip from the one that is bearing weight when walking, running, or standing, assisting the gluteus medius. It also contributes to hip internal rotation, hip flexion, and knee stabilization by affecting the amount of tension in the iliotibial band.[29] The test position described in Fig 6.59 will minimize the contribution of the gluteus medius. There are no test positions below grade 3 because of the inability to isolate the TFL. The ilio-tibial band is not a muscle in that it does not contact.[29]

Grade 5, Grade 4, and Grade 3

Position of Patient: Side lying. Uppermost leg (test leg) is flexed to 45° and lies across the lowermost leg with the foot resting on the table (Fig. 6.59).

Instructions to Clinician: Stand behind patient at level of pelvis. Ask patient to flex hip and lift leg to 30°. If successful, place hand for resistance on lateral surface of the thigh just above the knee. Hand providing stabilization is placed on the crest of the ilium (Fig. 6.60).

Test: Patient abducts hip through approximately 30° of motion with hip flexed 45°. Resistance is given downward (toward floor) from the lateral surface of the distal femur.

Instructions to Patient: "Lift your leg. Hold it! Don't let me push it down."

Grading

Grade 5: Holds test position against maximum resistance.

Grade 4: Holds test position against strong to moderate resistance.

Grade 3: Completes movement; holds test position but without resistance (Fig. 6.61).

FIGURE 6.60

FIGURE 6.59

FIGURE 6.61

(Adductor magnus)

Adductor brevis

Pectineus

Adductor longus

Adductor magnus

Gracilis

ANTERIOR

FIGURE 6.62

FIGURE 6.63

Femoral n.
To: Pectineus
L2-L3

Obturator n.
To: Adductor magnus
L2-L4
Adductor brevis
L2-L4
Adductor longus
L2-L4
Gracilis
L3-L4

FIGURE 6.64

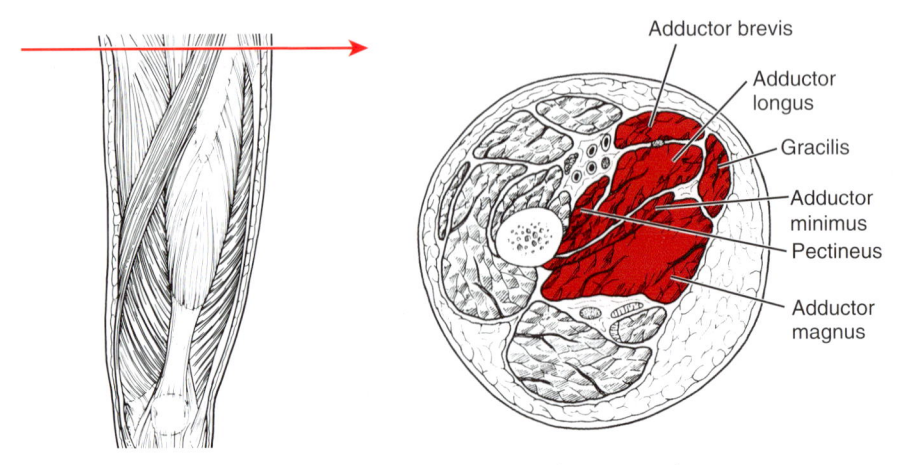

Adductor brevis

Adductor longus

Gracilis

Adductor minimus

Pectineus

Adductor magnus

FIGURE 6.65 Arrow indicates level of cross section.

Range of Motion

0°–15°–20°

Table 6.8 HIP ADDUCTION

I.D.	Muscle	Origin	Insertion	Function
181	Adductor magnus	Ischial tuberosity (inferolateral) Ischium (inferior ramus) Pubis (inferior ramus) Fibers from pubic ramus to femur (gluteal tuberosity), often named the Adductor minimus	Femur (linea aspera via aponeurosis, medial supracondylar line, and adductor tubercle on medial condyle)	Hip adduction Hip extension from a position of hip flexion toward extension (inferior fibers) Hip flexion (superior fibers; weak) if the hip is moving from extension toward flexion[5] The role of the adductor magnus in rotation of the hip is dependent on the position of the thigh
180	Adductor brevis	Pubis (body and inferior ramus)	Femur (via aponeurosis to linea aspera)	Hip adduction Hip flexion
179	Adductor longus	Pubis (anterior aspect between crest and symphysis)	Femur (linea aspera via aponeurosis)	Hip adduction Hip flexion (accessory) Hip rotation (depends on position of thigh)
177	Pectineus	Pubic pectin Fascia of pectineus	Femur (on a line from lesser trochanter to linea aspera)	Hip adduction Hip flexion (accessory)
178	Gracilis	Pubis (body and inferior ramus) Ischial ramus	Tibia (medial shaft distal to condyle) Pes anserinus Deep fascia of leg	Hip adduction Knee flexion Internal (medial) rotation of knee (accessory)
Others				
188	Obturator externus			
182	Gluteus maximus (posterior fibers)			
192	Biceps femoris (long head)			
196-200	Quadratus femoris			

The adductor muscles are organized into three layers. The pectineus adductor longus and gracilis occupy the superficial layer. The middle layer is occupied by the adductor brevis. The deep layer is occupied by the massive adductor magnus. The adductor magnus comprises 63% of the mass of adductor volume.[30] The hip adductors function in all three planes of the hip and are required to work under both closed-chain (e.g., in the stance leg, with the axial compression forces from gravity) and open-chain conditions (e.g., during kicking). The adductor longus may be more active than the adductor magnus during open-chain activities. The adductor magnus is most active in weight-bearing tasks such as sit to stand and walking up stairs and during loading and initial contact phases of gait.[31]

HIP ADDUCTION

(Adductor magnus)

Grade 5, Grade 4, and Grade 3

Position of Patient: Side lying with test leg (lowermost) resting on the table.

Instructions to Clinician: Stand behind patient at knee level. Support uppermost leg (non-test leg) in 25° of abduction with forearm, the hand supporting the leg on the medial surface of the knee (Fig. 6.66). Alternatively, the upper leg can be placed on a padded stool straddling the test leg and approximately 9 to 12 inches high (not shown). Ask patient to lift the bottom leg to the uppermost one. If successful, place hand giving resistance on the medial surface of the distal femur of the lower leg, just proximal to the knee joint. Resistance is directed straight downward toward the table (Fig. 6.67).

Test: Patient adducts hip until the lower leg contacts the upper one.

Instructions to Patient: "Lift your bottom leg up to your top one. Hold it! Don't let me push it down."

For Grade 3: "Lift your bottom leg up to your top one. Don't let it drop!"

Grading

Grade 5: Holds test position against maximal resistance.

Grade 4: Holds test position against strong to moderate resistance.

Grade 3: Completes full range; holds test position but without resistance (Fig. 6.68).

FIGURE 6.66

FIGURE 6.68

FIGURE 6.67

Grade 2

Position of Patient: Supine. The non-test leg is positioned in some abduction to prevent interference with motion of the test leg.

Instructions to Clinician: Stand at side of test leg at knee level. One hand supports the ankle and elevates it slightly from the table surface to decrease friction as the leg moves across the table (Fig. 6.69). Clinician uses this hand neither to assist nor resist motion. The opposite hand palpates the adductor mass on the inner aspect of the proximal thigh. In the supine test position for Grades 2, 1, and 0, the weight of the opposite leg stabilizes the pelvis, so there is no need for manual stabilization of the non-test hip.

Test: Patient adducts hip without rotation. Toes stay pointed toward the ceiling.

Instruction to Patient: "Bring your leg in toward the other one."

Grading

Grade 2: Patient adducts leg through full range with gravity minimized.

FIGURE 6.69

(Adductor magnus)

Grade 1 and Grade 0

Position of Patient: Supine.

Instructions to Clinician: Stand on side of test leg. One hand supports the leg under the ankle. The other hand palpates the adductor mass on the proximal medial thigh (Fig. 6.70).

Test: Patient attempts to adduct hip.

Instruction to Patient: "Try to bring your leg in."

Grading

Grade 1: Palpable contraction, no leg movement.

Grade 0: No discernable palpable contraction.

FIGURE 6.70

Substitution

Hip flexor substitution: The patient may attempt to substitute the hip flexors for the adductors by internally rotating the hip (Fig. 6.71). The patient will appear to be trying to turn supine from side lying. Maintenance of true side lying is necessary for an accurate test.

FIGURE 6.71

Clinical Relevance

- Greater atrophy of the adductor magnus muscle occurs with bed rest, alluding to its function as a hip stabilizer.[31]
- The adductor muscles produce an extensor torque when the hip is markedly flexed, assisting the primary hip extensors. When the hip is flexed, the adductors augment the other extensor muscles.[5] As an example, when runners were permitted to use foot blocks in the Olympics during the 1930s (or dig a trough to permit a crouch position), times for the 100-m race were notably reduced (improved), as the adductors contributed explosive force to bring the femur from flexion toward extension.

Suggested Strengthening Exercises for Hip Adductors

- Ball squeeze with hip in neutral (long lever)[32]
- Copenhagen exercise[33] (side lying, top leg is stabilized on weight bench, perform side bridge on elbow, then adduct bottom leg to top leg)
- Side-lying hip adduction

Suggested Strengthening Exercise for Pectineus
- Supine hip flexion[34]

L4

L5

S1

S2

S3

Common
peroneal

Sciatic

Tibial

Sciatic (tibial) n.
To: Semimembranosus
L5-S2
Semitendinosus
L5-S2
Biceps femoris (long head)
L5-S2

Sciatic (common peroneal) n.
To: Biceps femoris (short head)
L5-S2

FIGURE 6.74

Biceps
femoris

Semitendinosus

Semimembranosus

POSTERIOR

FIGURE 6.72

FIGURE 6.73

Range of Motion
0°–135°

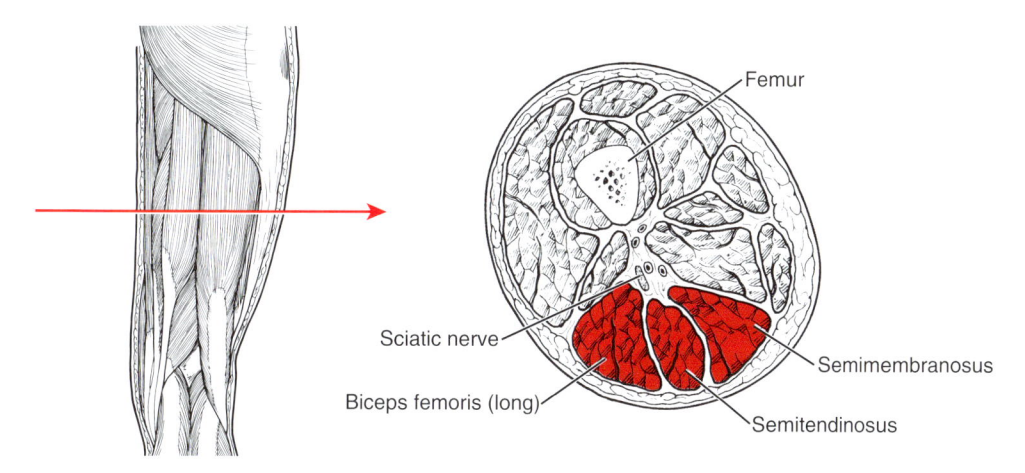

Femur

Sciatic nerve

Biceps femoris (long)

Semimembranosus

Semitendinosus

FIGURE 6.75 Arrow indicates level of cross section.

KNEE FLEXION

(All hamstring muscles)

Table 6.9 **KNEE FLEXION**

I.D.	Muscle	Origin	Insertion	Function
192	**Biceps femoris**			Knee flexion Hip extension Knee external rotation
	Long head	Ischium (tuberosity) Sacrotuberous ligament	Aponeurosis (posterior) Fibula (head, lateral aspect) Fibular collateral ligament	Hip extension and external rotation (long head)
	Short head	Femur (linea aspera and lateral condyle) Lateral intermuscular septum	Tibia (lateral condyle)	Knee flexion
193	**Semitendinosus**	Ischial tuberosity (inferior medial aspect) Tendon via aponeurosis shared with biceps femoris (long)	Tibia (proximal shaft) Pes anserinus Deep fascia of leg	Knee flexion Knee internal rotation Hip extension Hip internal rotation (accessory)
194	**Semimembranosus**	Ischial tuberosity Sacrotuberous ligament	Distal aponeurosis Tibia (medial condyle) Oblique popliteal ligament of knee joint	Knee flexion Knee internal rotation Hip extension Hip internal rotation (accessory)
Others				
178	Gracilis			
185	Tensor fasciae latae (knee flexed more than 30°)			
195	Sartorius			
202	Popliteus			
205	Gastrocnemius			
207	Plantaris			

The hamstring muscle group is comprised of three individual muscles, the semitendinosus, semimembranosus, and biceps femoris that originate at the hip and attach at the tibia and fibula by crossing the knee and thus are considered two-joint muscles. The hamstrings play a prominent role in hip extension (especially in control of the pelvis and trunk over the femur) and knee flexion and are activated during the final 25% of the swing phase of gait. They also provide dynamic stabilization of the knee joint. The maximal-effort knee flexion torque is greatest in the last 20° of full extension and declines steadily as the knee is progressively flexed, with the greatest flexor leverage at 50° to 90° of knee flexion.[35]

Grade 5, Grade 4, and Grade 3

There are three basic muscle tests for the hamstrings at Grades 5 and 4. The clinician should test first for the aggregate of the three hamstring muscles (with the foot in midline). Only if there is deviation (or asymmetry) in the movement or a question in the clinician's mind is there a need to test the medial and lateral hamstrings separately. The hamstrings are two-joint muscles and should be tested in midrange (50° to 90° of knee flexion).

HAMSTRING MUSCLES IN AGGREGATE

Position of Patient: Prone with legs straight and toes hanging over the edge of the table. A towel roll placed just above the knee may make this position more comfortable (not shown in Fig. 6.76).

Instructions to Clinician: Stand next to leg to be tested. Ask patient to flex the knee as far as possible. Observe possible tightness in the rectus femoris that may be indicated by limited knee flexion or hip flexing. If sufficient range is present, place leg between 50° and 90° of knee flexion (midrange). Hand provides resistance on posterior surface of the leg just above the ankle (Fig. 6.76). The other hand provides stabilization over the hamstring tendons on the posterior thigh (optional). Firm pressure with the stabilizing hand may offset any cramping of the hamstring muscles. Resistance is applied in the direction of knee extension for Grades 5 and 4.

Test: Patient holds knee between 50° and 90° of knee flexion while maintaining leg in neutral rotation.

Instructions to Patient: "Hold it! Don't let me straighten it."

MEDIAL HAMSTRING TEST (SEMITENDINOSUS AND SEMIMEMBRANOSUS)

Position of Patient: Prone with knee flexed to between 50° and 90° of knee flexion. Leg in internal rotation (toes pointing toward midline).

Instructions to Clinician: Clinician resists knee flexion at the ankle using a downward and outward force (Fig. 6.77).

Test: Patient flexes knee, maintaining the leg in internal rotation (heel toward clinician, toes pointing toward midline).

Instructions to Patient: "Hold it! Don't let me straighten it."

FIGURE 6.76

FIGURE 6.77

KNEE FLEXION

(All hamstring muscles)

Grade 5, Grade 4, and Grade 3 Continued

LATERAL HAMSTRING TEST (BICEPS FEMORIS)

Position of Patient: Prone with knee flexed between 50° and 90° of knee flexion. Leg is in external rotation (toes pointing laterally).

Instructions to Clinician: Clinician resists knee flexion at the ankle using a downward and inward force (Fig. 6.78).

Test: Patient flexes knee, maintaining leg in external rotation (heel away from clinician, toes pointing toward clinician) (see Fig. 6.76).

Instructions to Patient: "Hold it! Don't let me straighten it."

Grading the Hamstring Muscles (Grade 5, Grade 4, and Grade 3)

Grade 5 for All Three Tests: Patient holds test position against maximal resistance.

Grade 4 for All Three Tests: Holds test position against strong to moderate resistance.

Grade 3 for All Three Tests: Patient completes full range of motion without external resistance (Fig. 6.79).

Grade 2

Position of Patient: Side lying with test leg (uppermost leg) supported by clinician or resting on suitable height stool. Lower leg flexed for stability.

Instructions to Clinician: Stand behind patient at knee level. One arm is used to cradle thigh, providing hand support at medial side of knee. Other hand supports the leg at the ankle just above the malleolus (Fig. 6.80).

Test: Patient flexes knee through available range of motion.

Instruction to Patient: "Bend your knee."

FIGURE 6.79

FIGURE 6.78

Grade 2

FIGURE 6.80

Grading

Grade 2: Completes available range of motion in side-lying position, with gravity minimized.

Grade 1 and Grade 0

Position of Patient: Prone. Legs are straight with toes extending over end of table. Knee is partially flexed and supported at ankle by clinician.

Instructions to Clinician: Stand next to test leg at knee level. (Clinician shown on opposite side to avoid obscuring test position.) One hand supports the flexed leg at the ankle (Fig. 6.81). The opposite hand palpates both the medial and the lateral hamstring tendons just above the posterior knee.

Test: Patient attempts to flex knee.

Instruction to Patient: "Try to bend your knee."

Grading

Grade 1: Tendons become prominent, but no visible movement occurs.

Grade 0: No discernable contraction of the muscles; tendons do not stand out.

FIGURE 6.81

Substitutions

- Hip flexion substitution: The prone patient may flex the hip to start knee flexion. The buttock on the test side will rise as the hip flexes, and the patient may appear to roll slightly toward supine (Fig. 6.82).
- Gastrocnemius substitution: Do not permit the patient to strongly dorsiflex in an attempt to use the tenodesis effect of the gastrocnemius.

FIGURE 6.82

Clinical Relevance

- Hamstring muscle strain injuries have the highest prevalence in sport and especially in track and field. One of the proposed risk factors for acute hamstring injuries in track and field athletes is muscle weakness during concentric and/or eccentric contractions. The hamstring muscles act as hip extensors and knee flexors during both stance and swing phase of sprinting, the most common mechanism of injury in track-and-field athletes. They work eccentrically during the late stance phase of gait and during the late swing phase of overground running.[36]
- If the biceps femoris is stronger than the medial hamstrings, the leg will externally rotate during knee flexion. Similarly, if the semitendinosus and semimembranosus are the stronger components, the leg will internally rotate during knee flexion. This is the situation that, when observed, indicates asymmetry and the need to test the medial and lateral hamstrings separately.
- If the hip flexes at the end of the knee flexion range of motion, check for a tight rectus femoris muscle because this tightness will limit the range of knee motion.
- The optimum quadriceps to hamstring strength ratio of 1:1 has been proposed as a rehabilitation goal in many types of knee injuries, especially the anterior cruciate ligament–deficient and repaired knee.

Suggested Strength Exercises for Hamstrings

- Single-leg deadlifts
- Slide leg curl[36]
- Good mornings with at least 25% body weight[37]
- Nordic hamstring exercise
- Eccentric leg curls

(Quadriceps)

Rectus femoris

FIGURE 6.83

Vastus intermedius

Vastus medialis*

Vastus lateralis

ANTERIOR

FIGURE 6.84

*Illustration does not differentiate the long and oblique heads of the vastus medialis.

L2

L3

L4

Femoral n.
To: Quadriceps femoris
(all five heads)
L2-L4

FIGURE 6.85

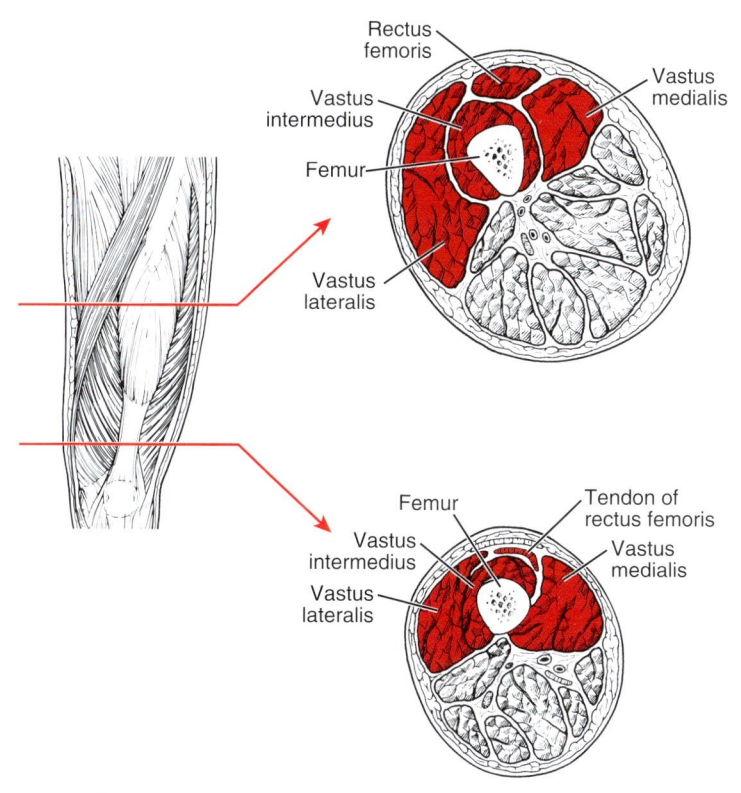

Range of Motion

135° to −2°15

FIGURE 6.86 Arrows indicate level of cross section.

Table 6.10 KNEE EXTENSION

I.D.	Muscle	Origin	Insertion	Function
196	Rectus femoris	Ilium (anterior inferior iliac spine) Acetabulum (groove above) Capsule of hip joint Aponeurosis (anterior)	Aponeurosis (posterior) Patella (base via quadriceps tendon) Tibial tuberosity via ligamentum patellae	Knee extension Hip flexion (by rectus femoris, which crosses the hip joint)
197	Vastus lateralis	Femur Linea aspera (lateral lip) Greater trochanter (inferior) Intertrochanteric line (via aponeurosis) Gluteal tuberosity (lateral lip) Lateral intermuscular septum	Aponeurosis (deep surface, distal) Patella (base and lateral border via quadriceps tendon) Lateral expansion to capsule of knee joint and iliotibial tract Tibial tuberosity via ligamentum patellae	Knee extension (none of the heads functions independently)
198	Vastus intermedius	Femur (shaft, upper 2/3 lateral and anterior surfaces) Intermuscular septum (lateral)	Aponeurosis (anterior forming deep quadriceps tendon) Patella (base, lateral aspect) Tibia (lateral condyle) Tibial tuberosity via ligamentum patellae	Knee extension (none of the heads function independently)
199	Vastus medialis longus (two parts)	Femur (linea aspera, medial lip; intertrochanteric line) Origin of vastus medialis oblique Tendon of adductor magnus Intermuscular septum (medial)	Aponeurosis (deep) Patella (medial border) Tibial tuberosity via ligamentum patellae	Knee extension (none of the heads functions independently)
200	Vastus medialis oblique (considered part of the vastus medialis) (see Fig. 6.86)	Femur: linea aspera (distal); supracondylar line Tendon of adductor magnus Intermuscular septum	Aponeurosis to capsule of knee joint Patella (medial aspect) Quadriceps tendon (medial) Tibial tuberosity via ligamentum patellae	Knee extension (none of the heads functions independently)

(Quadriceps)

The vastus group of muscles produces about 80% of the total extension torque of the knee, and the rectus femoris produces about 20%.[5] The vastus lateralis is the strongest member of the vastus group, estimated to contribute 40% of the overall strength of the quadriceps.[38] Together, the quadriceps muscles produce about two-thirds greater torque than the knee flexor muscles.[5] Maximal knee extension torque occurs between 45° and 70° of knee flexion (midrange), with less torque produced at the near extremes of flexion and extension.[5]

The quadriceps femoris muscles are tested together as a functional group. None of the four muscle heads can be separated from any other by manual muscle testing. The rectus femoris may be partially isolated from the other quadriceps during a hip flexion test. At one time, the vastus medialis was thought to be activated during the terminal 15° of knee extension; however, this has been conclusively disproven.[39-41]

Grade 5, Grade 4, and Grade 3

Position of Patient: Short sitting. Place a towel roll under patient's distal thigh for comfort. Patient's hands rest on the table on either side of the body for stability or may grasp the table edge. Patient should be allowed to lean backward slightly to relieve hamstring muscle tension. Do not allow patient to hyperextend the knee because this may lock the knee into position, thus masking weakness.

Note: The authors recommend the use of 30° of knee flexion, which is the lower end of midrange where the quadriceps generate the most force. Because this muscle group can be difficult to resist in a break test, the recommended joint angle may provide a slight advantage to the clinician to generate maximum patient force while achieving a break test.

Instructions to Clinician: Stand at side of leg to be tested. Ask patient to straighten the knee. If sufficient range is present, position the knee in approximately 30° of knee flexion (midrange). Place the palm of the hand providing resistance over the anterior surface of the distal leg just above the ankle, using a straight-arm technique because of the potential strength of these muscles.

For Grades 5 and 4, resistance is applied in a downward direction toward the floor (Fig. 6.87).

Test: Patient extends knee through available range of motion but not beyond 0°.

Instructions to Patient: "Hold it! Don't let me bend it."

Helpful Hint

To prevent the patient's pelvis from rising (a common occurrence in a Grade 4 or 5 test), the patient may be secured to the testing surface by a belt or strap (not shown).

Grading

Grade 5: Holds test position against maximal resistance. Clinician should not be able to break the Grade 5 knee extensors.

Grade 4: Holds test position against strong to moderate resistance.

Grade 3: Completes available range, including the last 15° (Fig. 6.88).

FIGURE 6.87

FIGURE 6.88

Grade 2

Position of Patient: Side lying with test leg uppermost. Lowermost leg may be flexed for stability. Leg to be tested is held in about 90° of knee flexion. The hip should be in full extension.

Instructions to Clinician: Stand behind patient at knee level. One arm cradles the test leg around the thigh with the hand supporting the underside of the knee (Fig. 6.89); alternatively, the test leg may be placed on a powder board. The other hand holds the leg just above the malleolus.

Test: Patient extends knee through the available range of motion. Clinician supporting the leg provides neither assistance nor resistance to patient's voluntary movement.

Instruction to Patient: "Straighten your knee."

Grading

Grade 2: Completes available range of motion.

Grade 1 and Grade 0

Position of Patient: Supine.

Instructions to Clinician: Stand next to leg to be tested at knee level. Hand used for palpation should be on the quadriceps tendon just above the knee with the tendon "held" gently between the thumb and fingers. Clinician also may want to palpate the patellar tendon just below the knee (Fig. 6.90).

Test: Patient attempts to extend knee.

As an alternate test, clinician may place one hand under the slightly flexed knee; palpate either the quadriceps or the patellar tendon while patient tries to extend the knee.

Instructions to Patient: "Push the back of your knee down into the table." OR "Tighten your kneecap" (quadriceps setting).

For Alternate Test: "Push the back of your knee down into my hand."

Grading

Grade 1: Contractile activity can be palpated in muscle through the tendon. No joint movement occurs.

Grade 0: No discernable contractile activity.

FIGURE 6.90

FIGURE 6.89

KNEE EXTENSION

(Quadriceps)

Clinical Relevance

- To assess functional strength, the quadriceps can be tested by a chair stand test (see description in Chapter 8, page 340) where strength equal to half the body weight is needed to rise from a chair unassisted (no arm use).[42]
- Knowledge of the patient's knee flexion range of motion is useful before conducting tests for knee extension strength because tight (shortened) hamstrings will limit knee extension. The shorter the hamstrings, the greater the backward trunk lean in short sitting.
- A combined force of 1.1 N/m/kg^{-1} is the minimum strength threshold of the knee extensors required for walking.[3] Knee extensor strength contributes to maximum walking speed; however, strength greater than a combined knee extensor force of 2.3 N/m/kg^{-1} is considered reserve and does not further increase maximum walking speed.
- To avoid overgrading the quadriceps, quantitative methods can be used such as handheld muscle dynamometry (Chapter 9) or a one-repetition maximum leg press (see Chapter 7). These tests have age- and sex-appropriate reference scores.

Suggested Strength Exercises for Quadriceps

- Squats (knee angle and hip position will selectively recruit different quad muscles)
- Back squats
- Split squats
- Single-leg press
- Lunges

Gastrocnemius

Soleus

POSTERIOR

FIGURE 6.91

FIGURE 6.92

L5

S1

S2

Sciatic

Tibial

Tibial n.
To: Soleus
S1-S2

Tibial n.
To: Gastrocnemius
S1-S2

FIGURE 6.93

Tibia

Fibula

Soleus

Gastrocnemius
(lateral)

Gastrocnemius
(medial)

FIGURE 6.94 Arrow indicates level of cross section.

Range of Motion
0°–45°

ANKLE PLANTAR FLEXION

(Gastrocnemius and Soleus)

Table 6.11 PLANTAR FLEXION

I.D.	Muscle	Origin	Insertion	Function
206	Soleus	Fibula (head, posterior aspect, and proximal 1/3 of shaft) Tibia (soleal line and middle 1/3 of medial shaft) Aponeurosis between tibia and fibula over popliteal vessels Aponeurosis (anterior)	Aponeurosis (posterior; tendinous raphe in midline of muscle) Tendo calcaneus when tendon of soleus joins tendon of gastrocnemius Calcaneus via Tendo calcaneus	Ankle plantar flexion Foot inversion
205	Gastrocnemius			Ankle plantar flexion Knee flexion (accessory) Foot eversion
	Medial head	Femur (medial condyle, popliteal surface) Capsule of knee joint	Anterior aponeurosis Tendo calcaneus (tendon of Achilles) formed when tendon of gastrocnemius joins tendon of soleus	
	Lateral head	Femur (lateral condyle, lateral surface, and supracondylar line) Capsule of knee joint Aponeurosis (posterior)	Calcaneus (posterior)	
Others				
204	Tibialis posterior			
207	Plantaris			
208	Fibularis longus			
209	Fibularis brevis			
213	Flexor digitorum longus			
222	Flexor hallucis longus			

The gastrocnemius and soleus muscles make up the triceps surae group. They differ in structure, anatomical position, function, and fiber-type characteristics. The medial gastrocnemius is the larger of the two heads. The gastrocnemius has 49% type 1 fibers compared to 80% in the soleus. This difference in fiber type makes the gastrocnemius more amenable to faster, more explosive movements, while the soleus is more active during lower-intensity and longer-duration activities.[43] Because of the architecture and size of the soleus, the soleus generates the most force of any skeletal muscle, generating 2.5 to 3 times the force as the gastrocnemius. The soleus is isolated by flexing the knee during heel rise (Fig. 6.95).

GASTROCNEMIUS AND SOLEUS COMBINED TEST

Grade 5, Grade 4, and Grade 3

Position of Patient: Patient stands on leg to be tested with knee extended, facing a wall. Patient is likely to need external support; thus, fingers can be placed on the wall, above shoulder height. Alternatively, no more than one or two fingers should be used on a table (or other horizontal surface) to avoid assisting the lifting motion. (Fig. 6.96).

Instructions to Clinician: Assess range of motion of the ankle to assure sufficient range is present. Demonstrate heel rise to patient. Then, stand or sit with a lateral view of test leg to ascertain height of heel rise. Ask patient to lift heel while keeping knee straight. If patient can clear the floor by 2 inches, ask patient to continue lifting the heel until patient can no longer achieve 1 inch of rise. This is when the test is terminated. Patient should not bear weight through arms.

FIGURE 6.95

FIGURE 6.96

(Gastrocnemius and Soleus)

Grade 5, Grade 4, and Grade 3 Continued

Test: Patient raises heel from floor consecutively through maximum available range at a rate of one rise every 2 seconds until patient no longer achieves 50% of initial plantar range (Fig. 6.97).

Instructions to Patient: "Stand on one leg. Lift your heel. Now lower. Repeat this as many times as possible, lifting your heel as high as you can." Repeat test for other leg, if both are tested.

FIGURE 6.97

Grading

Grade 5: Patient successfully completes 25 heel rises through full range of motion without a rest between rises.[44,45] Twenty-five heel rises elicit approximately 60% of the maximum electromyographic activity of the plantar flexors.[20] In the current standardized tests that have been in use for many years, 25 repetitions is the accepted reference score. However, a more recent study suggests that the average number of repetitions in the sample studied is less than 25 repetitions (Table 6.12).[46] Clinicians should be aware that strength deficits in the plantar flexors are common, particularly with advancing age, and strength deficits will affect the heel rise portion of the gait cycle and thus reduce gait speed.

Grade 4: A grade of 4 is conferred when patient completes between 2 and 24 heel rises of at least 50% of initial heel raise height at a consistent rate of one rise every 2 seconds using correct form in all repetitions. The criterion for Grade 4 is not well defined.

Grade 3: Able to hold body weight once in a heel-up position with full range, but unable to raise body weight from neutral more than one time.

If patient cannot complete at least one correct full-range heel rise in the standing position, the grade must be less than 3. Regardless of the force of resistance in a nonstanding position for any reason, patient must be given a grade of less than 3.[44]

Table 6.12 AVERAGE VALUES OF UNTRAINED SUBJECTS

	MALES (BY AGE)				FEMALES (BY AGE)			
	Lunsford and Perry[46]	Jan et al.[47]	Jan et al.[47]	Jan et al.[47]	Lunsford and Perry[46]	Jan et al.[47]	Jan et al.[47]	Jan et al.[47]
Age (mean or range)	34.7 (8.5)	21–40	41–60	61–80	29.3 (5.0)	21–40	41–60	61–80
Mean repetitions	27.8 (11.5)	22.1 (9.8)	12.1 (6.6)	4.1 (1.9)	28.4 (9.8)	16.1 (6.7)	9.3 (3.6)	2.7 (1.5)
Range of repetitions	6–70	9–46	4–30	0–7	7–51	6–30	5–19	0–5
80th percentile		17	7	2		10	5	1

(Gastrocnemius and Soleus)

Grade 2

Position of Patient: Prone with feet off end of table.

Instructions to Clinician: Stand at foot of patient. Ask patient to flex and extend ankle to assure sufficient range is present. Hand giving resistance is placed against the plantar surface at the level of the metatarsal heads with foot in 80° of dorsiflexion. These muscles are capable of tremendous force, which is why a more stable point of resistance is needed (Fig. 6.98).

Test: Patient plantar flexes ankle against manual resistance.

Instructions to Patient: "Point your foot down, like a ballet dancer. Don't let me push them up."

Grading

Grade 2: Holds test position against maximal manual resistance. Because of the functional strength of these muscles, clinician should not expect to break the contraction in a Grade 2 prone test.

Grade 1 and Grade 0

Position of Patient: Prone with feet off end of table.

Instructions to Clinician: Stand at end of table in front of foot to be tested. One hand palpates gastrocnemius-soleus activity by monitoring tension in the Achilles tendon just above the calcaneus (Fig. 6.99). The muscle bellies of the two muscles also may be palpated (not illustrated).

Test: Patient attempts to plantar flex the ankle.

Instruction to Patient: "Point your toes down, like a ballet dancer."

Grading

Grade 1: Able to move through partial range. Contractile activity may be palpated in muscle bellies. The best location to palpate the gastrocnemius is at midcalf with thumb and fingers on either side of the midline but above the soleus. Palpation of the soleus is best done on the posterolateral surface of the distal calf. In most people with calf strength of Grade 3 or better, the two muscles can be observed and differentiated during plantar flexion testing because their definition is clear.

Grade 0: No discernable palpable contraction.

FIGURE 6.98

FIGURE 6.99

ANKLE PLANTAR FLEXION

(Gastrocnemius and Soleus)

Clinical Relevance

- Patient may try to flex knee and rock forward to ball of foot to raise heel from floor in standing test, which indicates weakness in the gastrocnemius (Grade 2 or less).
- If, for any reason patient cannot lie prone for Grades 2, 1, or 0, an alternative for any of these tests is to use the supine position for non–weight-bearing testing. The highest grade awarded in this case is a Grade 2.
- During standing plantar flexion tests, the tibialis posterior and the fibularis longus and brevis muscles must be of sufficient strength (Grades 5 or 4) to stabilize the forefoot to attain and hold the tip-toe position.
- It may be advantageous to use a wall to brace clinician while resisting plantar flexion in the prone position. However, even with clinician stabilization, manual testing or handheld dynamometry of this muscle group in prone or supine is not reliable.
- Care must be taken to avoid transferring weight through the fingertips used for balance. Therefore, it is recommended to place patient's arms at shoulder height or higher on the wall in front of patient. Patient should maintain a fully erect posture. If patient leans forward or flexes the knee, such posture can bring the heel off the ground, creating a testing artifact.
- Reference data for children (5 to 12) are[47]:
- Ages 5 to 6: 12.5 ± 5.4
- Ages 7 to 8: 18.1 ± 3.6
- Ages 9 to 10: 22.3 ± 8.0
- Ages 11 to 12: 31.6 ± 12.5
- Young women who wear shoes with a heel height of at least 5 cm for 40 hours or more per week for 1 year demonstrate decreased strength and power in the soleus and reduced ankle range.[48]
- Updated results of the heel rise test of 600 subjects of various physical activity levels performed on a 10° incline demonstrated median number of heel rise repetitions decreased with age in younger individuals (<age 60 years) but not in older individuals (60 to 80 years). Median number of repetitions also decreased with lower physical activity levels and higher body mass index, and the median number of heel raises are substantially higher for older individuals than the data shown in Table 6.12.[49]
- The medial gastroc generates more force than the lateral gastroc (79.2% MVIC, 68.9% MVIC respectively) in a standing heel raise the toe out position.[49a]

Suggested Strength Exercises for Gastrocnemius and Soleus

- Straight leg heel raises for gastrocnemius[43]
- Seated calf raise for soleus[43]
- Agility drills on toes

CROSS SECTIONS OF THE LEG

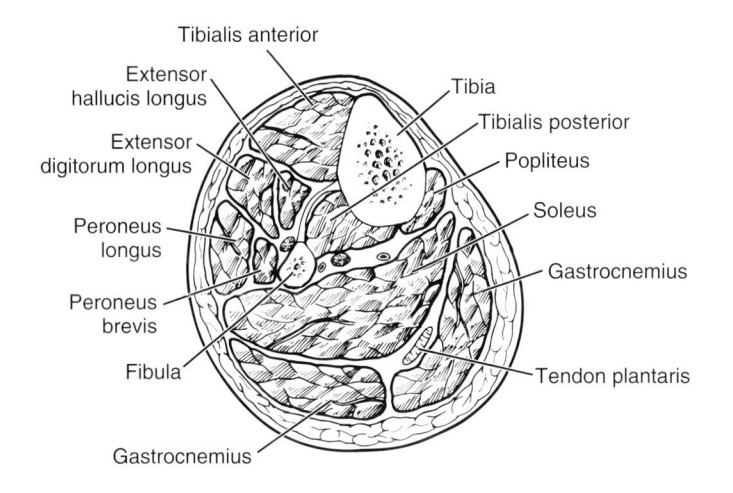

MID LEG
AT UPPER PORTION OF
GASTROCNEMIUS AND
SOLEUS AT LARGEST
CIRCUMFERENCE OF CALF

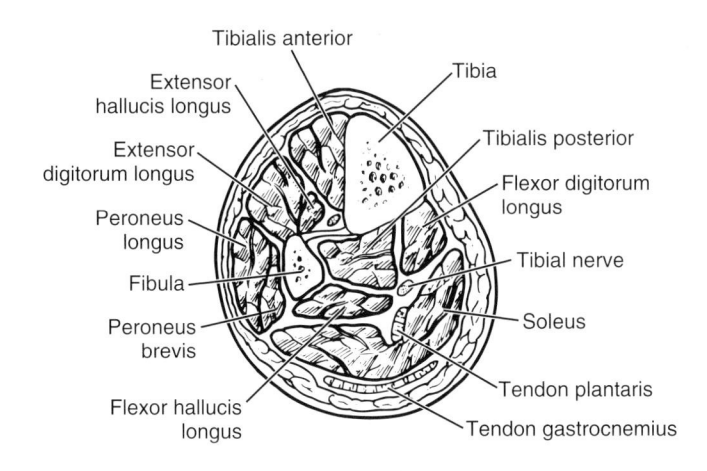

LOWER LEG
NEAR END OF MUSCULAR
PORTIONS OF TRICEPS
SURAE. GASTROCNEMIUS
IS ALL TENDINOUS.

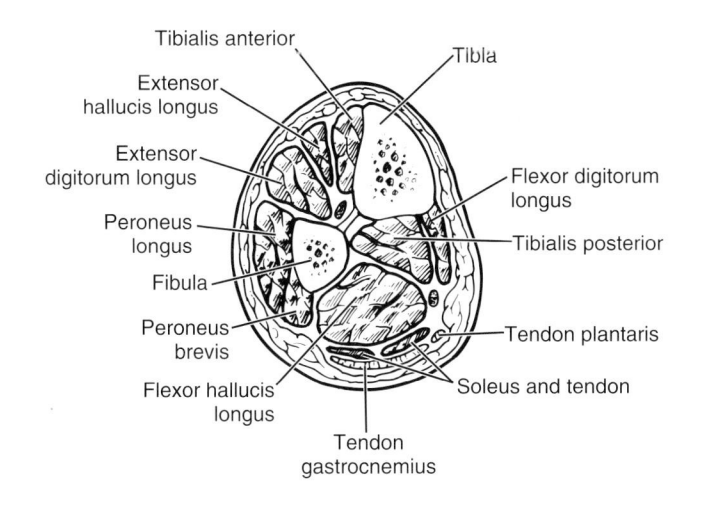

HIGH ANKLE
LOWER LEG WHERE
GASTROCNEMIUS,
SOLEUS, AND PLANTARIS
ARE TENDINOUS

PLATE 7

(Tibialis anterior)

Tibialis anterior

ANTERIOR

FIGURE 6.100

L4
L5
S1

Deep peroneal n.
To: Tibialis anterior
L4-S1

FIGURE 6.101

Tibialis anterior   Tibia

FIGURE 6.102 Arrow indicates level of cross section.

(Tibialis anterior)

Range of Motion

0°–25°[15]

Table 6.13 FOOT DORSIFLEXION AND INVERSION

I.D.	Muscle	Origin	Insertion	Function
203	Tibialis anterior	Tibia (lateral condyle and proximal 2/3 of lateral shaft) Interosseous membrane Fascia cruris (deep) Intermuscular septum	1st (medial) cuneiform (on medial and plantar surfaces) 1st metatarsal (base)	Ankle dorsiflexion (talocrural joint) Foot inversion and adduction (supination) at subtalar and midtarsal joints Supports medial-longitudinal arch of foot in walking
Others				
210	Fibularis (peroneus) tertius			Ankle dorsiflexion Foot eversion (accessory)
211	Extensor digitorum longus			
221	Extensor hallucis longus			

Ankle dorsiflexion strength and range are critical functions of gait and balance[50] and, therefore, of mobility. Many diseases and conditions, such as stroke, some types of cancer, idiopathic peripheral neuropathy, diabetes mellitus, and cerebral palsy, can produce ankle dorsiflexion weakness. Extreme weakness can result in foot drop. Reduced ankle strength, power, and range are factors in falls in people of all ages, especially in older adults. Reduced ankle strength and power are also factors in ankle instability that can increase risk for ankle sprains.

All Grades

Position of Patient: Supine. (Note: The authors recommend the supine position for this test, rather than an antigravity position, because of the mechanical advantage it affords the clinician when providing adequate resistance to this very strong muscle.)

Instructions to Clinician: Stand at foot of patient with patient's heel resting on table. Ask patient to bring the foot up and in, toward the body (Fig. 6.103). If sufficient range exists, place hand providing resistance on the medial aspect of the foot over the first ray. Resistance is

FIGURE 6.103

(Tibialis anterior)

All Grades Continued

provided down and out (Fig. 6.104). This is a strong muscle, so applying resistance with the hand and flexed forearm can help provide enough resistance for a valid test. Additionally, this position is not against gravity, so this test should be graded stringently.

Test: Patient dorsiflexes ankle and inverts foot, keeping toes relaxed.

Instructions to Patient: "Bring your foot up and in. Hold it! Don't let me pull it down."

Grading

Grade 5: Holds test position against maximal resistance.

Grade 4: Holds test position against strong to moderate resistance.

Grade 3: Completes available range of motion without resistance (see Fig. 6.103).

Grade 2: Completes only a partial range of motion.

Grade 1: Clinician will be able to detect some contractile activity in the muscle, or the tendon will "stand out." There is no joint movement.

 Palpate the tendon of the tibialis anterior on the anteromedial aspect of the ankle at about the level of the malleoli (Fig. 6.105). Alternatively, palpate the muscle for contractile activity over its belly just lateral to the "shin" (not shown).

Grade 0: No discernable palpable contraction.

FIGURE 6.105

FIGURE 6.104

Substitution

Substitution by the extensor digitorum longus and the extensor hallucis longus muscles results in toe extension. Instruct patient to keep the toes relaxed so they are not part of the test movement.

Clinical Relevance

- In the sitting and supine positions, make sure the knee is flexed to put the gastrocnemius on slack. If the knee is extended and there is gastrocnemius tightness, patient will not be able to achieve full dorsiflexion range.
- Because the supine position is not against gravity, clinician should expect to give maximum resistance, utilizing body weight of the clinician. A pull force will be more protective of clinician's shoulder than a push force.
- The authors sometimes use the forearm rather than the hand to provide resistance, which can be more comfortable for the patient and clinician and assist with providing sufficient resistance.

Suggested Strength Exercises for Tibialis Anterior

- Resisted dorsiflexion using elastic resistance or pulling against a pedal or other object
- Foot taps
- Heel walking

Tibialis posterior

POSTERIOR VIEW OF LEG
PLANTAR VIEW OF FOOT

FIGURE 6.106

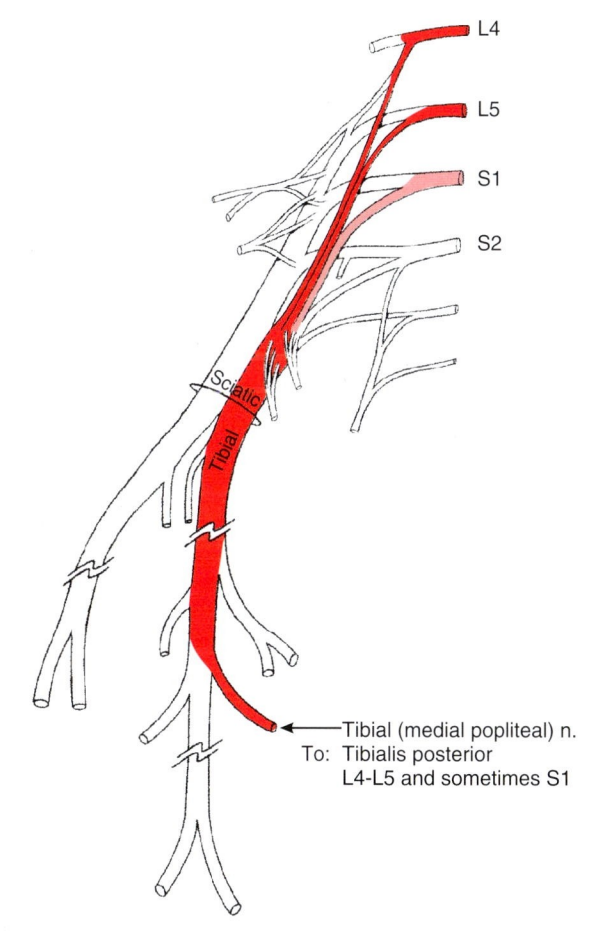

L4

L5

S1

S2

Sciatic

Tibial

Tibial (medial popliteal) n.
To: Tibialis posterior
L4-L5 and sometimes S1

FIGURE 6.107

Tibia

Tibialis
posterior

Fibula

FIGURE 6.108 Arrow indicates level of cross section.

Range of Motion

0°–35°

FOOT INVERSION

(Tibialis posterior)

Table 6.14 FOOT INVERSION

I.D.	Muscle	Origin	Insertion	Function
204	Tibialis posterior	Tibia (proximal 2/3 of posterior lateral shaft below soleal line) Interosseous membrane (posterior) Fibula (shaft, proximal posterior medial 2/3) Deep transverse fascia Intermuscular septa	Navicular bone (tuberosity) Cuneiform bones Sustentaculum tali (distal) Metatarsals 2–4 (via tendinous band)	Foot inversion (supination) Ankle plantar flexion (accessory)
Others				
203	Tibialis anterior			
213	Flexor digitorum longus			
222	Flexor hallucis longus			
206	Soleus			
221	Extensor hallucis longus			

The tibialis posterior muscle is active primarily during the stance phase of gait, providing an inversion moment at the subtalar joint and stabilizing the medial longitudinal arch. Dysfunction of the tibialis posterior tendon, a more recently recognized degenerative and progressive condition, is a common cause of adult-acquired flat-footedness and tendon rupture.

Grade 5, Grade 4, Grade 3, and Grade 2

Position of Patient: Sitting with ankle in slight plantar flexion.

Instructions to Clinician: Sit on low stool in front of patient or on side of test leg (antigravity position). With patient's heel resting on clinician's thigh, ask patient to move the foot down and in. Perform this movement passively if needed. If sufficient active range exists, place stabilizing hand on the posterior calf just above the malleoli (Fig. 6.109). The majority of resistance is toward forefoot abduction (up-and-out direction). Hand providing resistance is placed on the foot with the hand providing resistance over the medial side of the forefoot.

Test: Patient inverts foot through available range of motion.

Instructions to Patient: "Turn your foot down and in. Hold it. Don't let me move it."

FIGURE 6.109

Grade 5, Grade 4, Grade 3, and Grade 2 Continued

Grading

Grade 5: Patient holds the test position against maximal resistance.

Grade 4: Patient holds the test position against strong to moderate resistance.

Grade 3: Patient will be able to invert the foot through the full available range of motion (Fig. 6.110).

Grade 2: Patient will be able to complete only partial range of motion.

FIGURE 6.110

FIGURE 6.111

Grade 1 and Grade 0

Position of Patient: Sitting or supine.

Instructions to Clinician: Sit on low stool or stand in front of patient. Palpate tendon of the tibialis posterior between the medial malleolus and the navicular bone (Fig. 6.111). Alternatively, palpate tendon above the malleolus.

Test: Patient attempts to invert foot.

Instructions to Patient: "Try to turn your foot down and in."

Grading

Grade 1: The tibialis posterior tendon will stand out if there is contractile activity in the muscle. If palpable activity occurs in the absence of movement, the grade is 1.

Grade 0: No discernable palpable contraction.

Substitution

Flexors of the toes should remain relaxed to prevent substitution by the flexor digitorum longus and flexor hallucis longus.

Clinical Relevance

- The single-leg heel raise is painful or impossible in the presence of tibialis posterior dysfunction.
- If heel inversion does not occur or is asymmetrical during the heel rise, insufficiency in the tibialis posterior may be present.
- The action of the tibialis posterior is to plantarflex and invert the ankle, having the effect of placing the forefoot into adduction. To isolate the tibialis posterior, resisted forefoot adduction should be the primary force with less force toward dorsiflexion (producing the up-and-out movement).

Suggested Strength Exercises for Tibialis Posterior

- Foot inversion exercise (pushing soles of feet together)
- Eccentric foot inversion exercise with elastic resistance
- Heel rise with inversion (heels together)

(Fibularis longus and brevis—previously called Peroneus longus and brevis)

ANTEROLATERAL

FIGURE 6.112

FIGURE 6.113

FIGURE 6.114

FIGURE 6.115 Arrow indicates level of cross section.

FOOT EVERSION WITH PLANTAR FLEXION

(Fibularis longus and brevis—previously called Peroneus longus and brevis)

Range of Motion

0°–25°

Table 6.15 FOOT EVERSION

I.D.	Muscle	Origin	Insertion	Function
With Plantar Flexion				
208	Fibularis longus (peroneus longus)	Fibula (head and proximal 2/3 of shaft, lateral aspect) Tibia (lateral condyle, occasionally) Fascia cruris Intermuscular septa	1st metatarsal (base and lateral aspect) Medial cuneiform (base and lateral aspect) Other metatarsals occasionally	Foot eversion Ankle plantar flexion (assist) Depression of 1st metatarsal Support of longitudinal and transverse arches
209	Fibularis brevis (peroneus brevis)	Fibula (distal and lateral 2/3 of shaft) Crural intermuscular septum	5th metatarsal (tuberosity at base, lateral aspect)	Foot eversion Ankle plantar flexion (accessory)
With Dorsiflexion				
211	Extensor digitorum longus	Tibia (lateral condyle on lateral side) Fibula (shaft: upper 3/4 of medial surface) Interosseous membrane (anterior surface) Deep crural fascia and intermuscular septum	Tendon of insertion divides into four tendon slips to dorsum of foot that form an expansion over each toe: Toes 2–5: middle phalanges (PIP joints) of the four lesser toes (intermediate slip to dorsum of base of each) Distal phalanges (two lateral slips to dorsum of base of each)	MP extension of four lesser toes PIP and DIP extension (assist) of four lesser toes Ankle dorsiflexion (accessory) Foot eversion (accessory)
210	Fibularis tertius	Fibula (distal 1/3 of medial surface) Interosseous membrane (anterior) Intermuscular septum	5th metatarsal (dorsal surface of base; shaft, medial aspect)	Ankle dorsiflexion Foot eversion (accessory)
Other				
205	Gastrocnemius			

DIP, Distal phalanges; *MP*, metatarsophalangeal; *PIP*, proximal phalanges.

The fibularis longus and brevis muscles provide the main source of active stability to the lateral side of the ankle and are active throughout the stance phase of walking.

FOOT EVERSION WITH PLANTAR FLEXION

(Fibularis longus and brevis—previously called Peroneus longus and brevis)

Grade 5, Grade 4, Grade 3, and Grade 2

Position of Patient: Sitting with ankle in neutral position (midway between dorsiflexion and plantar flexion). Test also may be performed with patient supine.

Instructions to Clinician: Sit on low stool in front of patient or stand at end of table if patient is supine. Ask patient to turn foot down and out (eversion). If sufficient range is present, place stabilizing hand at the ankle just above the malleoli. Take care not to squeeze the distal tibia. Hand providing resistance is contoured around the dorsum and lateral border of the forefoot (Fig. 6.116). Resistance is directed toward inversion and slight dorsiflexion (up and in).

Test: Patient everts foot with depression of first metatarsal head and some plantar flexion.

Instructions to Patient: "Turn your foot down and out. Hold it! Don't let me move it in."

Grading

Grade 5: Patient holds test position against maximal resistance.

Grade 4: Patient holds test position against strong to moderate resistance.

Grade 3: Patient completes available range of eversion but without resistance (Fig. 6.117).

Grade 2: Patient will be able to complete only a partial range of eversion motion.

FIGURE 6.116

FIGURE 6.117

(Fibularis longus and brevis—previously called Peroneus longus and brevis)

Grade 1 and Grade 0

Position of Patient: Short sitting or supine.

Instructions to Clinician: Sit on low stool or stand at end of table. To palpate the fibularis longus, place fingers on the lateral leg over the upper one-third just below the head of the fibula. The tendon of the muscle can be felt posterior to the lateral malleolus but behind the tendon of the fibularis brevis.

To palpate the tendon of the fibularis brevis, place index finger over the tendon as it comes forward from behind the lateral malleolus, proximal to the base of the fifth metatarsal (Fig. 6.118). The belly of the fibularis brevis can be palpated on the lateral surface of the distal leg over the fibula.

Test: Patient attempts to evert foot.

Instruction to Patient: "Try to move your foot down and out."

FIGURE 6.118

Grading

Grade 1: Palpation will reveal contractile activity in either or both muscles, which may cause the tendon to stand out. No motion occurs.

Grade 0: No discernable palpable contractile activity.

Isolation of Fibularis Longus

Give resistance against the plantar surface of the head of the first metatarsal in a direction toward inversion and dorsiflexion.

Clinical Relevance

- Foot eversion is accompanied by either dorsiflexion or plantar flexion. The toe extensors are the primary dorsiflexors accompanying eversion because the fibularis tertius is not always present.
- The fibularis brevis cannot be isolated if both longus and brevis are innervated and strong.

  If there is a difference in strength between the fibularis longus and the fibularis brevis, the stronger of the two can be ascertained by the relative amount of resistance taken in eversion versus the resistance taken at the first metatarsal head. If greater resistance is taken at the first metatarsal head, the fibularis longus is the stronger muscle.

Suggested Strength Exercise for Foot Eversion

Lateral hop[51]

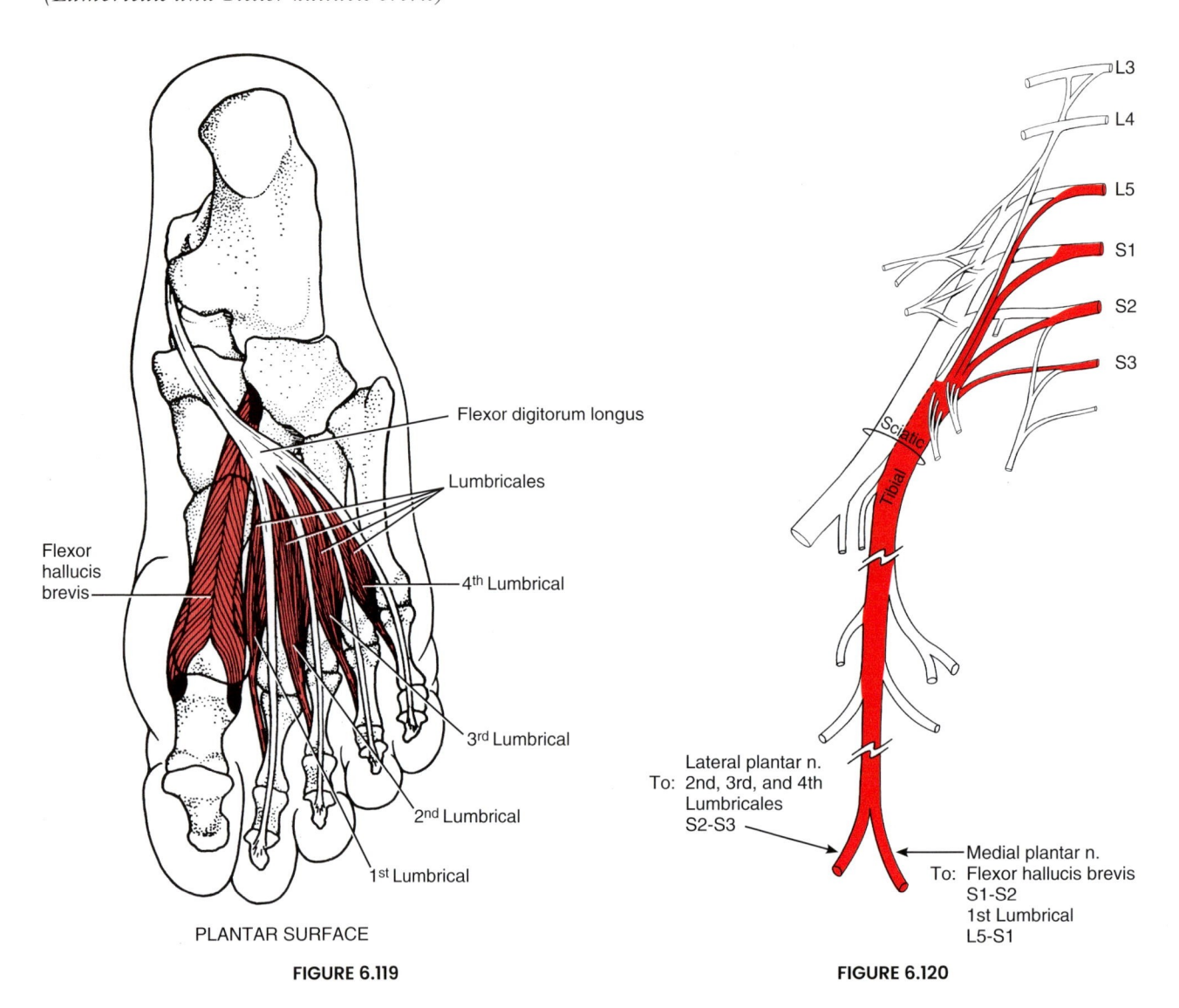

Flexor digitorum longus

Lumbricales

4th Lumbrical

Flexor hallucis brevis

3rd Lumbrical

2nd Lumbrical

1st Lumbrical

PLANTAR SURFACE

FIGURE 6.119

L3
L4
L5
S1
S2
S3

Sciatic

Tibial

Lateral plantar n.
To: 2nd, 3rd, and 4th
Lumbricales
S2-S3

Medial plantar n.
To: Flexor hallucis brevis
S1-S2
1st Lumbrical
L5-S1

FIGURE 6.120

Range of Motion
Great toe, 0°–45°
Lateral four toes, 0°–40°

(Lumbricals and Flexor hallucis brevis)

Table 6.16 FLEXION OF MP JOINTS OF TOES AND HALLUX

I.D.	Muscle	Origin	Insertion	Function
Toes				
218	**Lumbricals**	Tendons of flexor digitorum longus near angles of separation 1st lumbrical (by a single head, tendon of flexor digitorum longus bound for toe 2) 2nd–4th lumbricals (arise by dual heads from adjacent sides of tendons of flexor digitorum longus bound for toes 3–5)	All: toes 2–5 (proximal phalanges and dorsal expansions of the tendons of extensor digitorum longus)	Toes 2–5: MP flexion Toes 2–5: PIP and DIP extension (assist)
Hallux				
223	Flexor hallucis brevis (rises by 2 heads)			Hallux abduction (away from toe 2) Hallux MP flexion
	Lateral head	Cuboid bone (plantar surface) Lateral cuneiform bone	Hallux (proximal phalanx on both sides of base) Blends with adductor hallucis	
	Medial head	Medial intermuscular septum Tibialis posterior (tendon)	Hallux (proximal phalanx on both sides of base) Blends with abductor hallucis	
216	Flexor digiti minimi brevis	5th metatarsal base Sheath of peroneus longus	Toe 5 (proximal phalanx, lateral aspect of base)	Toe 5 MP flexion
Others				
219, 220	Interossei, dorsal and plantar			
213	Flexor digitorum longus			
214	Flexor digitorum brevis			
222	Flexor hallucis longus			
224	Abductor hallucis			
225	Adductor hallucis			

DIP, Distal interphalangeal; *MP*, metatarsophalangeal; *PIP*, proximal interphalangeal.

HALLUX AND TOE METATARSOPHALANGEAL (MP) FLEXION

(Flexor hallucis brevis)

HALLUX MP FLEXION *(Flexor hallucis brevis)*

Grades 5 to 0

Position of Patient: Sitting (alternate position: supine) with legs hanging over edge of table. Ankle is in neutral position (midway between dorsiflexion and plantar flexion).

Instructions to Clinician: Sit on low stool in front of patient. Alternate position: stand at side of table near patient's foot. Test foot rests on clinician's lap. Ask patient to bend the big toe over finger. If sufficient range is present, place stabilizing hand over the dorsum of the foot just below the ankle (Fig. 6.121). The index finger of the other hand is placed beneath the proximal phalanx of the great toe. Alternatively, the tip of the finger (with very short fingernails) is placed up under the proximal phalanx.

Test: Patient flexes great toe.

Instructions to Patient: "Bend your big toe over my finger. Hold it. Don't let me straighten it."

FIGURE 6.121

Grading

Grade 5: Patient holds position against strong resistance.

Grade 4: Patient holds test position against moderate to mild resistance.

Grade 3: Patient completes available range of MP flexion of the great toe without resistance.

Grade 2: Patient completes only partial range of motion.

Grade 1: Clinician may note contractile activity but no toe motion.

Grade 0: No discernable contractile activity.

Clinical Relevance

- The muscle and tendon of the flexor hallucis brevis cannot be palpated.
- When the flexor hallucis longus is not functional, the flexor hallucis brevis will flex the metatarsophalangeal joint but without flexion of the interphalangeal (IP) joint. In the opposite condition, when the flexor hallucis brevis is not functional, the IP joint flexes, and the metatarsophalangeal joint may hyperextend. (When this condition is chronic, the posture is called hammer toe.)
- Loss of the flexor hallucis longus results in balance instability, as it stabilizes the big toe against the ground during each step.

(Flexor hallucis brevis)

TOE MP FLEXION

Grades 5 to 0

Position of Patient: Sitting with foot on clinician's lap. Alternate position: supine. Ankle is in neutral (midway between dorsiflexion and plantar flexion).

Instructions to Clinician: Sit on low stool in front of patient. Alternate position: stand next to table beside test foot. Ask patient to bend the toes over clinician's fingers. If sufficient range is present, place stabilizing hand over the dorsum of the foot (as in test for flexion of the hallux) (Fig. 6.122). The index finger of the other hand is placed under the MP joints of the four lateral toes to provide resistance to flexion.

FIGURE 6.122

Test: Patient flexes lateral four toes at the MP joints, keeping the interphalangeal (IP) joints neutral.

Instructions to Patient: "Bend your toes over my finger. Hold it!"

Grading

Grading is the same as that used for the great toe.

Clinical Relevance

- In actual practice, the great toe and the lateral toes are rarely tested independently. Many patients cannot separate hallux motion from motion of the lateral toes, nor can they separate metatarsophalangeal and interphalangeal motions.
- The clinician could test each toe separately because the lumbricals are notoriously uneven in strength. This may not, however, be practical.

Suggested Strength Exercises for Hallux and Toe MP Flexion

- Picking up marbles with the toes (occurs in conjunction with flexor halluces and flexor digitorum longus)
- Scrunching a towel with the toes

HALLUX AND TOE DIP AND PIP FLEXION

(Flexor digitorum longus, Flexor digitorum brevis, Flexor hallucis longus)

Flexor digitorum longus

POSTERIOR VIEW OF LEG

FIGURE 6.123

Flexor hallucis longus

Flexor digitorum brevis

PLANTAR VIEW OF FOOT

FIGURE 6.124

Common peroneal

Sciatic

Tibial

L5

S1

S2

Tibial n.
To: Flexor digitorum longus
L5-S2

Flexor hallucis longus
L5-S2

Medial plantar n.
To: Flexor digitorum brevis
S1-S2

FIGURE 6.125

Tibia

Flexor digitorum longus

Tibial nerve

Fibula

Flexor hallucis longus

FIGURE 6.126 Arrow indicates level of cross section.

(Flexor digitorum longus, Flexor digitorum brevis, Flexor hallucis longus)

Range of Motion

PIP flexion, four lateral toes:
0°–35°

DIP flexion, four lateral toes:
0°–60°

IP flexion of hallux: 0°–90°

Table 6.17 FLEXION OF IP JOINTS OF HALLUX AND TOES

I.D.	Muscle	Origin	Insertion	Function
DIP, Toes				
213	Flexor digitorum longus	Tibia (shaft, posterior aspect of middle 2/3) Fascia over tibialis posterior	Toes 2–5 (distal phalanges, plantar surfaces, and base)	Toes 2–5: MP, PIP, and DIP flexion Ankle plantar flexion (accessory) Foot inversion (accessory)
PIP, Toes				
214	Flexor digitorum brevis	Calcaneus (tuberosity, medial process) Plantar aponeurosis Intermuscular septum	Toes 2–5 (by 4 tendons to middle phalanges, both sides)	Toes 2–5 MP and PIP flexion
IP, Hallux				
222	Flexor hallucis longus	Fibula (shaft, 2/3 of posterior aspect) Interosseous membrane Intermuscular septum (posterior crural) Fascia over tibialis posterior	Slip of tendon to flexor digitorum longus Hallux (distal phalanx, base, plantar aspect)	Hallux IP flexion Hallux MP flexion (accessory) Ankle plantar flexion and foot inversion (accessory)
Others				
DIP, Toes				
217	Quadratus plantae			
PIP, Toes				
213	Flexor digitorum longus			

DIP, Distal interphalangeal; *IP*, interphalangeal; *MP*, metatarsophalangeal; *PIP*, proximal interphalangeal.

HALLUX AND TOE DIP AND PIP FLEXION

(Flexor digitorum longus, Flexor digitorum brevis, Flexor hallucis longus)

Grades 5 to 0

Position of Patient: Sitting with foot on clinician's lap or supine.

Instructions to Clinician: Sit on a short stool in front of patient or stand at the side of table near patient's foot. Ask patient to curl toes (or big toe). If sufficient range is present, place stabilizing hand over anterior foot with fingers placed across the dorsum of foot and thumb under the proximal phalanges or distal phalanges or under the IP of the hallux (Figs. 6.127, 6.128, and 6.129). The other hand applies resistance using the four fingers or the thumb under the middle phalanges (for the IP test) (see Fig. 6.127), under the distal phalanges for the DIP test (see Fig. 6.128), and with the index finger under the distal phalanx of the hallux (see Fig. 6.129). Resistance will be minimal.

Test: Patient flexes the toes or hallux.

Instructions to Patient: "Curl your toes; hold it. Curl your big toe and hold it."

Grading

Grade 5 and Grade 4: Patient holds test position of toes and then hallux; resistance in both tests may be minimal.

Grade 3 and Grade 2: Patient holds test position without resistance (Grade 3) or completes only a partial range (Grade 2).

Grade 1 and Grade 0: Minimal to no palpable contractile activity occurs. Tendon of the flexor hallucis longus may be palpated on the plantar surface of the proximal phalanx of the great toe.

FIGURE 6.127

FIGURE 6.129

Clinical Relevance

- As with all toe motions, patient may not be able to move one toe separately from another or separate MP from IP activity among individual toes.
- Some people can separate hallux activity from toe motions, but fewer can separate MP from IP hallux activity.
- Many people can "pinch" with their great toe (adductor hallucis), but this is not a common clinical test.
- The abductor hallucis is not commonly tested because it is only rarely isolated. Its activity can be observed by resisting adduction of the forefoot, which will bring the great toe into abduction, but the lateral toes commonly extend at the same time.

FIGURE 6.128

(Extensor digitorum longus and brevis, Extensor hallucis longus)

Extensor digitorum longus

Extensor hallucis longus

Extensor digitorum brevis

ANTEROLATERAL VIEW

FIGURE 6.130

FIGURE 6.131

L4

L5

S1

Common peroneal
Sciatic
Tibial

Deep peroneal n.
To: Extensor digitorum longus
L5-S1
Extensor digitorum brevis
L5-S1
Extensor hallucis longus
L5

FIGURE 6.132

Extensor hallucis longus

Extensor digitorum longus

Fibula

Tibia

FIGURE 6.133 Arrow indicates level of cross section.

HALLUX AND TOE MP AND IP EXTENSION

(Extensor digitorum longus and brevis, Extensor hallucis longus)

Table 6.18 EXTENSION OF METATARSOPHALANGEAL JOINTS OF TOES AND INTERPHALANGEAL JOINT OF HALLUX

I.D.	Muscle	Origin	Insertion	Function
211	**Extensor digitorum longus**	Tibia (lateral condyle) Fibula (shaft, proximal 3/4 of medial surface) Fascia cruris (deep) Interosseous membrane (anterior) Intermuscular septum	Toes 2–5 (to each middle and each distal phalanx, dorsal surface)	MP extension of four lesser toes PIP and DIP extension (assist) of four lesser toes Ankle dorsiflexion (accessory) Foot eversion (accessory)
212	Extensor digitorum brevis	Calcaneus (anterior superolateral surface) Lateral talocalcaneal ligament Extensor retinaculum (inferior)	Ends in four tendons: hallux (proximal phalanx, dorsal surface [may be named extensor hallucis brevis]) Toes 2–4: join tendons of extensor digitorum longus (lateral sides)	Hallux (great toe): MP extension Toes 2–4: MP extension Toes 2–4: IP extension (assist)
221	Extensor hallucis longus	Fibula (shaft, middle 1/2 of medial aspect) Interosseous membrane	Hallux (distal phalanx, dorsal aspect of base) Expansion to proximal phalanx	Hallux: MP and IP extension Ankle dorsiflexion (accessory) Foot inversion (accessory)

DIP, Distal interphalangeal; *IP*, interphalangeal; *MP*, metatarsophalangeal; *PIP*, proximal interphalangeal.

Grades 5 to 0

Position of Patient: Sitting with foot on clinician's lap. Alternate position: supine. Ankle in neutral (midway between plantar flexion and dorsiflexion).

Instructions to Clinician: Sit on low stool in front of patient or stand beside table near patient's foot. Ask patient to straighten big toe or all the toes.

Lateral Toes: One hand stabilizes the metatarsals with the fingers on the plantar surface and the thumb or index finger on the dorsum of the foot (Fig. 6.134). The other hand is used to give resistance, with the thumb placed over the dorsal surface of the proximal phalanges of the toes.

FIGURE 6.134

(Extensor digitorum longus and brevis, Extensor hallucis longus)

Hallux: Stabilize the metatarsal area by contouring the hand around the plantar surface of the foot, with the thumb curving around to the base of the hallux (Fig. 6.135). The other hand stabilizes the foot at the heel. For resistance, place thumb over the MP joint (see Fig. 6.134) or over the IP joint (Fig. 6.136).

Test: Patient extends lateral four toes or extends hallux.

Instructions to Patient: "Straighten your big toe. Hold it." OR "Straighten your toes and hold it."

Grading

Grade 5 and Grade 4: Patient can extend the toes fully against variable resistance (which may be small).

Grade 3 and Grade 2: Patient can complete range of motion with no resistance (Grade 3) or can complete a partial range of motion (Grade 2).

Grade 1 and Grade 0: Tendons of the extensor digitorum longus can be palpated or observed over dorsum of metatarsals. Tendon of the extensor digitorum brevis often can be palpated on the lateral side of the dorsum of the foot just in front of the malleolus.

Palpable contractile activity is a Grade 1; no discernable palpable contractile activity is a Grade 0.

FIGURE 6.135

Clinical Relevance

- Many (if not most) patients cannot separate great toe extension from extension of the four lateral toes. Nor can most separate metatarsophalangeal (MP) from interphalangeal (IP) activity.
- The test is used not so much to ascertain strength as to determine whether the toe muscles are active.
- Normal strength in the ankle and foot muscles allows us to walk on uneven surfaces and supplies the major muscle forces needed for balance.
- Bilateral extensor digitorum brevis wasting is a reliable clinical bedside marker while assessing for underlying lumbar central canal stenosis.[52]

FIGURE 6.136

HALLUX AND TOE MP AND IP EXTENSION

(Extensor digitorum longus and brevis, Extensor hallucis longus)

Supplemental Video Resources

Visit Elsevier eBooks+ (eBooks.Health.Elsevier.com) to access supplemental videos about the following tests:

- Scapular Abduction and Upward Rotation
- Scapular Adduction
- Scapular Depression and Adduction
- Scapular Adduction and Downward Rotation
- Scapular Depression
- Preliminary Examination
- Shoulder Abduction
- Shoulder Horizontal Abduction
- Shoulder Horizontal Adduction
- Shoulder External Rotation
- Elbow Extension
- Wrist Flexion
- Wrist Extension
- PIP Tests
- DIP Tests
- Finger MCP Extension
- Finger MCP Flexion
- Finger Abduction
- Finger Adduction
- Thumb MCP and IP Flexion
- Thumb MCP and IP Extension
- Thumb Abduction
- Abductor Pollicis Longus
- Abductor Pollicis Brevis
- Opposition
- Hip Flexion, Abduction, and External Rotation with Knee Flexion
- Hip Extension Test to Isolate Gluteus Maximus
- Hip Extension Tests Modified for Hip Flexion Tightness
- Supine Hip Extension Test
- Hip Abduction from Flexed Position
- Hip Adduction
- Hip External Rotation
- Hip Internal Rotation
- Lateral Hamstring Test (Biceps Femoris)
- Ankle Plantar Flexion
- Foot Inversion
- Foot Eversion with Plantar Flexion
- Hallux MP Flexion
- Hallux and Toe DIP and PIP Flexion
- Hallux and Toe MP and IP Extension

1. Singh D, Agarwal S. Morphological study of psoas minor muscles with embryological basis and clinical insights. *J Clin Diagn Res.* 2021;15(4):AC10–AC14. https://www.jcdr.net/articles/PDF/14782/47305_CE[Ra1]_F[SK]_PF1(ShG_SL)_PFA(Pr_KM)_PN(KM).pdf.

2. Gottschall JS, Kram R. Energy cost and muscular activity required for leg swing during walking. *J Appl Physio.* 2005;99:23–30.

3. Rantanen T, Guralnik JM, Izmirlian G, et al. Association of muscle strength with maximum walking speed in disabled older women. *Am J Phys Med Rehabil.* 1998;77(4):299–305.

4. Yokozawa T, Fujii N, Ae M. Muscle activities of the lower leg during level and uphill running. *J Biomech.* 2007;40:3467–3475.

5. Neumann DA. Kinesiology of the hip: a focus on muscular action. *J Orthop Sports Phys Ther.* 2010;40(2):82–94.

5a. Neumann DA. Kinesiology of the hip: a focus on muscular actions. *J Orthop Sports Phys Ther.* 2010;40(2):39–128. https://www.jospt.org/doi/10.2519/jospt.2010.3025.

6. Ikezoe T, Tsuboyama T, Tabara Y, et al. Weak hip flexor strength predicts progression of functional capacity decline due to locomotor system dysfunction in community-older adults: a longitudinal cohort study. *Arch Gerontol Geriatr.* 2021;97:104499.

7. Sato H, Kondo S, Saito M, Saura R. Effects of strengthening the hip flexor muscles on walking ability and the locomotive syndrome rank test: an intervention study. *J Orthop Sci.* 2020;25:892–896.

8. LaBan M. Iliopsoas weakness: a clinical sign of lumbar spinal stenosis. *Am J Phys Med Rehabil.* 2004;83(3):224–225. https://journals.lww.com/ajpmr/pages/articleviewer.aspx?year=2004&issue=03000&article=00015&type=Fulltext.

9. Winter D. *Biomechanics and Motor Control of Human Movement.* Hoboken, NJ: John Wiley & Sons; 2005.

10. Reinman MP. A literature review of studies evaluating gluteus maximus and gluteus medius activation during rehabilitation exercises. *Physiother Theory Pract.* 2012;28(4):257–268.

11. Waters RL, Perry J, McDaniels JM, et al. The relative strength of the hamstrings during hip extension. *J Bone Joint Surg Am.* 1974;56:1592–1597.

12. Perry J, Weiss WB, Burnfield JM, et al. The supine hip extension manual muscle test: a reliability and validity study. *Arch Phys Med Rehabil.* 2004;85(8):1345–1350.

13. Youdas JW, Hartman JP, Murphy BA, et al. Electromyographic analysis of gluteus maximus and hamstring activity during the supine resisted hip extension exercise versus supine unilateral bridge to neutral. *Physiother Theory Pract.* 2017;33(2):124–130.

14. Macadam P, Feser EH. Examination of gluteus maximum electromyographic excitation associated with dynamic hip extension during body weight exercise: a systematic review. *Int J Sports Phys Ther.* 2019;14(1):14. https://pubmed.ncbi.nlm.nih.gov/30746289/.

15. McKay MJ, Baldwin JN, Ferreira P, et al. Normative reference values for strength and flexibility of 1,000 children and adults. *Neurology.* 2017;88(1):36–43.

16. Delp SL, Hess WE, Hungerford DS, et al. Variation of rotation moment arms with hip flexion. *J Biomech.* 1999;32:493–501.

17. Cibulka MT, Strube MJ, Meier D, et al. Symmetrical and asymmetrical hip rotation and its relationship to hip rotator muscle strength. *Clin Biomech (Bristol, Avon).* 2010;25(1):56–62.

18. Hoglund LT, Wong AL, Rickards C. The impact of sagittal plane hip position on isometric force of hip external rotator and internal rotator muscles in healthy young adults. *Int J Sports Phys Ther.* 2014;9:58–67.

19. Dawson, H. Multibriefs. The importance of hip internal rotation. 2014. http://exclusive.multibriefs.com/content/the-importance-of-hip-internal-rotation/medical-allied-healthcare. [Accessed 12 November 2023].

20. Bolgla LA, Uhl TL. Electromyographic analysis of hip rehabilitation exercises in a group of healthy subjects. *J Orthop Sports Phys Ther.* 2005;35:487–494.

21. Boudreau SN, Dwyer MK, Mattacola CG, et al. Hip-muscle activation during the lunge, single-leg squat, and step-up-and-over exercises. *J Sport Rehabil.* 2009;18:91–103.

22. Bergmann G, Graichen F, Rohlmann A. Hip joint loading during walking and running, measured in two patients. *J Biomech.* 1993;26(8):969–990. https://doi.org/10.1016/0021-9290(93)90058-m. PMID: 8349721.

22a. Soderberg G.L., Dostal W.F. Electromyographic study of three parts of the gluteus medius muscle during functional activities. *Phys Ther.* 1978;58:691–696.

23. Bennell KL, Hunt MA, Wrigley TV, et al. Hip strengthening reduces symptoms but not knee load in people with medial knee osteoarthritis and varus malalignment: a randomized controlled trial. *Osteoarthritis Cartilage.* 2010;18:621–628.

24. Chi AS, Long SS, Zoga AC, et al. Association of gluteus medius and minimus muscle atrophy and fall-related hip fracture in older individuals using computed tomography. *J Comput Assist Tomogr.* 2016;40(2):238–242.

25. Jacobs CA, Lewis M, Bolgla LA, et al. Electromyographic analysis of hip abductor exercises performed by a sample of total hip arthroplasty patients. *J Arthroplasty.* 2009;24(7):1130–1136.

26. Anderson LL, Magnusson SP, Nielsen M, et al. Neuromuscular activation in conventional therapeutic exercises and heavy resistance exercises: implications for rehabilitation. *Phys Ther.* 2006;86(5):683–697.

27. Ekstrom RA, Donatelli RA, Carp KC. Electromyographic analysis of core trunk, hip, and thigh muscles during 9 rehabilitation exercises. *J Orthop Sports Phys Ther.* 2007;37(12):754–762.

28. Moore D, Semciw AI, Pizzari T. A systematic review and meta-analysis of common therapeutic exercises that generate highest muscle activity in the gluteus medius and gluteus minimus segments. *Int J Sports Phys Ther.* 2020;15(6):856. https://pubmed.ncbi.nlm.nih.gov/33344003/.

29. Hutchinson LA, Lichtwark GA, Willy RW, Kelly LA. The iliotibial band: a complex structure with versatile functions. *Sports Med.* 2022;52:995–1008.

30. Takizawa M, Suzuki D, Ito H, et al. Why adductor magnus muscle is large: the function based on muscle morphology in cadavers. *Scand J Med Sci Sports.* 2014;24(1):197–203.

31. Hides JA, Beall P, Franettovich Smith MM, et al. Activation of the hip adductor muscles varies during a simulated weight-bearing task. *Phys Ther Sport.* 2016;17:19–23.

32. Light N, Thorborg K. The precision and torque production of common hip adductor squeeze tests used in elite football. *J Sci Med Sport.* 2016;19(11):888–892.

33. Ishøi L, Sørensen CN, Kae NM, et al. Large eccentric strength increase using the Copenhagen Adduction exercise in football: a randomized controlled trial. *Scand J Med Sci Sports.* 2016;26(11):1334–1342.

REFERENCES

34. Giphart JE, Stull JD, Laprade RF, et al. Recruitment and activity of the pectineus and piriformis muscles during hip rehabilitation exercises: an electromyography study. *Am J Sports Med.* 2012;40(7):1654–1663.

35. Frey-Law LA, Laake A, Avin KG, et al. Knee and elbow 3D strength surfaces: peak torque-angle-velocity relationships. *J Appl Biomech.* 2012;28(6):726–737.

36. Malliaropoulos N, Mendiguchia J, Pehlivanidis H, et al. Hamstring exercises for track and field athletes: injury and exercise biomechanics, and possible implications for exercise selection and primary prevention. *Br J Sports Med.* 2012;46(12):846–851.

37. Schellenberg F, Lindorfer J, List R, et al. Kinetic and kinematic differences between deadlifts and good mornings. *BMC Sports Sci Med Rehabil.* 2013;5(1):27.

38. Farahmand F, Senavongse W, Amis AA. Quantitative study of the quadriceps muscles and trochlear groove geometry related to instability of the patellofemoral joint. *J Orthop Res.* 1998;16(1):136–143.

39. Mirzabeigi E, Jordan C, Gronley JK, et al. Isolation of the vastus medialis oblique muscle during exercise. *Am J Sports Med.* 1999;27:50–53.

40. Bronikowski A, Kloda M, Lewandowska M, et al. Influence of various forms of physical exercise on bioelectric activity of quadriceps femoris muscle. Pilot study. *Orthop Traumatol Rehabil.* 2010;12:534–541.

41. Davlin CD, Holcomb WR, Guadagnoli MA. The effect of hip position and electromyographic biofeedback training on the vastus medialis oblique: vastus lateralis ratio. *J Athl Train.* 1999;34:342–346.

42. Eriksrud O, Bohannon RW. Relationship of knee extension force to independence in sit-to-stand performance in patients receiving acute rehabilitation. *Phys Ther.* 2003;83:544–551.

43. Signorile JF, Applegate B, Duque M, et al. Selective recruitment of the triceps surae muscle with changes in knee angle. *J Strength Cond Res.* 2002;16(3):433–439.

44. Mulroy S. Functions of the triceps surae during strength testing and gait. In: *PhD Dissertation, Department of Biokinesiology and Physical Therapy.* Los Angeles: University of Southern California; 1994.

45. Lunsford BR, Perry J. The standing heel-rise test for ankle plantar flexion: criterion for normal. *Phys Ther.* 1995;75:694–698.

46. Jan MH, Chai HM, Lin YF, et al. Effects of age and sex on the results of an ankle plantar-flexor manual muscle test. *Phys Ther.* 2005;85:1078–1084.

47. Yocum A, McCoy SW, Bjornson KF, Mullens P, Burton GN. Reliability and validity of the standing heel-rise test. *Phys Occup Ther Pediatr.* 2010;30(3):190–204. https://doi.org/10.3109/01942631003761380. PMID: 20608857.

48. Farrag A, Elsayed W. Habitual use of high-heeled shoes affects isokinetic soleus strength more than gastrocnemius in healthy young females. *Foot Ankle Int.* 2016;37(9):1008–1016.

49. Hebert-Losier K, Wessman C, Alricsson M, Svantesson U. Updated reliability and normative values for the standing heel-rise test in healthy adults. *Physiotherapy.* 2017;103(4):446–452.

49a. Cibulka M., Wenthe A., Boyle Z., Callier D., Schwerdt A., Jarman D., Strube M.J. Variation in medial and lateral gastrocnemius muscle activity with foot position. *Int J Sports Phys Ther.* 2017;12(2):233–241. PMID: 28515978; PMCID: PMC5380866.

50. Fujimoto M, Hsu WL, Woollacott MH, et al. Ankle dorsiflexor strength relates to the ability to restore balance during a backward support surface translation. *Gait Posture.* 2013;38(4):812–817.

51. Yoshida M, Taniguchi K, Katayose M. Analysis of muscle activity and ankle joint movement during the side-hop test. *J Strength Cond Res.* 2011;25(8):2255–2264.

52. Munakomi S, Kumar BM. Wasting of extensor digitorum brevis as a decisive preoperative clinical indicator of lumbar canal stenosis: a single-center prospective cohort study. *Ann Med Health Sci Res.* 2016;6(5):296–300. (PMC free article).

CHAPTER 7

Alternatives to Manual Muscle Testing

Alternatives to Manual Muscle Testing

Introduction

General Testing Considerations

One-Repetition Maximum Test

Equipment-Based Strength Testing

Interpretation of

Equipment-Based Strength Testing Data

Sitting Unilateral Knee Extension Test

Power Testing

Body Weight Testing

Cyriax Method of Testing Contractile Lesions

INTRODUCTION

Manual muscle testing is a foundational measure of strength that is widely used across the health professions for both diagnosis and rehabilitation. Yet manual muscle testing has specific limitations, as discussed in Chapter 2. Consequently, alternative strength measures are needed in certain cases. Examples include when strength exceeds a functional threshold, strength of the patient is greater than that of the clinician, subtle asymmetries exist between sides or between the agonist and antagonist, and power or endurance needs to be measured. Equipment-based tests are the most commonly used alternatives to manual muscle testing.

There are many options for equipment-based testing, and each has its advantages and disadvantages. Choosing the best option depends on clinic space constraints, available budget, individual characteristics of the patient, goals of treatment, and how comprehensive the evaluation needs to be. For example, in a small outpatient clinic where most patients have low back or neck pain, the approach to equipment-based testing will differ substantially from that required in most acute care settings or most high-performance clinics focused on elite athletic performance. Strength-testing instruments that can be used effectively for children and older adults will differ from those used for elite athletes. The equipment-based tests presented in this chapter represent the more popular approaches, are appropriate for adults regardless of age, and have demonstrated reliability and validity.

GENERAL TESTING CONSIDERATIONS

It is presumed that any clinician conducting a strength-testing session will perform a prescreening exam for red flag conditions. Maximal strength testing for the trunk flexors in a patient with back pain, severe osteoporosis, or recent compression fracture, for example, may not be appropriate. Likewise, patients with unstable blood pressure may have an adverse reaction while exerting maximum effort on a leg press, particularly if the patient does so while performing a Valsalva maneuver by holding his or her breath. The typical warm-up includes completing three to five submaximal contractions at 40% to 50% of maximum using the muscle or muscle group that is being tested.[1] Active range of motion should be assessed to determine if adequate joint range and muscle length will allow maximum effort in the correct test position.

Tips for Achieving Optimal Results in Alternative Muscle Testing

Before starting any of the alternative muscle tests described in this chapter, have all the tools and data collection materials ready so assessments proceed smoothly. Efficiency in testing will grow with clinical experience.

1. Calibrate device (if appropriate). Any device that records force or torque will lose accuracy over time. All testing devices should be routinely calibrated as per the manufacturer's recommendations (which may recommend from daily to monthly calibrations, depending on the device).
2. Provide a conducive test environment. The more distractions there are (such as background noise or crowding), the more unlikely it is that an optimal effort will be made.
3. Once the patient is settled, the first thing to do is educate the patient. Demonstrate each test while explaining it in terminology the patient can easily understand. Allow the patient to practice using light weights. This practice could be incorporated into the warm-up (see later in text). Patient cooperation and understanding are critical for achieving accurate results.
4. Provide a warm-up to the muscles that will be assessed. This warm-up may include walking on a treadmill, pedaling a stationary bicycle, or cycling with an arm ergometer for 5 min before muscles are

tested. It is also feasible to warm up cold muscles by performing the test with three to five submaximal contractions at 40% to 50% of the patient's maximum using the muscle or muscle group that is being tested, as described previously.

5. If there is suspected asymmetry in muscle performance, test the less involved side first. Side-to-side comparisons are critical, and testing the less involved side also permits the patient to "feel" what the test is going to entail on their weaker limb.
6. Stabilize body part and patient. Depending on the test, each patient may need a seat belt, a stabilizing belt across the pelvis, and/or towels to position the arm or leg. After a part or extremity is stable, the test can be performed easily and accurately.
7. Standardize clinician commands to ensure that the test is performed the same way each time.
8. Allow patient to rest between efforts. A minimum rest period of 1 to 3 minutes is needed between attempted repetitions of maximal effort.[2]
9. Provide feedback on the test. It is part of human nature to desire knowing if side-to-side differences exist, if test 1 is different from test 2, and so forth. Including the patient in the results or outcome optimizes their participation and enhances their compliance.

ONE-REPETITION MAXIMUM TEST

The one-repetition maximum (1-RM) test is regarded as the standard for dynamic muscle strength testing. The 1-RM refers to the amount of load a patient can move 1 time (and 1 time only) through full range in a controlled manner with good form.[1] It is a safe technique, perhaps safer than a submaximum strength test, even though muscle soreness may occur and blood pressure may spike during a maximum exertion test.[3] One-repetition maximum tests are highly reliable when specific procedures are followed, more so than any other type of strength assessment.[4] In addition, the fundamental method for establishing 1-RM is the same for each muscle group, and thus, the 1-RM test is more precise than most.

One-repetition maximum testing serves several functions. Obtaining a patient's maximum strength ability may serve to establish the amount of resistance needed for an exercise prescription, it may help to determine the progress of a progressive, resistive exercise program, or it may be used to compare a patient to established reference scores. Many reference scores for men and women of all ages exist for movements such as bench press, latissimus dorsi pull-down, leg press, and knee extension and are included throughout this chapter.

Technique

There are several methods that can be used to determine a 1-RM. For patients with certain health conditions (e.g., known cardiovascular disease, pulmonary diseases, or metabolic disorders), a conservative approach is recommended, such as a multiple-RM, described later in this section. The technique described below is chosen because it works well in the clinic and is recommended by the American College of Sports Medicine (ACSM).[1] The basic steps for performing a 1-RM are as follows[1]:

1. Testing should be completed only after the patient has participated in familiarization/practice sessions.
2. A warm-up should be done by having the patient complete a number of submaximal repetitions for the specific exercise that will be used to determine the 1-RM.
3. Determine the 1-RM (or any multiple of 1-RM) within four trials with rest breaks of 1 to 3 minutes between trials.

4. Select an initial weight that is within the patient's perceived capacity (~50% to 70% of capacity).
5. Resistance is progressively increased by 5% to 10% for upper body or 10% to 20% for lower body exercise from the previous successful attempt until the individual cannot complete the selected repetition(s); all repetitions should be performed at the same speed of movement and range of motion to instill consistency between trials.
6. The final weight lifted successfully when no other repetition can be performed is recorded as the absolute 1-RM (or multiple-RM).

Selecting the Starting Weight

Selecting the amount of the starting weight is crucial because the fewer repetitions to reach 1-RM the better to avoid muscular fatigue and to prevent an underestimation of the true 1-RM. It is helpful for the tester to have knowledge of reference scores for the test. For example, standing from a chair requires quadriceps strength of nearly half a person's body weight, regardless of the age. Therefore, when performing a 1-RM using a leg press to test the quadriceps of a person who can stand without using one's arms successfully, but with difficulty, a starting weight might be 60% of patient's body weight. Alternatively, reference scores exist for the leg press based on age. These scores might be a starting point for establishing a 1-RM. Other variables that can be factored into the clinical decision of initial load are body size (muscular versus thin), fitness level, the presence of pain, and patient's self-perception of ability.

Other considerations that should be attended to during 1-RM testing include breathing, form, and pain. First and foremost, patients should *not* hold their breath during the test. Thus, breath control should be practiced during the warm-ups. Second, the patient should maintain correct form throughout the test. For example, the patient should not be permitted to pitch the trunk forward during the knee extension test, avoid muscle substitution, or use momentum. Joint movements during the test should be executed smoothly and consistently throughout the entire concentric and eccentric phase in a controlled manner without jerking the bar or weight. If the test causes pain, an alternative to the 1-RM test should be selected, such as a multiple-RM test.

Multiple-Repetition Maximum Test

A multiple-RM test is based on the principles of a 1-RM test. The multiple-RM test is the number of repetitions performed using good form and proper breath technique at the point of muscle failure. Although not as exact as a 1-RM, a multiple-RM test may be desirable for certain situations. For example, some untrained adults are not comfortable exerting the kind of effort necessary for a true 1-RM. A multiple-RM test may be a safer option when joint or soft tissues are compromised (e.g., connective tissue disease, rotator cuff tear, ligamentous injury, or post-surgery). For individuals without an exercise history and for patients who cannot tolerate high joint compression forces, such as those with osteoarthritis and rheumatoid arthritis, or with systemic weakness, the multiple-RM test, such as an 8- or 10-RM test, is safer than the 1-RM test. A 10- to 15-RM test is recommended if the patient has a health condition such as cardiovascular disease or a pulmonary or pulmonary condition.[1]

A 1-RM test can be estimated from a multiple-RM test (Table 7.1),[5] although this estimation has been shown to be quite variable (Table 7.2), with the 5 RM shown to be the most reliable.[6,7,8] The general principle is as the percentage of 1-RM increases, the number of repetitions decreases (Table 7.3). Large muscle group exercises allow the completion of more repetitions than small muscle groups at the same relative intensity.[9] Because the volume of work is greater with a 10-RM than a 1-RM, fatigue will be a factor. The 1-RM and multiple-RM tests can be performed using the same equipment.

The number of repetitions performed at a given percent of 1-RM is influenced by the amount of active muscle mass. For example, more repetitions can be performed during the back squat than either the bench press or arm curl.[9] The 4- to 6-RM is more accurate than the 10-RM. Variability in RM increases with lighter loads.[10]

Table 7.1 ESTIMATING ONE-REPETITION MAXIMUM FROM A MULTIPLE-REPETITION MAXIMUM TEST

Number of Repetitions Performed	Percent of 1-Repetition Maximum	Multiply Weight Lifted By:
1	100	1.00
2	95	1.05
3	93	1.08
4	90	1.11
5	87	1.15
6	85	1.18
7	83	1.20
8	80	1.25
9	77	1.30
10	75	1.33
11	70	1.43
12	67	1.49
15	65	1.54

Chapman, P. P., Whitehead, J. R., & Binkert, R. H. (1998). The 225-lb reps-to-fatigue test as a submaximal estimate of 1RM bench press performance in college football players. *J Strength Cond Res.* 12(4), 258–261; Lander, J. (1984). Maximum based on reps. *NSCA J.* 6(6), 60–61; Mayhew, J. L., Ball, T. E., Arnold, M. E., & Bowen, J. C. (1992). Relative muscular endurance performance as a predictor of bench press strength in college men and women. *J Appl Sport Sci Res.* 6(4), 200–206; Morales, J., & Sobonya, S. (1996). Use of submaximal repetition tests for predicting 1-RM strength in class athletes. *J Strength Cond Res.* 10(3), 186–189.

Definition of Terms

The kinetic chain refers to all the muscles and joints that are involved in producing a given movement. For example, in gait, the kinetic chain consists of the trunk, hip, knee, and ankle. Most exercises and tasks involve more than one muscle group and joint, which work simultaneously to produce the movement. Exercises in the kinetic chain can be performed two ways, open and closed, referred to as open chain and closed chain.

Open-chain exercises are performed such that the distal end of the kinetic chain is free to move. An example of an open-chain activity is quadriceps knee extension sitting on a plinth where the leg moves from 90° of flexion to full extension.

Closed-chain exercises are performed with the distal end of the kinetic chain fixed. An example of a closed-chain exercise for the quadriceps is squatting. The knee is again moving through 90° of movement, but the leg is fixed in place and the thigh is moving over the fixed leg.

Table 7.2 NUMBER OF REPETITIONS PERFORMED AT 80% OF THE ONE-REPETITION MAXIMUM[6]

| Exercise | TRAINED | | UNTRAINED | |
	Men	Women	Men	Women
Leg press	19	22	15	12
Lat pull-down	12	10	10	10
Bench press	12	14	10	10
Leg extension	12	10	9	8
Sit-up	12	12	8	7
Arm curl	11	7	8	6
Leg curl	7	5	6	6

Hoger, W. W., Hopkins, D. R., Barette, S.L., et al. (1990). Relationship between repetitions and selected percentages of one repetition maximum: a comparison between untrained males and females. *J Strength Cond Res.* 4,47–54.

Table 7.3 MAXIMUM WEIGHT THAT CAN BE LIFTED DECREASES WITH THE NUMBER OF REPETITIONS

Given:	1-RM	2-RM	3-RM	4-RM	5-RM	6-RM	7-RM	8-RM	9-RM	10-RM
The load would be (lb.)	100	95	93	90	87	85	83	80	77	75
Number of repetitions	1	2	3	4	5	6	7	8	9	10

RM, Repetition maximum.

Because practice patterns have changed extensively since the advent of manual muscle testing, methods to identify muscle weakness have also evolved. The days of poliomyelitis are behind us, and the need to identify deficiencies related to sports-related injuries, trauma, aging, and a host of other clinical conditions has resulted in the development of new and more specific testing techniques for the characterization of muscle weakness. This chapter segment will present an overview of some of the more popular approaches.

Equipment-based strength tests offer many advantages. The main advantage of using equipment (such as a strength-testing device) for RM testing is that the stability afforded by the device is far greater than in manual muscle testing and thus allows for highly controlled, single-plane movements and increased patient safety. In addition, reference scores for many movements are available with equipment-based testing. The disadvantages of using equipment for testing are they take up space, may not be readily available, can be expensive, can test only one plane of movement, and can test only a finite number of muscle groups.

INTERPRETATION OF EQUIPMENT-BASED STRENGTH TESTING DATA

Equipment-based strength testing data are informative only if used in context with other clinical findings. For example, the correlation between identified side-to-side strength differences for shoulder flexion and difficulty lifting or the presence of pain on the weaker side enhances the clinician's clinical decision making, and treatment can be confidently and competently applied. If gait speed is slow or there is evidence of gait deviation, equipment-based strength testing may help to inform the clinician of the reasons for the gait slowness or deviation and thus enhance treatment planning. Equipment-based strength testing, as with manual muscle testing, is only as good as the technique applied and is useful only in conjunction with other important functional findings. *Clinical competence develops with practice, practice, and more practice*, which includes all testing procedures, particularly those that provide information about strength deficits. Investing the time to learn correct testing procedures results in improved treatment planning, more targeted goal setting, better documentation of the patient's status and rate of improvement, and greater success in receiving reimbursements from health insurance providers.

SITTING UNILATERAL KNEE EXTENSION TEST

Purpose: The sitting unilateral knee extension test is used primarily to determine quadriceps strength when the strength of the patient's knee extensors exceed the strength or stabilization abilities of the clinician providing resistance. The sitting unilateral knee extension test can be used to distinguish side-to-side differences in quadriceps force output and elicit a true maximum effort.

Position of Patient: Seated comfortably on a knee extension machine that has been adjusted for leg length. If necessary, padding may be placed beneath the thigh being tested for patient's comfort.

The resistance pad should be positioned at distal third of tibia (Fig. 7.1). A seat belt may be placed around the patient's pelvis, if needed, to provide stability (seat belt not shown in figure).

Instructions to Clinician: To achieve a 1-RM, select an initial weight from the weight stack, based on the screening exam. A good place to start is approximately 25% of

FIGURE 7.1

body weight if the screening exam verifies the patient can stand unassisted. Note that the weight lifted will be less than on a leg press machine. Standing at the side of patient, with patient sitting and arms at sides and hands holding the handles, have patient completely extend the knee through full range of motion with the selected weight. If successful, after a minimum 1- to 3-minute rest, another repetition with a higher weight is performed through full range of motion. After the load cannot be moved through full range or patient loses form, patient is asked to perform another repetition at that weight, after the appropriate rest period, to verify muscle failure and confirm that patient cannot complete another repetition.

Instructions to Patient: "Lift the weighted bar, completely straightening your knee."

Scoring

Record the highest weight the patient lifted one time only (was not able to lift a second time) to reach full knee extension for a 1-RM. The multiple-RM is recorded as the weight lifted at last repetition and the number of repetitions the patient performed at that weight to achieve muscle failure. (Note: Knee extension through full range of motion, particularly the last 15° to 0°, must be achieved for a successful test.)

Clinical Relevance

- A patient will move less weight on a single-joint machine, such as a unilateral knee extension machine, than on a multiple-joint machine, such as a unilateral leg press, because of the amount of muscle mass involved (e.g., quadriceps only versus quadriceps, gastrocnemius/soleus, and gluteals combined) and because only one leg is being used.

Leg Press Test

The leg press machine is one of the most useful devices in a clinic, as it is a closed-chain activity, thus mimicking a component of standing, walking, and rising from a chair. The force output generated by a patient will tell the clinician whether a patient has enough strength to be functional in activities of daily living or with sport activities requiring a large amount of strength, such as soccer.

Purpose: The leg press assesses force output of all extensor muscles in the lower extremities (hip and knee extensors and plantar-flexors).

Position of Patient: Seated comfortably on leg press machine, with head and spine in contact with seat back, both feet on the foot plate, approximately 12 in. apart, knees bent approximately 90° over the hips and in line with feet (avoid knees dropping toward each other in hip adduction), and hands on grab bars (Fig. 7.2). Feet on the footplate in either the low position (Fig. 7.3) or the high foot position (see Fig. 7.2).

FIGURE 7.2

FIGURE 7.3

Instructions to Clinician: Ensure patient has painless and sufficient hip, knee, and ankle range to perform the test and is warmed up sufficiently. Select the initial weight that is ~50% to 70% of capacity (see Table 7.4 for leg press reference values) and ask the patient to fully extend the legs with feet against the footplate so that shins are parallel with the floor. The knees should be softly extended at the end of the push (avoid a "locked out" position). Note: Some leg press machines require clinician to place weights on either side of the footplate bar (e.g., two 25-lb weights) and lock the weights in place. Other machines will require the patient to sit upright. Obtain 1-RM.

Instructions to Patient: "Push the plate until your legs are straight. Don't hold your breath during the test or lock your knees out. Keep your knees in line with your feet. Let the weight back slowly; don't slam the weight."

Scoring

Record the highest weight patient can push 1 time (for 1-RM) or, for a multiple-RM, the weight achieved and number of repetitions with the end weight that produced muscle failure.

Clinical Relevance

- The leg press uses the closed-chain approach (distal end of the kinetic chain is fixed).
- Foot position low on the plate (see Fig. 7.3) elicits greater muscle activity from the rectus femoris and gastrocnemius at 80% 1-RM than high foot position (see Fig. 7.2), suggesting that the feet should routinely be positioned low on the plate when using a 40% or 80% 1-RM.[11]
- The high foot position elicits gluteus maximus more than low foot position.[11]
- Not all patients can comfortably assume a low foot position; in terms of importance, comfort should outweigh desired muscle activation.
- There are established reference scores for leg press for men and women ages 20 through early 60s that are expressed as a ratio of force output to body weight. Thus, a typical ratio of weight to body weight for a young woman in her twenties is 2.05, meaning that she should be able to generate force equivalent to twice her body weight.
- Reference scores for the leg press compiled from hundreds of men and women that have been tested by the Cooper Institute are presented in Table 7.4.
- Absolute leg press reference scores for men and women 60 to 85 years by half decades using a Keiser pneumatic leg press are also available.[12]

Table 7.4 LEG PRESS NORMS FOR MEN AND WOMEN IN VARIOUS AGE GROUPS; VALUES REFLECT ONE-REPETITION MAXIMUM/BODY WEIGHT

Percentile[a]	20–29 YEARS		30–39 YEARS		40–49 YEARS		50–59 YEARS		60+ YEARS	
	Men	Women	Men	Women	Men	Women	Men	Women	Men	Women
90th	2.27	2.05	2.07	1.73	1.92	1.63	1.80	1.51	1.73	1.40
80th	2.13	1.00	1.93	1.50	1.82	1.46	1.71	1.30	1.62	1.25
70th	2.05	1.42	1.85	1.47	1.74	1.35	1.64	1.24	1.56	1.18
60th	1.97	1.36	1.77	1.32	1.68	1.26	1.58	1.18	1.49	1.15
50th	1.91	1.32	1.71	1.26	1.62	1.19	1.52	1.09	1.43	1.08
40th	1.83	1.25	1.65	1.21	1.57	1.12	1.46	1.03	1.38	1.04
30th	1.74	1.23	1.59	1.16	1.51	1.03	1.39	0.95	1.30	0.98
20th	1.63	1.13	1.52	1.09	1.44	0.94	1.32	0.86	1.25	0.94
10th	1.51	1.02	1.43	0.94	1.35	0.76	1.22	0.75	1.16	0.84

[a]Descriptors for percentile rankings: 90, well above average; 70, above average; 50, average; 30, below average; 10, well below average.

Data for men provided by Heyward, V. H. (2005). *The Physical Fitness Specialist Manual*. The Cooper Institute for Aerobics Research. http://hk.humankinetics.com/AdvancedFitnessAssessmentandExercisePrescription/IG/269618.indd.pdf; and Data for women provided by the Women's Exercise Research Center, The George Washington University Medical Center, Washington, DC, 1998.

Latissimus Dorsi Pull-Down Test

The latissimus dorsi pull-down test (lat pull-down test) is a general measure of bilateral scapular adduction and scapular downward rotation. The lat pull-down machine is commonly available in clinics, wellness centers, and workout facilities. The test is one of the safest and easiest to perform of all upper extremity exercises. This test is feasible for most adults without shoulder or neck problems.

Purpose: To measure the collective force of the latissimus dorsi muscles, pectoralis major, rhomboids, and middle and lower trapezius.

Position of Patient: Seated, facing the weight stack, feet flat on floor. Arms overhead with hands on bar in overhand grip (pronation) with a wide hand position (Fig. 7.4). Head position should be over shoulders, with attention to avoiding a forward head position.

FIGURE 7.4

Instructions to Clinician: Ensure the patient has no shoulder pain and sufficient shoulder and elbow range to perform the test. Bring the overhead bar to the patient. Hands placed on the bar should be in an overhand grip with hands slightly wider than shoulders. Select a weight based on the initial screening that is relatively easy, such as 20 lb. for a woman and 40 lb. for a man. Adjust the soft pad above the thighs so that it is comfortable and contributes to stability. The clinician then stands behind the patient to monitor the position of the scapulae. Correct form is when the bar is pulled down to shoulder height in front of the body with shoulders retracted (scapular adduction and downward rotation), flexed elbows driving back, and trunk leaning slightly backward. The position of pulling down in front of the head provides the greatest activation of the latissimus dorsi and pectoralis major.[13,14] Depending on performance of the first repetition, increase or decrease weight as indicated to achieve a 1- or multiple-RM.

Instructions to Patient: "In a smooth manner, pull the bar down in front of you level with your shoulders while pulling your shoulder blades back and down. Don't hold your breath."

Scoring

Record the highest weight and number of repetitions the patient performs without losing form for a 1-RM or multiple-RM. Norms for the latissimus pull-down activity are typically 66% of body weight for young men and 50% of body weight for young women.[15] Reference scores for men and women who are middle-aged and older have not been established.

Clinical Relevance

The front neck lat pull-down is more comfortable and has greater pectoralis major activation without sacrificing latissimus dorsi activation compared to the behind-the-neck position.[13]

Free Weight Testing

Free weights are the gold standard for reliability and validity of the 1-RM method because of their ease of application and specificity. They offer important advantages for muscle testing, such as permitting the clinician to assess strength in both the concentric and eccentric modes. Free weights are readily available in most clinical settings and are easily accessible for home use, where some household items can be substituted for weights when testing weaker patients. They can also be used through full range and through multiple planes.

Moreover, movements with free weights require greater motor coordination and better balance (if standing), resulting in greater muscle recruitment. They use important stabilizing muscles to complete a lift compared with machines, which do not emphasize the stabilizing musculature because movements occur in only one plane of motion. They also allow the clinician freedom to test different movement variations that can better inform an exercise prescription. Strengthening exercise that allows multiple planes of motion such as with free weights has demonstrated greater strength gains than equipment-based strengthening with fixed ranges of motion in which patients are unable to deviate from the intended range.[16]

However, several disadvantages of using free weights exist. Greater control is required through all planes of movement because of stabilization required. Free weights can challenge the entire kinetic chain, thus stressing the "weakest link" rather than the targeted muscle or movement unless proper stabilization is provided. Maximum muscle loading occurs only at the weakest point in the range, thus requiring an attentive clinician. Proper positioning is critical for safety and test reliability. Spotting is necessary because the patient may lose control of the weight, potentially causing injury.

Examples of Free Weight Testing

Biceps Curl

The biceps curl is an example of using free weights to determine a 1-RM or multiple-RM. In this instance, the biceps, brachialis, and brachioradialis are the muscles that will be challenged, particularly the biceps and brachialis. This test can easily discern side-to-side differences and whether strength is adequate for lifting during work.

Purpose: To determine the maximum force capability of the biceps brachii and brachialis, as well as the brachioradialis and, to a lesser extent, the pronator teres muscles.

Position of Patient: Either standing or seated comfortably in a standard chair with no arms. Provide seat belt if needed. Elbow should be straight, with arm at the side, forearm supinated. Standing requires stabilization of the trunk, which may be a more functional position, although more difficult.

Instructions to Clinician: Based on prescreening, which may include questions such as "can you easily carry a bag of groceries" (approximately 10 lb.) or "how much do you normally curl?" and determination that full range of motion can be achieved painlessly; the clinician should select a weight that is reasonably challenging, generally 50% more than what is routinely lifted. Standing next to the patient, place weight in patient's hand with forearm supinated and ask patient to flex elbow through full range of motion in a supinated position (Fig. 7.5). After a rest of a minimum of 1 to 3 minutes, increase or decrease weight in appropriate intervals based on performance to achieve a 1-RM or multiple-RM.

Instructions to Patient: "While holding the weight, bend your elbow until the weight touches your upper arm, keeping your hand facing your face."

Scoring

Record 1-RM or multiple-RM. Reference scores are approximately 25% of body weight for women and 33% of body weight for men.[10]

Note: The incremental increase in weight lifted is far less for the upper extremity compared with the lower extremity because of the difference in muscle mass.

A hammer curl is performed in the same manner but keeping the forearm in a neutral position with thumb toward body. The hammer curl primarily works the long head of the biceps brachii and brachialis, and therefore, the patient is able to lift more weight than in a biceps curl.

Bench Press Test

The bench press is one of the most popular tests of upper extremity strength because it provides a composite value for many muscles, similar to the leg press.

FIGURE 7.5

Purpose: To determine the maximum force capability of the larger anterior scapulohumeral muscles that include the pectoralis major, pectoralis minor, anterior deltoid, infraspinatus, serratus anterior, and upper and lower trapezius. In addition, the triceps brachii is critical to extend the elbow.

Position of Patient: Supine on the testing bench, back flat against bench with feet flat on the floor. Nipple line is directly below the weight bar. Hand position is pronated (overhand grip) and slightly wider than shoulders (Fig. 7.6).

Instructions to Clinician: Prescreen patient to ensure the presence of full, painless range of motion. Observe patient's muscle bulk, and ask prescreening questions such as "Do you chest press regularly?" Then, select two equal-weight plates and place them at each end of the bench press bar, locking weights in place. Provide for a warm-up period. Once warmed up, adjust weight to approximately 40% of body weight for women and 50% body weight for men. Be sure to consider weight of the bar itself.

FIGURE 7.6

Stand at patient's head to "spot" the patient throughout the movement (see Fig. 7.6). Have patient grasp bar with a pronated grip. At a signal from the patient, assist patient in moving bar off the supports and lowering bar directly over chest. Release bar smoothly after you are confident the patient is in control of the bar. Ask patient to lower bar to the nipple level, keeping head flat against bench. Then, ask patient to push bar overhead until elbows are fully extended. The back should not come off bench. Weight is either decreased (if first attempt is not successful) or increased if patient indicates multiple repetitions can be performed. Provide the patient a minimum of 1 to 3 minutes of rest between lifts. Test failure is observed when the patient is unable to complete full range of motion. At test failure, grasp the bar with alternating overhand and underhand grips (see Fig. 7.6), and place it on the rack supports.

Instructions to Patient: "Lower weight slowly and smoothly, then push bar straight up overhead until your elbows are completely straight. Do not hold your breath. Be sure to tell me if you need assistance with the bar."

Scoring

Record 1-RM or multiple-RM. Reference scores for men and women are listed in Table 7.5.

Clinical Relevance

The standard bench press bars weigh 45 lb. The weight of the bar must be taken into consideration when determining ultimate load.

- It may be necessary for the clinician to take weight bar away from the patient at test failure, so the clinician should be sure (in advance) that he or she is physically capable of handling the weight bar being lifted.
- If there is no weight bench and patient is lying on a plinth, the clinician must place fully loaded lifting bar into position above the patient, approximately 6 in. above chest at nipple level. Help may be needed if the clinician is unable to handle the loaded weight bar. "Spotting" patient is an even more important safety consideration in this adaptation of the bench press.

Table 7.5 BENCH PRESS NORMS BY SEX AND AGE VALUES REFLECT ONE-REPETITION MAXIMUM/BODY WEIGHT (IN POUNDS)

Per-centile	20–29 YEARS		30–39 YEARS		40–49 YEARS		50–59 YEARS		60+ YEARS		70+ YEARS
	Men	Women	Men	Women	Men	Women	Men	Women	Men	Women	Women
90th	1.48	0.54	1.24	0.49	1.10	0.46	0.97	0.40	0.89	0.41	0.44
80th	1.32	0.49	1.12	0.45	1.00	0.40	0.90	0.37	0.82	0.38	0.39
70th	1.22	0.42	1.04	0.42	0.93	0.38	0.84	0.35	0.77	0.36	0.33
60th	1.14	0.41	0.98	0.41	0.88	0.37	0.79	0.33	0.72	0.32	0.31
50th	1.06	0.40	0.93	0.38	0.84	0.34	0.75	0.31	0.68	0.30	0.27
40th	0.99	0.37	0.88	0.37	0.80	0.32	0.71	0.28	0.66	0.29	0.25
30th	0.93	0.35	0.83	0.34	0.76	0.30	0.68	0.26	0.63	0.28	0.24
20th	0.88	0.33	0.78	0.32	0.72	0.27	0.63	0.23	0.57	0.26	0.21
10th	0.80	0.30	0.71	0.27	0.65	0.23	0.57	0.19	0.53	0.25	0.20

Descriptors for percentile rankings: 90, well above average; 50, average; 30, below average; and 10, well below average.

Data for women are derived from the Women's Exercise Research Center, The George Washington University Medical Center, Washington, DC, 1998; and data for men were provided by Heyward, V. H. (2005). *The Physical Fitness Specialist Manual*. The Cooper Institute for Aerobics Research. http://hk.humankinetics.com/Advanced-FitnessAssessmentandExercisePrescription/IG/269618.indd.pdf.

Isokinetic Testing

Isokinetic testing was developed in the 1960s and is now primarily used for research because of its objectivity. Advantages of isokinetic testing for evaluating muscle strength and contraction speed include testing through a spectrum of movement speeds (e.g., 0° to 400° per second), providing highly reliable data, and providing safety in testing by ensuring movement control. Most importantly, isokinetic machines (e.g., Cybex, Biodex, Kin Com) allow maximal resistance throughout the entire range of motion, something that no other testing method can provide. Eccentric strength can also be objectively assessed.

The disadvantages of isokinetic testing include:
- Prohibitive cost and space requirements of the oversized testing equipment
- Time required to set up the tests
- Only single planes of movement can be tested
- Many sports-specific movements are faster than any isokinetic machine
- Isokinetic contractions are nonphysiological

Isokinetic machines allow speed to remain constant, but the force generated through the range is not consistent, which means that muscle demand (percentage of force required) is highly variable throughout the range of motion. To use the knee extensors as an example, under physiological conditions, quadriceps strength demand is greatest at the end of the range, where length tension and the patella lever arm are poorest. Therefore, isokinetic peak torque and strength from 1-RM are not equivalent when evaluating muscle strength changes in patients.[17]

Although setup for isokinetic testing is protocol driven, the actual test execution requires skill, computer interaction, and know-how that is beyond the scope of this book. For complete instruction in isokinetic testing, the reader is referred to the remarkable amount of material on the internet and the instruction booklets from the makers of isokinetic machines and instrumentation.

Elastic Band Testing

Elastic band testing is a common form of strength testing that uses elastic resistance that is color coded according to level of resistance. Resistance of the band is based on the amount and kind of material used in the band. Thicker bands provide more resistance. Some bands use a polymerized synthetic rubber, whereas others use a natural rubber latex (TheraBand) that may provide better elasticity and lower susceptibility to rupture. The force of elastic resistance depends on its percentage of elongation, regardless of initial length. The elastic band should be the same length as the lever arm being tested to ensure elongation remains less than 200%.[18] For example, if the length of the patient's leg, from hip to heel, is 50 in., then a band of 50 in. should be used. Force elongation in pounds for 100% elongation of TheraBand elastic bands is listed in Table 7.6.

In addition to elastic band availability in nearly all clinics and ease of application for home use, there are several other advantages to elastic band testing. Elastic bands produce a curvilinear length-tension profile, which can be used to challenge the end range, potentially producing a higher peak force than might be achieved with a free weight or machine.[19] Elastic bands increase the agonist-antagonist co-contraction, challenging stability.

Eccentric contractions are especially challenged with elastic bands. Patients receive immediate feedback about their progress because the color of band changes according to strength increases. The cost of bands is low compared with other methods of strength testing. Any movement can be tested, with a little creativity.

Disadvantages of elastic band testing include the need for stabilization and the amount of force-generated changes throughout the range. Greater force is required as the band elongates, which may alter form. There is difficulty standardizing elements of band elongation and the patient and/or extremity positioning, and quantifying test interpretation is dependent on the manufacturer. For example, if you have two patients and one patient abducts the hip only 10° against a gray elastic band (high strength demand), whereas another abducts the hip 20° against a green elastic band (low strength demand), which patient has more strength? Strength indexes help to standardize this issue; however, they are widely known only for TheraBand elastic bands.[20] Different manufacturers use different color codes, and published strength indexes are not interchangeable.

For safety, test positions can be adapted. For example, testing of the elbow flexors can be done with the patient sitting or standing. Fig. 7.7A (start position) and Fig. 7.7B (end position illustrate the use of elastic band testing for shoulder abduction strength.

Table 7.6 FORCE ELONGATION FOR THERABAND ELASTIC BANDS AT 100% ELONGATION (VALUE = FORCE IN POUNDS)

Elongation (%)	Yellow	Red	Green	Blue	Black	Gray	Gold
100 (twice the length of the band)	3	3.7	4.6	5.8	7.3	10.2	14.2

The percentage of elongation (change in length) is calculated with the following formula:

Percentage of elongation

$= ($final length$) - ($resting length$)/($resting length$] \times 100$.

Page, P. *Can I assess strength with elastic bands?* Thera-Band Academy. http://www.thera-bandacademy.com/resource/x-showResource.aspx?id=5534. (Last accessed 21 October 2023).

FIGURE 7.7

Example of Elastic Band Testing

Testing the Shoulder Abductors

Purpose: To test maximum strength of shoulder abductors (deltoid and rotator cuff). Muscles also involved are serratus anterior and upper/lower trapezius that upwardly rotate the scapula to support the humerus.

Position of Patient: Standing (or sitting, not shown).

Instructions to Clinician: Before patient testing, shoulder abduction should be assessed for available range and the absence of pain. To assess strength, an elastic band of a resistance based on prescreening is selected for use. In general, a medium resistance band is feasible for most trained patients who do not have shoulder pain. Measure the band so that it is the same length as the length of the arm. Secure one end to an immovable object or knot the end and have the patient stand on the end of the band with knot secured on the inside of the foot. Stand to the side and slightly behind patient. Ask patient to hold the other end of band, with any slack in band removed. Ask the patient to lift the arm into 90° of abduction to height of shoulder, keeping the hand/forearm pronated and the elbow straight. At this position, the band should be elongated 2× (100%) its original length. Then, ask the patient to slowly lower the arm (generally 3× slower than the lifting phase). Decrease resistance color of the band if patient is unable to complete full range or has discomfort and increase resistance if patient can perform multiple repetitions. Clinician should monitor form to include stabilization of trunk, head, and neck position, pronation of the forearm/hand, and scapular adduction and downward rotation.

Instructions to Patient: "Lift your arm out and away from the side of your body to the height of your shoulder. Keep your elbow straight and hand pointed down. Don't hold your breath during the test."

Scoring

Record the color of the band used to complete a full 90° of abduction and how many repetitions were performed

Clinical Relevance

- Most companies sell handles to attach to the end of the band, thus making it easier for patients to use the band.
- With repeated use and age of the band, elastic bands lose their elasticity and/or become brittle and should be replaced. Bands should always be inspected for small tears or holes that may weaken the band and cause it to break during elongation. Periodic inspections will determine if it is time to discard the original band.
- If the clinician underestimated the strength of the patient, the patient's force may overcome the elastic properties of the band and cause it to break, creating a potentially unpleasant and unsafe condition. Therefore, care must be used when familiarizing a patient with this type of resistance for exercise testing.

to muscle failure if more than one repetition was completed. Consult appropriate chart for force in pounds (depending on manufacturer of band). Force elongation for 100% elongation of TheraBand elastic bands as described by the manufacturer is listed in Table 7.6.

POWER TESTING

Power testing, also known as maximal anaerobic power testing, was initially developed to assess explosive strength in a sports setting. Maximal power is defined as force per unit of time, and thus, a power measure includes not just muscular force production but the rate of force development. The specific formula for power is:

$$Power = work/seconds$$

Powerful athletes can accelerate rapidly with explosive force output (e.g., the Olympic 100-m dash). In addition, the rate of force development may be the critical determinant of a person's safety, especially in unexpected or emergent situations. For example, a patient must go from gas pedal to brake quickly enough to prevent a vehicular crash. Another important reason for rapid force development is to prevent a fall. Once a person loses balance, only the power of rapid limb movement can rescue the individual. Power is a major determinant of functional impairment in older adults and is considered even more important than strength (e.g., in the chair rise).[21] Thus, power is an important aspect of muscle performance even for acute hospitalized older adults.[22]

When following guidelines for power testing that includes two to three familiarization sessions and an adequate warm-up before each testing session, muscle power testing appears to be a safe procedure even for older people with a broad range of health and functional states.[23]

The power tests in the next section have been selected because they do not require special equipment or extensive preparation. In addition, these tests require maximum muscle power. Because maximal muscular activity is involved in performing power tests, they are anaerobic and are of short duration.

Margaria-Kalamen Stair Sprint Test[24]

Since the early 1960s, numerous adaptations of the original Margaria stair sprint test[24] have been made as the relevance and importance of power testing have become evident. Modified versions include running two stairs at a time and shortening the starting distance. Regardless, the test is of short duration (lasting less than 5 seconds). It is considered a standard test for determining peak power. A disadvantage of the test is that typically only the young and healthy can perform it.

Purpose: To measure maximal anaerobic strength and power of the lower extremities.

Test Instructions[5]: Ensure patient can safely negotiate nine stairs, three steps at a time. Weigh patient in kilograms. Each stair should be 17.5 cm (~7 in.) tall. The clinician should stand at the bottom of the stairs to monitor the effort. A timer start switch mechanism is placed on the third step, and a stop switch mechanism is placed on the ninth step. With patient positioned 6 m (20 ft) from the bottom stair, ask the patient to run towards stairs, taking three steps at a time at maximal speed. Repeat the test 2× with a 3-minute recovery period between each trial.

Scoring

The time from third- to ninth-step contact is determined to the nearest 0.01 second using the timing system. Power in watts is calculated according to the following formula:

$$\text{Power (in watts)} = \text{weight (body weight in kg)} \times 9.807$$
$$\times \text{vertical height of six stairs in meters}$$
$$\left(\text{step } 3 - \text{step } 9\right)/\text{time} \left(\text{seconds}\right)$$

Example: Mark weighs 210 lb. and scored a best attempt of 1.2 seconds when climbing six steps with a combined height of 49.5 inches.

$$210 \text{ lb.} = 95.25 \text{ kg}$$

$$\text{Vertical height} = 17.5 \text{ cm stairs} \times 6 = 1.05 \text{ meters}$$

$$\text{Power} = \left(92.25 \times 9.807\right) \times 1.05/1.2 = 831 \text{ watts}$$

Reference scores are described in Table 7.7.

Table 7.7 MARGARIA–KALAMEN STAIR SPRINT TEST REFERENCE SCORES (WATTS)

| Classifi-cation | AGE GROUPS (YEARS) | | | | | | | | | |
| | 15–20 | | 20–30 | | 30–40 | | 40–50 | | OVER 50 | |
	M	F	M	F	M	F	M	F	M	F
Excellent	Over 2197	Over 1785	Over 2059	Over 1648	Over 1648	Over 1226	Over 1226	Over 961	Over 961	Over 736
Good	1844–2197	1491–1785	1726–2059	1383–1648	1383–1648	1040–1226	1040–1226	814–961	814–961	608–736
Average	1471–1824	1187–1481	1373–1716	1098–1272	1098–1373	834–1030	834–1030	647–804	647–804	481–598
Fair	1108–1461	902–1177	1040–1363	834–1089	834–1088	637–824	637–824	490–637	490–637	373–471
Poor	Under 1108	Under 902	Under 1040	Under 834	Under 834	Under 637	Under 637	Under 490	Under 490	Under 373

Data from Hoffman, J. (2006). *Norms for fitness, performance, and health*. Human Kinetics. Adapted from Fox, E., Bowers, R., & Foss, M. (1993). *The Physiological Basis for Exercise and Sport* (p. 676) (5th ed.). William C. Brown Company with permission of the McGraw-Hill Companies; based on data from Kalamen, J. (1968). *Measurement of maximum muscular power in man*. [Doctoral dissertation, The Ohio State University]; and Margaria, R., Aghemo, I., & Rovelli, E. (1966). Measurement of muscular power (anaerobic) in man. *J Appl Physiol*. 21, 1662-1664.

Medicine Ball Throw Test

Purpose: To determine strength of flexion, extension, and rotational strength and power of important scapulothoracic and glenohumeral muscles, particularly pectoralis major and minor, anterior deltoid, supraspinatus, and infraspinatus.

Test Instructions: With patient seated, assess ability of patient to throw a medicine ball from chest.[25] Weight of the ball usually ranges from 1.5 to 4 kg. Athletes perform this test seated on the floor with legs extended in front and back against the wall (not shown). If patient can perform the task, place a 1- to 4-kg ball in patient's hands close to the chest (like a basketball) (Fig. 7.8A). Ask patient to push ball forward as rapidly as possible. An alternate method of throwing the ball from behind the head is depicted in Fig. 7.8B. In this instance, patient throws the ball using an overhead technique. Either technique is acceptable.

Scoring

The test is repeated three times. Record the maximum or average distance from front of the chair to where the medicine ball lands. No reference values exist, and scores depend on weight of the ball. However, the top score in the 2013 NHL Combine using a 4-kg ball was 6.25 m (sitting on the floor).[26] Older men and women (mean age, 72.4 years) threw a 1.5-kg ball a range of 2 to 6 m and a 3-kg ball a range of 2 to 4.5 m.[25]

Shot Put Test

Purpose: As with the medicine ball throw, the shot put test challenges the musculature of the glenohumeral and scapulothoracic muscles. However, the test is unilateral, which permits side-to-side comparisons. Because the test is done standing, it also challenges balance. The test can also be done sitting, similar to the two-handed medicine ball throw test.

Test Instructions: Assess patient's ability to throw a shot put from overhead. If patient can perform the test, select a "shot" that is appropriate for patient (1 to 7 kg). The clinician then places the shot put in the patient's hand. Ask patient to bring the shot put to the shoulder and then rapidly thrust shot put away from body as far as possible. The technique requires patient momentarily balancing the shot put on the shoulder and chin (Fig. 7.9). The trial is repeated three times, and the farthest distance is recorded.

FIGURE 7.8A AND B

Scoring

The trial is repeated three times, and the farthest distance is recorded. No reference values exist; however, distances of more than 20 m have been recorded for female and male athletes.

Alternative Shot Put Test: Standing and using two hands, patient leans forward, brings the shot down between legs, and throws the shot forward as far as possible. The throw is underhand instead of overhand and involves both arms instead of just one. This test is easier for the patient to perform. To score, record the distances of the effort.

Vertical Jump Test

Purpose: The vertical jump test assesses maximum muscle power and strength. It specifically challenges the extensors of the lower extremity, particularly the gluteus maximus and minimus, hamstrings, quadriceps, gastrocnemius, and soleus. Only those with adequate balance can perform the test.

Test Instructions: Tape a yardstick or piece of paper with height markings onto the wall. The clinician chalks the patient's fingers on the dominant hand. Ask the patient to reach as high as possible with the dominant hand, touching the wall while keeping the feet flat. Note chalk mark that serves as starting position. Standing flat-footed without preparation, ask patient to jump as high as possible, swinging arms backward before reaching overhead, touching dominant, chalked hand to wall (Fig. 7.10). The patient may flex knees and hips with jump. Repeat test.

Scoring

The total distance jumped is recorded, which is the highest mark minus the initial mark. Score the best of the two trials. Reference values are listed in Table 7.8 for athletes in various sports.

FIGURE 7.9

FIGURE 7.10

Table 7.8 VERTICAL JUMP DESCRIPTIVE DATA FOR VARIOUS GROUPS

Group, Sport, or Position	Vertical Jump (in./cm)
NCAA Division I college football split ends, strong safeties, offensive and defensive backs	31.5/80
NCAA Division I college football wide receivers and outside linebackers	31/79
NCAA Division I football linebackers, tight ends, and safeties	29.5/75
NCAA Division I college football quarterbacks	28.5/72
NCAA Division I college basketball players (men)	28/71
High school football backs and receivers	24/61
College baseball players (men)	23/58
College tennis players (men)	23/58
17-year-old boys	20/51
NCAA Division I college basketball (girls)	17.5–19/44–48
18- to 34-year-old men	16/41
18- to 34-year-old sedentary women	8/20
17-year-old girls	13/33

NCAA, National Collegiate Athletic Association.

Baechle, T.R., & Earle, R.W. NSCA Essentials of Strength Training and Conditioning (3rd ed., p. 278). Champaign, IL: Human Kinetics.

Hop and Standing Long Jump Tests

There are several variations on long jump power tests. As depicted in Fig. 7.11, the tests can be done on one leg, alternating from side to side or on both (Fig. 7.12). For a more challenging examination (done frequently in athletic training centers), patient is required to clear an obstacle with each jump, with some obstacles being ≥18 in.

Purpose: To test the power of the lower extremity extensors and pelvic stabilizers, particularly gluteals, quadriceps, and plantar flexors. Patients require adequate abdominal strength and balance control.

Test Instructions: For both tests, measure a 20-foot-long line. Add line on the floor as the starting position.
Single hop test: Ensure that patient can balance easily on dominant leg. If able, ask patient to stand on the line with feet just behind the line. Then ask patient to leap upward and forward on dominant leg, completing three consecutive single-leg hops (see Fig. 7.11). The total distance achieved in the three hops is measured and recorded.
Standing long jump: With both feet behind the starting line, ask patient to jump 1 time, as far forward as possible (see Fig. 7.12). Patient must land on both feet for the jump to be scored. Measure from the starting line to the patient's heel. Repeat for two trials.

Scoring

Hop Jump: The cumulative total distance achieved in the three hops is recorded.
Standing long jump: Best of two trials is the score. Long jump scores for young athletes range from 1.88 m to 3.76 m. (1.2 to 2× body height for a 5- and 6-ft individual, respectively). The long jump is an item on the Fullerton Advanced Balance Scale with full (a 4/4) scoring achieved if greater than twice the length of the patient's feet was achieved.[27]

More difficult power tests are available, but it is rarely appropriate to use tests that are at the higher end of physical performance capacity in active rehabilitation. For more definitive work on this aspect of testing, the reader is referred to other sources.[28,29] Most power tests were developed for the young athlete. However, clinician judgment regarding patient's abilities should be the key element, not age alone, in deciding whether a test is appropriate. Extreme care should be exercised in choosing a power test for those with significant weakness (Grade 3 or lower) or patients with painful conditions.

FIGURE 7.11

FIGURE 7.12

BODY WEIGHT TESTING

Using body weight as resistance provides important information about the ability of patients to use the strength they possess to move their bodies in space. These tests are also effective exercises for strengthening the core as well as specific muscle groups. Several functional tests presented in Chapter 8 use body weight resistance. Presented next are other tests that use body mass as resistance. These tests are highly demanding and should not be used for patients with specific weakness.

Pull-Up (Chin-Up) Test

Purpose: The pull-up test uses patient's body weight to challenge the shoulder extensors (latissimus dorsi, teres major, triceps brachii, and posterior deltoid). The middle and lower trapezius, pectoralis minor, and rhomboids pull the scapula down. To pull the body up to the chin-up bar, the biceps brachii, brachialis, and brachioradialis are contracting vigorously at the elbow. The wrist and finger flexors must also contract to hold the body on the bar.

Test Instructions: Assess patient's ability to fully flex the shoulders and extend the elbows. If adequate range is present and no complaints of pain are presented, ask patient to stand below an overhead bar that should be higher than patient's outstretched arms. Have patient stand on a stool if unable to reach the bar. Ask patient to grasp bar with an underhand (supinated) grip and hang from the bar with the elbows fully extended. Then, ask patient to lift the entire body multiple times to muscle failure. For each repetition to count, body must be raised so that the chin is brought above the bar. Subsequently, body is lowered to the original starting position with each repetition.

Scoring

The number of pull-ups that can be performed successfully is recorded. Reference scores for men and women are listed in Table 7.9.

Clinical Relevance

- Norms for young boys and girls can be found at http://www.exrx.net/Testing/YouthNorms.html#anchor581034
- Norms used by the Marine Corps can be found at http://www.military.com/military-fitness/marine-corps-fitness-requirements/usmc-physical-fitness-test

Table 7.9 NORMS FOR ADULTS FOR THE PULL-UP BY SEX

Sex	Excellent	Above Average	Average	Below Average	Poor
Male	>13	9–13	6–8	3–5	<3
Female	>6	5–6	3–4	1–2	0

Adapted from Davis, B. et al. (2000). *Physical Education and the Study of Sport* (p. 124) (4th ed.). Harcourt.

Push-Up Test

Purpose: A test of strength for shoulder flexors, scapular stabilizers (especially serratus anterior), and triceps brachii. Push-ups are used not only as a test of strength but as a test of endurance, particularly in the US Armed Forces.

Test Instructions: Ensure that patient does not have shoulder or any upper extremity pain and that adequate range of the shoulder, elbow, and wrist is present. Then, on the floor or other low surface, ask patient to assume the starting position or "up" position with hands shoulder width apart, back straight, head up, and using the toes as the pivotal point. Patient then lowers the body until the arms are parallel to the floor (Army standard) or until the chest touches the clinician's fist held vertically against the ground (ACSM standard). The Army uses the same position on toes for men and women. The ACSM allows women to perform push-ups on bent knees with ankles crossed. For both men and women, the back should be straight at all times, and the patient must push up to a straight arm position.[1]

Scoring

The Army standard is as many repetitions as possible within a timed 2-minute period. The patient may only pause in the up position. For the ACSM standard, as many repetitions as possible are performed until failure. Reference scores for the ACSM and Army personnel are listed in Tables 7.10 and 7.11.[3,30]

CYRIAX METHOD OF TESTING CONTRACTILE LESIONS

A common reason for strength testing in orthopedics is to diagnose the tissues contributing to musculoskeletal pain lesions. Because manual muscle testing typically requires completion of full range of motion to assign a grade, an alternative system is needed. James Cyriax developed a system to differentiate between painful contractile and noncontractile (inert) soft tissues.[31] Contractile tissues are parts of the muscle (belly, tendon, and their bony insertions). Inert tissues are those without the capacity to contract or relax, such as joint capsule, ligaments, nerve roots, and the dura mater. The clinician

Table 7.10 CONVERTING THE PUSH-UP SCORE (NUMBER) TO A HEALTH BENEFIT RATING

Age	Zone	Male	Female	Age	Zone	Male	Female
15–19	Excellent	≥39	≥33	40–49	Excellent	≥25	≥24
	Very Good	29–38	25–32		Very Good	17–24	15–23
	Good	23–28	18–24		Good	13–16	11–14
	Fair	18–22	12–17		Fair	10–12	5–10
	Poor	≤17	≤11		Poor	≤9	≤4
20–29	Excellent	≥36	≥30	50–59	Excellent	≥21	≥21
	Very Good	29–35	21–29		Very Good	13–20	11–20
	Good	22–28	15–20		Good	10–12	7–10
	Fair	17–21	10–14		Fair	7–9	2–6
	Poor	≤16	≤9		Poor	≤6	≤1
30–39	Excellent	≥30	≥27	60–69	Excellent	≥18	≥17
	Very Good	22–29	20–26		Very Good	11–17	12–16
	Good	17–21	13–19		Good	8–10	5–11
	Fair	12–16	8–12		Fair	5–7	2–4
	Poor	≤11	≤7		Poor	≤4	≤1

Table 7.11 PUSH-UP STANDARDS FOR US ARMY PERSONNEL[a]

Age Range	PUSH-UP STANDARDS FOR US ARMY PERSONNEL REPETITIONS IN 2 MINUTES																			
	M	F	M	F	M	F	M	F	M	F	M	F	M	F	M	F	M	F	M	F
17–21	6		13		20	2	28	8	35	13	42	19	49	25	57	31	64	36	71	42
22–26		5		14		23	2	31	11	40	17	49	24	58	32	66	39	75	46	
27–31		1		11		20		30	10	39	17	49	25	58	34	68	42	77	50	
32–36				7		17		26	9	36	15	46	23	56	30	65	38	75	45	
37–41				5		15		24	7	34	13	44	20	54	27	63	33	73	40	
42–46						12		21	6	30	12	39	18	48	25	57	31	66	37	
47–51						8		17		25	10	34	16	42	22	51	28	59	34	
52–56								11		20	9	29	15	38	20	47	26	56	31	
57–61								9		18	8	27	13	36	18	44	23	53	28	
62+								8		16	7	25	12	33	16	42	21	50	25	
Points Awarded	10		20		30		40		50		60		70		80		90		100	

[a]60 points is passing; 90 points is excellent. Men and women start in up position on toes.

F, Female; M, male.

http://www.military.com/military-fitness/army-fitness-requirements/army-physical-fitness-test-score-chart.

selects passive movements to specifically test inert tissue and resisted movements to specifically stress contractile tissue. If passive movement is painful, it may be that inert tissues are at fault. If resisted movement is painful, the contractile tissue may be at fault. Active movement stresses both inert and contractile tissue. As an example, if a patient has biceps tendonitis (long head), then resisted flexion (isometric, midrange) will provoke pain. Passive movement through the flexion range of motion should not provoke pain because the biceps is relaxed. Theoretically, after the specific tissue is identified, the clinician can provide the appropriate treatment.

To test a muscle and its components (e.g., a contractile tissue), the clinician uses an isometric force on an immobilized limb segment so that the joint does not move. The joint is held in midrange to keep from compromising the inert tissue. No joint movement should occur to direct the tension on the contractile tissue. If a contractile lesion is present, the resisted movement may provoke pain or demonstrate weakness, occasionally both. Normal contractions are strong and painless.

Because of the inherent strength of a normal muscle, the clinician should stand in a position of maximum advantage with proper hand placement to exert the strongest possible force as appropriate. In addition, the following rules, similar to manual muscle testing, should be followed:

- Muscles must be tested in such a way that the clinician's and patient's strength are evenly matched.
- The clinician uses one hand for resistance and the other hand for stabilization.

- Muscles other than those being tested must not be included. Proper hand placement should help to isolate the muscle(s) (e.g., preventing supination when isolating the brachialis muscle).
- The joint that the muscles control must not move and should be held at near midrange.
- The patient must be encouraged to try as hard as possible.

In one small study examining the reliability of the Cyriax selective tissue tension (STT) method of otherwise healthy individuals between the ages of 20 and 40 years, with either unilateral shoulder or knee pain of undiagnosed origin, intrarater reliability for the knee ranged from 0.74 to 0.82, and interrater reliability ranged from 0.42 to 0.46.[32] Both intrarater and interrater reliability were highest for knee flexion. For the shoulder, intrarater reliability ranged from 0.44 to 0.67, and interrater reliability ranged from 0.00 to 0.45, with the highest values for shoulder abduction.[32] Nearly all the disagreements between clinicians came from whether a contraction was painful or not. The authors concluded that intrarater reliability for the knee was acceptable, but for the shoulder, it was not. Interrater reliability was not acceptable for either joint. More recently, others examined the intertester reliability of the Cyriax STT method to diagnose shoulder complaints.[33] They found kappa scores higher for individual diagnoses (0.84 to 0.97) than for individual tests (0.46 to 0.68). The authors recommend future research investigate the diagnostic validity of functional shoulder examination by the STT method.

REFERENCES

1. *ACSM's Guidelines for Exercise Testing and Prescription.* 11th ed. Philadelphia, PA: Wolters Kluwer; 2022.

2. Willardson JM. A brief review: factors affecting the length of the rest interval between resistance exercise sets. *J Strength Cond Res.* 2006;20(4):978–984. https://doi.org/10.1519/R-17995.1. PMID: 17194236.

3. Lovell DI, Cuneo R, Gass GC. The blood pressure response of older men to maximum and submaximum strength testing. *J Sci Med Sport.* 2011;14:254–258.

4. LeBrasseur NK, Bhasin S, Miciek R, et al. Tests of muscle strength and physical function: reliability and discrimination of performance in younger and older men and older men with mobility limitations. *J Am Ger Soc.* 2008;56:2118–2123.

5. Haff GG, Triplett ND. *Essentials of Strength Training and Conditioning.* Human Kinetics Champaign; 2016. ISBN: 978-1492501626.

6. Hoger WW, Hopkins DR, Barette SL, et al. Relationship between repetitions and selected percentages of one repetition maximum: a comparison between untrained males and females. *J Strength Cond Res.* 1990;4:47–54.

7. Androulakis-Korakakis P, Fisher JP, Steele J. The minimum effective training dose required to increase 1RM strength in resistance-trained men: a systematic review and meta-analysis. *Sports Med.* 2020;50(4):751–765. https://doi.org/10.1007/s40279-019-01236-0. PMID: 31797219.

8. Reynolds JM, Gordon TJ, Robergs RA. Prediction of one repetition maximum strength from multiple repetition maximum testing and anthropometry. *J Strength Cond Res.* 2006;20(3):584–592. https://doi.org/10.1519/R-15304.1. PMID: 16937972.

9. Shimano T, Kraemer WJ, Spiering BA, et al. Relationship between the number of repetitions and selected percentages of one repetition maximum in free weight exercises in trained and untrained men. *J Strength Cond Res.* 2006;20:819–823.

10. Dohoney P, Chromiak JA, Lemire K, et al. Prediction of one repetition maximum (1-RM) strength from a 4-6 RM and a 7-10 RM submaximal strength test in healthy young adult males. *JEP online. J Exercise Physiol.* 2002;5(3):54–59. https://www.asep.org/asep/asep/Dohoney.doc.

11. Da Silva EM, Brentano MA, Cadore AL, et al. Analysis of muscle activation during different leg press exercises at submaximum effort levels. *J Strength Cond Res.* 2008;22:1059–1065.

12. Parrino RL, Strand KL, Hockman AC, Signorile JF. Leg press and chest press strength normative values by half-decades in older persons. *Exp Gerontol.* 2021;150:111401. https://doi.org/10.1016/j.exger.2021.111401. Epub 2021 May 9. PMID: 33974938.

13. Sperandei S, Barros M, Silveria-Junior PCS, Oliveria CG. Electromyographic analysis of three different types of lat pull-down. *J Strength Cond Res.* 2009;23(7):2033–2038.

14. Signorile JF, Zink AJ, Szwed SP. A comparative electromyographical investigation of muscle utilization patterns using various hand positions during the lat pull-down. *J Strength Cond Res.* 2002;16:539–546.

15. Gibson AL, Wagner DR, Heyward VH. *Advanced Fitness Assessment & Exercise Prescription.* 8th ed. Champaign, IL: Human Kinetics; 2019.

16. Spennewyn KC. Strength outcomes in fixed versus free-form resistance equipment. *J Strength Cond Res.* 2008;22(1):75–81. https://doi.org/10.1519/JSC.0b013e31815ef5e7. PMID: 18296958.

17. Gentil P, Del Vecchio FB, Paoli A, et al. Isokinetic dynamometry and 1RM tests produce conflicting results for assessing alterations in muscle strength. *J Hum Kinet.* 2017;56:19–27. https://doi.org/10.1515/hukin-2017-0019. PMID: 28469740; PMCID: PMC5384049.

18. Arborelius UF, Ekholm J. Mechanics of shoulder locomotion system using exercises resisted by weight-and-pulley circuit. *Scand J Rehabil Med.* 1978;10:171–177.

19. Soria-Gila MA, Chirosa IJ, Bautista IJ, et al. Effects of variable resistance training on maximal strength: a meta-analysis. *J Strength Cond Res.* 2015;29(11):3260–3270.

20. Page P, Ellenbecker TS, eds. *The Scientific and Clinical Application of Elastic Resistance.* Champaign IL: Human Kinetics; 2003.

21. Bean JF, Kiely DK, LaRose S, et al. Are changes in leg power associated with clinically meaningful improvements in mobility in older adults? *J Am Soc Geriatr.* 2010;58:2363–2368.

22. Carneiro MAS, Franco CMC, Silva AL, et al. Resistance exercise intervention on muscular strength and power, and functional capacity in acute hospitalized older adults: a systematic review and meta-analysis of 2498 patients in 7 randomized clinical trials. *Geroscience.* 2021;43(6):2693–2705. https://doi.org/10.1007/s11357-021-00446-7. Epub 2021 Aug 28. PMID: 34453666; PMCID: PMC8602450.

23. Alcazar J, Guadalupe-Grau A, García-García FJ, Ara I, Alegre LM. Skeletal muscle power measurement in older people: a systematic review of testing protocols and adverse events. *J Gerontol A Biol Sci Med Sci.* 2018;73(7):914–924. https://doi.org/10.1093/gerona/glx216. PMID: 29309534.

24. Margaria R, Aghemo P, Rovelli E. Measurement of muscular power (anaerobic) in man. *J Appl Physiol.* 1966;5:1662–1664.

25. Harris C, Wattles A, DeBeliso M, et al. The seated medicine ball throw as a test of upper body power in older adults. *J Strength Cond Res.* 2011;25(8):2344–2348.

26. Wood R. *NHL Draft Combine Results;* 2013. Topend Sports Website http://www.topendsports.com/sport/ichockey/nhl-combine-results-2013.htm. Accessed March 7, 2023.

27. Rose DJ, Lucchese N, Wiersma LD. Development of a multidimensional balance scale for functionally independent older adults. *Arch Phys Med Rehabil.* 2006;87:1478–1485.

28. Sietsema KE, Sue DY, Stringer WW, Ward SA. *Wasserman and Whipp's Principles of Exercise Testing and Interpretation.* 6th ed. Philadelphia, PA: Wolters Kluwer; 2020. ISBN: 9781975136437.

29. Lawton TW, Cronin JB, McGuigan MR. Strength testing and training of rowers: a review. *Sports Med.* 2011;41(5):413–432. https://doi.org/10.2165/11588540-000000000-00000. PMID: 21510717.

30. McArdle WD, Katch FI, Katch FL, et al. *Exercise Physiology.* 7th ed. Baltimore: Lippincott, Williams & Wilkins; 2010:518.

31. Cyriax J. *Textbook of Orthopedic Medicine.* Vol. 1. London: Bailliere Tindall; 1982.

32. Hayes KW, Petersen CM. Reliability of classifications derived from Cyriax's resisted testing in subjects with painful shoulders and knees. *J Orthop Sports Phys Ther.* 2003;33:235–246.

33. Storheil B, Klouman E, Holmvik S, Emaus N, Fleten N. Intertester reliability of shoulder complaints diagnoses in primary health care. *Scand J Prim Health Care.* 2016;34(3):224–231. https://doi.org/10.1080/028134 32.2016.1207139. Epub 2016 Jul 12. PMID: 27404451; PMCID: PMC5036011.

Testing Functional Performance

Testing Functional
Performance

Introduction

Chair Stand

Gait Speed

Physical Performance
Test and Modified
Physical Performance
Test

Timed Up and Go

Stair Climb

Floor Rise

Gait

Current clinical practice presents a growing need to emphasize the relationship between strength and functional movement, especially in older adults. Each person has a threshold of strength that is minimal for the performance of activities of daily living (ADLs). The larger or taller the person is, for example, the more strength will be needed. Third-party payers require that clinicians show a relationship between strength and function in their treatment plans, frequently denying payment if their assessments fail to show this relationship. It has always been important for clinicians to show that patients have strength deficits, but it is now critical for them to show that strength deficits are tied to the patient's ability, or lack thereof, to independently complete ADLs, perform a job task (such as bricklaying), participate in hobbies/sports, or play with their children or grandchildren. This chapter presents a series of functional tests, particularly relevant to older individuals, that require strength to be of a minimum threshold. Once a specific weakness is pinpointed, a strengthening program can be designed to help patients achieve their functional goals.

The functional assessment tests described in this chapter have been correlated with specific essential muscles. The list of muscles for each task is not comprehensive, but it provides a starting point for the beginning clinician to design a plan for muscle tests when a functional deficit is observed. Reference scores are provided when available. Specific exercises for each muscle are listed after each muscle test in Chapters 5 and 6. In some cases, patients may be able to accomplish a task by compensating for a specific muscle weakness, so the clinician should be observant to accurately identify specific muscle weaknesses.

INTRODUCTION

Functional abilities represent a broad range of movements that require muscles to act in highly specific ways to achieve a desired purpose. These abilities include ADLs such as dressing, eating, bathing, transferring, and walking, as well as other tasks of mobility such as rising from a chair, climbing stairs, lifting, and rising from the floor. These functional activities are basic tasks of mobility that are required for all individuals to be independent in the home and community. Functional activity performance is especially important for older adults who may be at risk for institutionalization. An inability to independently perform specific functional tasks may lead to institutionalization. Many higher-level functional abilities, such as those required for sports and work, are discussed in Chapter 7, Alternatives to Manual Muscle Testing.

The Nagi Model of Disablement[1] and the International Classification of Functioning (ICF) disablement model[1] describe the impact of disease and pathology within the context of both function and societal roles and provide a conceptual model to guide clinical practice. In these models, diminished muscle strength is an impairment that affects a person's ability to perform functional tasks or to fulfill societal roles. Muscle strength testing takes place at the impairment level, whereas testing functional task performance occurs at the function level. One goal of this chapter is to integrate impairment (strength deficit) and physical performance (function).

It is generally accepted that in previously unaffected individuals, performance of basic functional tasks requires a relatively small amount of muscle strength in relation to the total amount of strength that existed before any injury, a lifestyle of inactivity, or passage of years. The minimum amount of strength required is referred to as a "functional threshold." If patients have strength above the required threshold amount, they are unlikely to show deficits in performance. The relationship of strength to function up to a functional threshold is illustrated in Fig. 8.1. According to the principle illustrated in this graph, if the patient's strength sufficiently improves to the point at which the curve flattens out, the patient should be strong enough to perform the task. For example, about 45% of one's body weight is required to rise from a chair without using the arms.[2] If a person is unable to rise from a chair unassisted because of weakness in the lower extremities, strengthening exercises will help to improve that function. Further strengthening will allow the person to rise more quickly and efficiently and will create a strength reserve to help preserve the ability to perform the task in the future.

Functional Testing

An analysis of any functional task shows that movements are multiplanar and asymmetrical, incorporate rotation, and are speed and balance dependent. Therefore, simply testing a muscle's maximum ability to generate force will not accurately represent its functional ability. Observation of the individual performing the functional task is the only way to accurately test functional ability. Such observation provides information about the quality of the performance, which, in turn, informs the clinician's clinical decision-making. Inferring that a specific muscle has functional strength without direct observation of the functional task is incorrect and should be avoided as noted in Chapter 2. Table 8.1 shows the key muscles required for some basic functional tasks.

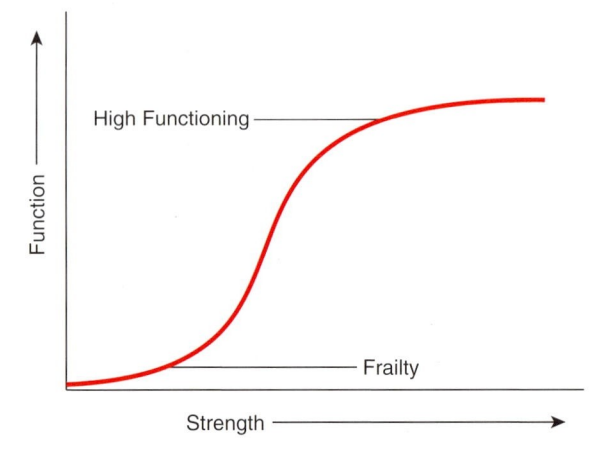

FIGURE 8.1 Conceptual Diagram of Curvilinear Relationship Between Strength and Function.

Table 8.1 KEY MUSCLES ESSENTIAL FOR FUNCTIONAL MOVEMENTS

Functional Movement	Key Muscles
Bed mobility	Abdominals, erector spinae, gluteus maximus
Transfers and squats	Gluteus maximus, medius, and obturator externus, piriformis, quadriceps
Ambulation and stair climbing	Abdominals, erector spinae, gluteus maximus and medius, obturator externus, piriformis, quadriceps, and anterior tibialis and gastroc soleus
Floor transfers	Abdominals, erector spinae, gluteus maximus and medius, obturator externus, piriformis, quadriceps and gastroc soleus
Fast gait and jumping	Gastrocsoleus, gluteus maximus and medius, quadriceps

Measurement

Functional task performance is measured in several ways. Ordinal scales showing hierarchical levels of performance are commonly used in both manual muscle testing and some functional tests. In ordinal scales, numbers are sequentially and hierarchically assigned in accordance with the difficulty of the task. However, ordinal scales are limited by their susceptibility to subjectivity and their lack of responsiveness to small changes in performance. Therefore, using ratio scales, such as time, to measure individual patient performance is the preferred method. Timing task performance provides a strong measure of reliability and responsiveness. However, when a functional task is timed, such as when a patient is instructed to rise from a chair as quickly as possible, it should be noted that power is a component of the task in addition to strength. Ratio measures such as time and distance allow the clinician to compare an individual patient's performance against available reference scores of similar individuals. This comparison aids in clinical decision-making.

Purpose: The chair stand test is a test of mobility specifically targeting the force production of the leg muscles. There are two versions: the number of completed sit-to-stand (STS) motions (chair rises) completed in 30 seconds (30s STS) and the time required to complete five chair rises (5T-STS).

Essential Muscle Movements for Task Performance: Hip extension, hip abduction from a flexed position, hip external rotation, knee extension, ankle plantar flexion, ankle dorsiflexion and inversion,[3] and trunk extension and flexion.

Reliability: Test-retest reliability is excellent for all versions of the chair stand test (intraclass correlation coefficient [ICC] = 0.95 to 0.99).[4,5]

Validity: The 30s STS test correlates with measures of lower extremity strength, walking speed, stair-climbing ability, and balance[6,7] and correlates with one-repetition maximum (1-RM) leg press (r = 0.78 for men, 0.71 for women).[8] The 30s STS has concurrent and convergent validity in assessing lower extremity muscle strength and can discriminate between sufficient and insufficient physical activity levels in young healthy adults.[9]

The 5T-STS is a valid measure of dynamic balance and functional mobility in older adults.[10] Inability to complete the 5T-STS in less than 13.7 seconds is highly predictive of future mobility disability.[11] The 30s STS and 5T-STS have similar correlations with poor exercise tolerance and lower extremity skeletal muscle strength and are both reasonable choices for use in clinical and research practices.[12]

Equipment: A standard, armless chair, 17 in. (43 cm) high, and a stopwatch.

Testing Procedure: Both test versions are *always* done without the use of the patient's arms. Assess the ability of the patient to stand without the use of arms. If able, proceed to testing. Clinician should demonstrate the STS movement before testing.

Thirty-Second Version: Patient rises from a sitting position and stands to a fully erect position as many times as possible in 30 seconds. Clinician starts timing when the patient begins to move (rather than on "Go!").

Timed Five-Repetition Version: Patient comes to a full standing position five times as quickly as possible. Clinician begins timing on the command "Go!" Clinician times the effort from the command "Go!" until patient returns to a seated position after five repetitions.

Position of Patient: Sitting with arms crossed over the chest. Feet are planted on the floor in the position chosen by the patient (Fig. 8.2).

Clinician Instructions: Standing to fully view the patient's quality of movement (Fig. 8.3). Begin counting (30-s version) or timing (timed five-repetition version) on the command "Go."

Instructions to Patient

Thirty-Second Version: "On 'Go,' stand up as many times as you can in 30 seconds without using your arms. I'll keep count. Make sure you stand all the way up."

Timed Five-Repetition Version: "On Go, stand up five times, as quickly as you can without using your arms. I will be timing you. Make sure you stand all the way up."

FIGURE 8.2

FIGURE 8.3

Scoring

Thirty-Second Version:
- The number of repetitions is the patient's score. Count the repetition if the patient is more than halfway standing. If patient cannot complete one repetition without the use of the arms, the score for the 30-second version is zero. The minimal detectable change (MDC) ranges from 1.8 to 3.3 repetitions[13,5]
- Tables 8.2 and 8.3 show reference value ranges for physically active older men and women in the United States. Eight repetitions may be the threshold for physical disability.[8]
- Mean scores for 81 young individuals (mean + standard deviation [SD] age, 25.1 + 3.4 years) were 34 + 5.2 repetitions in sufficiently active group and 31.5 + 5.5 in insufficiently active group.[9]
- In a group of 775 community-dwelling older adults (60 to 70 years old) in Singapore, repetitions were 17.6 (5.1) seconds for women and 18.0 (5.4) seconds

for men.[14] The lack of difference between men and women in this sample is hypothesized to be because of similarities in height between men and women.
- The Women's Health and Aging Study (of moderately to severely disabled women) found a mean time of 15.3 seconds for women ages 65 to 85 and older.[15] The more time required, the more likely it is that the individual is frail.[16]

Timed Five-Repetition Version: The time taken to complete five repetitions is the score. If 60 seconds elapse before five repetitions are accomplished, the test is terminated and the score of 60 seconds is recorded with a notation. The odds of being disabled increase 1.4 times for every 1-second increase in the 5T-STS test. The MDC ranges from 1.1 to 2.5 seconds.[10,5] Scores of greater than 10 seconds increase the risk of developing disability within 2 years.[17]
- Mean scores for healthy adults (<60 years) in the United States are 5.98 seconds for males and 5.60 seconds for females, and for >60 years: 8.23 seconds for males and 9.00 seconds for females).[18]
- Mean scores for 81 young individuals (mean age, 25.1 [3.4] years) performed five repetitions of STS in 4.3 (0.6) seconds in sufficiently active group and 4.5 (0.8) seconds in insufficiently active group.[9]
- In a group of 775 community-dwelling older adults (60 to 70 years old) in Singapore, chair rise time was 9.3 (2.9) seconds for women and 9.1 (2.7) seconds for men.[14] The lack of difference between men and women in this sample is hypothesized to be because of similarities in height between men and women.
- Mean scores for 604 community-dwelling adults with mean age of 74 years old from Japan were 8.2 (2.6) seconds for men and 8.2 (2.9) seconds for women.[19]
- Mean scores for 12,605 population-based individuals (>40 years old) in China had mean time of 10.13 seconds in men and 11.03 seconds in women of all age categories.[20]

Table 8.2 NORMAL RANGE OF CHAIR STANDS BY SEX AND AGE (MIDDLE 50% OF POPULATION)

Age	M	F
60–64	14–19	12–17
65–69	12–18	11–16
70–74	12–17	10–15
75–79	11–17	10–15
80–84	10–15	9–14
85–89	8–14	8–13
90–94	7–12	4–11

F, Female; *M*, male.

From Jones, C. J., & Rikli, R. E. (2002). Measuring functional fitness of older adults. *The Journal of Active Ageing*, 24–30.

Table 8.3 REFERENCE SCORES[a] FOR 30-SECOND CHAIR STAND TEST FROM 1000 AUSTRALIANS

Age	3–9		10–19		20–59		60+	
	M	F	M	F	M	F	M	F
Mean (SD)	23.1 (6.6)	23.4 (6.1)	25.5 (5.7)	24.2 (5.9)	24.2 (6.0)	22.6 (6.2)	18.3 (5.73)	15.9 (4.8)

[a]Each decade included 100 people (20 to 80+).

F, Female; *M*, male; *SD*, standard deviation.

Data from McKay, M. J., Baldwin, J. N., Ferreira, P., et al. (2017). Normative reference values for strength and flexibility of 1,000 children and adults. *Neurology*, 88(1):36–43.

- Use a chair with a firm seat. Avoid the use of a folding chair, a very soft chair, a deep chair, or a chair on wheels for testing purposes. The chair should be placed against the wall for safety purposes.
- Chair heights from 80% to 90% of the patient's lower (tibia) leg length are optimal for the test.[21]
- Allow the patient to perform the sit-to-stand (STS) movement first, without coaching. If the patient has difficulty rising, then offer tips such as scooting to the edge of the chair, leaning forward, etc.
- It is useful to observe the position of the hips while the patient is attempting to stand and sit. If the hips are adducted and/or internally rotated, this may indicate weakness, and specific muscle testing is indicated, especially of the gluteus medius (Fig. 8.4).
- Excessive bending forward of the trunk to stand may indicate that the patient has weak quadriceps (Fig. 8.5).
- Although it is preferable to have the patient cross arms over chest, some patients may need to extend their arms forward to help them stand. If this occurs, it could indicate that the patient's legs are weak or balance is impaired (Fig. 8.6).
- If you suspect the patient will not be able to complete five repetitions, the 30s STS version is the preferred

test because the patient is required to only complete a minimum of one repetition for a successful test. A cutoff point of 300 N for knee extensor strength is needed to independently stand from a chair without use of upper extremities.[22]

FIGURE 8.5

FIGURE 8.4

FIGURE 8.6

Purpose: Gait speed is a functional test of one's ability to walk at a comfortable (usual) speed. A fast-paced walk can demonstrate available reserve and the ability to accelerate rapidly, such as in the need to get across a street. Possible gait speed times range from the fastest sprinters to the slowest possible gait, often seen in individuals residing in nursing homes. Gait speed has been called the sixth vital sign because of its validity in predicting functional ability, frailty, nursing home placement, and the ability to walk in the community.[23] It can be measured in any person who can walk, even those using assistive devices. A person's height is a significant predictor of gait speed.[24]

Essential Muscle Movements for Task Performance: Core; hip extension, abduction, and adduction; quadriceps and hamstrings; ankle plantar flexion; and ankle dorsiflexion with inversion.[25,26] Hip flexion also contributes to walking velocity.[27] The reader is referred to the gait section of this chapter for a more specific list of muscles that are imperative for smooth and normal gait.

Reliability: r = 0.715 to 0.92 for usual speed and 0.837 to 0.933 for fast gait speed.[28] There is also excellent test-retest reliability in chronic ambulatory stroke survivors (intraclass correlation coefficient [ICC]$_{2,1}$ = 0.991 to 0.992).[29]

Validity: Gait speed is related to age (Fig. 8.7) and muscle mass.[23,28] Gait speed at "usual pace" was found to be a consistent predictor of disability, cognitive impairment, institutionalization, falls, and/or mortality.[30] Fast gait speed is a robust predictor of disability when the annual decline exceeds –0.22 m/s.[31] A speed of less than 0.8 m/s is a predictor of 8-year mortality in predisabled women 75 years or older.[32] Women who had gait speeds of less than 0.60 m/s were 2.5 times more likely to die prematurely than those with faster gait speeds.[33] A speed of less than 1.2 m/s is highly predictive of future mobility disability.[11]

Equipment: A 4- to 10-m-long walkway and a stopwatch. It is helpful to have 1 to 2 m or so before and after the 4-m test course to allow for acceleration and deceleration, especially in people with stroke.[34] However, although this extra distance is desirable, it is not necessary to perform the test in people without pathology. Each

test should be performed the same way for consistency of results and accuracy of interpretation. The length of the walkway does not influence the consistency of results.[35]

Testing Procedure: First, describe the test clearly to the individual. Assure the patient is safe to walk independently (without another person). Demonstrate the test if needed, taking care not to walk too fast. Then, have the patient perform two trials with adequate rest in between, scoring the faster one. Test both comfortable (usual) and fast gait speeds. Begin timing the individual when the first foot crosses the line at the beginning of the course (Fig. 8.8A), and stop timing when the first foot crosses the end line (Fig. 8.8B). Any part of the foot will do; it is just important to be consistent.

Position of Patient: Standing, facing a marked-off walkway. Patient may use an assistive device if needed.

Walking Speed by Gender and Age

FIGURE 8.7 Self-Selected Walking Speed Categorized by Sex and Age.

A   B

FIGURE 8.8

Clinician Instructions: Stand and hold the stopwatch perpendicular to the starting line. Clinician should walk slightly behind the patient to obtain an accurate view of when the first foot crosses the finish line with care to not pace the patient. Clinician begins timing when the patient's first foot (or part of the first foot) crosses the start line of the 4-m walkway (see Fig. 8.8A).

Patient Instructions: "Walk at your usual and comfortable speed from this line to past the other line on the floor (indicate which line). I will be timing you. The first trial is for practice and then we'll time you. OK? Ready, go!" Two trials are given. The same directions are given for the fast-paced walk, with the patient instructed to walk as quickly, but as safely, as possible. Adequate rest should be provided as needed between trials.

Scoring

To determine a result in meters per second (m/s), the walkway distance is divided by the time taken (in seconds) to cover that distance. There are many gait speed standards. High-functioning adults have usual gait speeds of 1.75 to 2.25 m/s, whereas usual gait speeds slower than 0.5 m/s are common in nursing home residents. In one study, the mean usual gait speed used by 139 pedestrians was 1.32 (SD, 0.31) m/s.[36] MDC for usual gait speed in adults 51 to 90 years of age is 0.23 m/s.[37]

Table 8.4 indicates some conversions from meters per second to feet per second and miles per hour. Tables 8.5 and 8.6 list reference values for usual and fast gait speed by age for US adults.

- In a group of nearly 5000 individuals from the Netherlands (mean age of 67 [9.54] years) had a usual gait speed over 5 meters of 1.23 (0.20) m/s in men and 1.17 (0.20) m/s in women.[24] In this sample, gait speed was higher in taller and younger individuals.
- In a group of 775 community-dwelling older adults (60 to 70 years old) in Singapore over a 10-m distance, the mean gait speed was 1.34 m/s (0.22) for women and 1.35 (0.26) for men.[14]

Table 8.4 CONVERSIONS FOR GAIT SPEED

Meters/ Second	Feet/ Second	Minutes/ Mile	Miles/ Hour
0.25	0.82	106.7	0.6
0.30	0.98	88.9	0.7
0.35	1.15	76.2	0.8
0.40	1.31	66.7	0.9
0.45	1.48	59.3	1.0
0.50	1.64	53.3	1.1
0.55	1.80	48.5	1.2
0.60	1.97	44.4	1.4
0.65	2.13	41.0	1.5
0.70	2.30	38.1	1.6
0.75	2.46	35.6	1.7
0.80	2.62	33.3	1.8
0.85	2.79	31.4	1.9
0.90	2.95	29.6	2.0
0.95	3.12	28.1	2.1
1.00	3.28	26.7	2.3
1.10	3.61	24.2	2.5
1.20	3.94	22.2	2.7
1.30	4.26	20.5	2.9
1.40	4.59	19.0	3.2
1.50	4.92	17.8	3.4
1.60	5.25	16.7	3.6
1.70	5.58	15.7	3.8
1.80	5.90	14.8	4.1
1.90	6.23	14.0	4.3
2.00	6.56	13.3	4.5

Clinical Relevance

- Gait speed can be measured in patients who use an assistive device. When retesting performance in the same patient, retest using the same assistive device.
- Studies have shown that additional distance for acceleration and deceleration is not necessary; however, we recommend using a further end-point target to prevent patients from slowing down as they approach the finish line or using the instructions "walk past the line" (see Fig. 8.8B).
- Reliability improves with longer distances up to 10 m.[28]
- If walking with the individual, be careful not to set the pace, but walk slightly behind the individual.

This will allow you to get a more realistic view of the patient's actual performance. While always maintaining a safe test situation, do not inhibit the individual by standing too close or providing too many instructions. Certainly, use a gait belt if it is warranted. Knowing when to start and stop timing requires skill and practice. It is recommended to use a specific "event," such as when the first foot crosses the line, as the moment to begin and end timing, but any such event will do; just be consistent!

- Gait speed increases with the number of walk trials performed, indicating averaging the trials is preferred.[24]

Table 8.5 MEAN FAST GAIT SPEED TIME FOR MEN AND WOMEN AGE 20 YEARS AND OLDER

| | MAXIMUM GAIT SPEED (M/S) | |
| | MEAN (SD) | |
Age	Men	Women
20s	2.53 (0.29)	2.47 (0.25)
30s	2.46 (0.32)	2.34 (0.34)
40s	2.46 (0.36)	2.12 (0.28)
50s	2.07 (0.45)	2.01 (0.26)
60s	1.93 (0.36)	1.77 (0.25)
70s	2.08 (0.36)	1.75 (0.28)

SD, Standard deviation.

Data from Bohannon, R. W. (1997). Comfortable and maximum walking speed of adults aged 20–79 years: Reference values and determinants. *Age and Ageing*, 26(1):15–19.

Table 8.6 REFERENCE SCORES OF USUAL GAIT SPEED FOR HEALTHY ADULTS AGES 20–99

| | GAIT SPEED (M/S) | |
Age	Men	Women
20–29	1.22–1.47	1.08–1.50
30–39	1.32–1.54	1.26–1.42
40–49	1.27–1.47	1.22–1.42
50–59	1.12–1.49	1.10–1.56
60–69	1.03–1.59	0.97–1.45
70–79	0.96–1.42	0.83–1.50
80–99	0.61–1.22	0.56–1.17

Data from Bohannon R. W. & Williams Andrews A. (2011). Normal walking speed: a descriptive meta-analysis. *Physiotherapy*, 97(3):182–189.

PHYSICAL PERFORMANCE TEST AND MODIFIED PHYSICAL PERFORMANCE TEST

Purpose: The physical performance test (PPT) measures aspects of physical function and ADLs in older adults using nine items that emphasize mobility tasks. There are two versions of the PPT test: one with seven items and one with nine; the nine-item version also includes stair-climbing tasks.

The modified physical performance test (M-PPT) includes most of the items of the PPT but substitutes three balance tests and a timed 5T-STS for the writing and eating task.

Essential Muscle Movements for Physical

Performance Test Task Performance

Writing Task: (If the arm is supported, only hand and wrist muscles may be essential.) Wrist flexion and extension, and finger metacarpophalangeal (MCP), proximal interphalangeal (PIP), and distal interphalangeal (DIP) flexion.

Eating Task: Shoulder flexion, shoulder internal rotation, elbow flexion, forearm supination and pronation, wrist flexion and extension, and finger MCP, PIP, and DIP flexion.

Essential Muscle Movements for Physical Performance Test and Modified Physical Performance Test

Task Performance

Lifting a Book: Scapular protraction and upward rotation; shoulder flexion; shoulder external rotation; elbow flexion and extension; forearm supination and pronation; wrist flexion and extension; and finger MCP, PIP, and DIP flexion.

Putting On and Taking Off a Garment (Depending on Technique): Scapular protraction and upward rotation; shoulder flexion; shoulder external rotation; elbow flexion and extension; forearm supination and pronation; wrist flexion and extension; and finger MCP, PIP, and DIP flexion. Core stability (for sitting or standing). If the task is performed while standing: hip extension and abduction, knee extension, ankle plantar flexion, and ankle dorsiflexion with inversion.

Picking Up a Coin: Back extension; hip extension, knee extension; ankle plantar flexion; elbow flexion and extension; forearm supination and pronation; wrist flexion and extension; and finger MCP, PIP, and DIP flexion.

360° Turn: Ankle dorsiflexion with inversion, plantar flexion, foot inversion, foot eversion with plantar flexion, knee extension, hip abduction and extension, and core stability.

Walking Task: Hip extension and abduction, knee extension, ankle plantar flexion, and ankle dorsiflexion with inversion.[25] Hip flexion also contributes to walking velocity.[26] The reader is referred to the gait section of this chapter for a more specific list of muscles that are imperative for smooth and normal gait.

Stair Climb Tasks: Ascent: hip flexion and extension, knee extension and flexion, ankle plantar flexion, ankle dorsiflexion, spine extension, and core stability. Descent: eccentric knee extension, hip flexion, and core muscles.[38] Balance is also a key component of successful stair ascent and descent.

Reliability: The ICC for interrater reliability is 0.96 for the eight-item version (omitting the last item of four flights of stairs).[39] The ICC of test-retest reliability in the eight-item version is 0.88.[39] Test-retest reliability for the M-PPT is 0.96.[40]

Validity: Predictive validity for classifying level of care as dependent or independent.[41] Construct validity based on self-reported ADL and instrumental ADL performance.[42] Predictive of major health outcomes such as death and nursing home placement.[43] Predictive of first-time fall (within 12 months)[44] and recurrent falls.[45] The M-PPT is significantly related to age, gait speed, knee extension strength, balance confidence, and functional self-report[46] and can indicate whether an individual is frail.[47]

Equipment for Both Versions

Scoring form
Stopwatch
Table and chair (PPT)
Bowl (PPT)
Spoon (PPT)
Coffee can (PPT)
Five dry (uncooked) kidney beans (PPT)
5.5-lb. book
Two adjustable shelves
Patient's jacket or front-button sweater or extra-large lab coat, hospital gown, or other front-opening garment
25-foot walkway
One flight of stairs (10 to 12 stairs)

Testing Procedure

Physical Performance Test and Modified Physical Performance Test: Both versions take about 10 minutes to complete. The test items can be done in any order; however, they will be described here in the order in which they appear on the scoring forms. Each task is timed except for the 360° turn and climbing four flights of stairs. Two trials of each task are performed except for the stair-climbing task.

An assistive device can be used for the walking and stair-climbing tasks, but not for the other tasks. All tasks are to be completed unassisted and without support. As in all tests, patient safety should be assured. Although assistance from the clinician is not permitted during performance of the test, the clinician should be vigilant for balance problems. A gait belt is always recommended during test performance.

The nine PPT tasks are:
1. Writing a sentence
2. Simulated eating
3. Lifting a book onto a shelf
4. Putting on and taking off a garment
5. Picking up a coin from the floor
6. 360° turn
7. 50-foot walk
8. Climbing one flight of stairs
9. Climbing four flights of stairs

The nine M-PPT tasks are:
1. Standing static balance
   a. Side-by-side stance
   b. Semi-tandem stance
   c. Full tandem stance
2. Chair stand (five repetitions)
3. Lifting a book onto a shelf
4. Putting on and taking off a garment
5. Picking up a coin from the floor
6. 360° turn
7. 50-foot walk
8. Climbing one flight of stairs
9. Climbing four flights of stairs

Physical Performance Test Tasks

1. Writing a Sentence

Testing Procedure: Patient writes a sentence. The sentence can be written on the back of the test form, so there will be a record of the result. The clinician writes the sentence first: "Whales live in a blue ocean." A period is placed at the end of the sentence. Then, on the command of "Go!" the patient writes the same sentence. Timing begins on Go! and ends when the period is placed at the end of the sentence. Clinician records the time it takes patient to write the sentence legibly (Fig. 8.9).

Instructions to Patient: "The first task is a writing task. I am going to write the sentence 'Whales live in a blue ocean.' Then I want you to write the same sentence while I time you. Are you ready? Go!"

2. Eating Task

Testing Procedure: The second task is a simulated eating task. Five kidney beans are placed in a bowl 5 in. from the edge of the table in front of the patient. An empty coffee can is placed on the table at the patient's nondominant side. A teaspoon is placed in the patient's dominant hand. Clinician may demonstrate the task. Patient is asked on the command "Go!" to pick up the beans, one at a time with the spoon, and place them in the coffee can (Fig. 8.10). Timing begins with the command "Go!" and ends when the last bean is heard hitting the bottom of the can. Patient can use the nondominant hand to steady the bowl but not to move it in any way. The nondominant hand cannot help steady the can or complete the task except to help pick up a dropped bean. If patient drops a bean, timing continues while the patient picks up the bean.

Instructions to Patient: "This next task is an eating task. When I say 'Go!' I want you to use your spoon to move one bean at a time from this can to the bowl. You cannot use your other hand except to steady the bowl. Are you ready? Go!"

PPT and M-PPT

FIGURE 8.9

FIGURE 8.10

3. Lifting a Book Onto a Shelf

Testing Procedure: This task is done with patient sitting on a chair (or other surface) (Fig. 8.11) or standing (Fig. 8.12), depending on whether you want to assess the patient's standing or sitting balance while lifting. Using an open cabinet with multiple and/or two adjustable shelves, usually available in a clinic, is recommended. Having multiple or two adjustable shelves helps accommodate patient's height. The countertop can serve as the starting position for the book placement.

Adjust the higher shelf so that it is 12 in. above the patient's shoulders. A book weighing ~5.5 lb. is placed on the edge of the counter, with the book hanging slightly off the edge of the counter to make it easy for the patient to grab. The patient is asked to lift the book from the lower shelf to the upper shelf while the effort is timed. Clinician should demonstrate this task to ensure understanding.

Timing is stopped when patient's hand is removed from the book after it is placed on the top shelf. In the original PPT test, the patient is seated during the task (see Fig. 8.11). However, the task can be performed standing if desired (see Fig. 8.12). Time is recorded on the scoring form.

Instructions to Patient: "For this task, I want you to lift this book to this shelf while I time you. Do you understand? Now, I'll demonstrate. OK, when I say 'Go!' you may begin."

4. Putting On and Taking Off a Garment

Testing Procedure: This task involves putting on and removing a garment in a standing position. An extra-large bathrobe, front-buttoned shirt, or hospital gown can be used and put on so that it opens in the front. If patient has a jacket or sweater that opens in the front, use that. Make sure the garment is large enough to put on over any clothes the patient is wearing. To start, the garment is held so the label inside the garment is facing the patient (Fig. 8.13).

FIGURE 8.12

FIGURE 8.11

FIGURE 8.13

Patient is instructed to start with arms at sides and on "Go!" to take the garment, put it on (Fig. 8.14), square it on the shoulders, and then remove it completely, holding it out to the clinician. Timing begins on "Go!" and ends when patient hands the jacket to the clinician.

Instructions to Patient: "This task involves putting on and taking off this jacket while I time you. When I say 'Go!' I want you to take the jacket from me, put it on so that it is square on your shoulders, and then take it off and hand it back to me. Now go!"

5. Picking Up a Coin from the Floor

Testing Procedure: This is a timed task of patient's ability to pick up a coin from the floor. A coin is placed approximately 12 in. from the patient's foot (usually the dominant side). On the command "Go!" the patient picks up the coin from the floor and returns to a fully upright position (Fig. 8.15). Timing will begin with the command "Go!" and end when patient is standing erect with coin in hand.

Instructions to Patient: "I'm going to put a coin on the floor and on 'go!' I want you to pick it up, completely stand up, and hand it to me. OK. Are you ready?"

Clinical Relevance

If working with a patient with low vision, someone who may not be able to see a coin on the floor, substitute a larger-sized item such as a pencil or pen. Substituting a larger item obviates the need for a patient to spend excess time with their head down near the ground because they can't find the coin.

FIGURE 8.14

FIGURE 8.15

6. 360° Turn

Testing Procedure: The 360° turn task examines patient's ability to turn in a complete circle in both directions (Fig. 8.16). This effort is not timed but, rather, scored for the quality and safety of the effort.

Demonstrate the task. Demonstration speed of turning should not be so fast that it encourages the patient to mimic it, thus compromising his or her safety. Ask patient to turn 360° at a comfortable pace (in either direction) beginning with the toes pointed forward and ending when the toes are pointed forward again. Performance is evaluated for continuity of movement and steadiness.

Instructions to Patient: "I want you to turn in a full circle so that your toes are back on this line. You can choose whichever direction you want to go toward first since I will ask you to go in the other direction next. I will not be timing you." Upon completion, ask the patient to turn in the other direction, evaluating for continuity of movement and steadiness.

FIGURE 8.16

Clinical Relevance

Both directions will be examined, so it does not matter which direction is performed first. Typically, the patient will choose his or her best direction to perform first.

7. Timed 50-Foot Walk

Testing Procedure: This is a timed 50-foot walk task designed to examine the speed and observe the quality of the patient's gait. The patient stands at the start of a 50-foot walk test course that consists of a walkway 25 feet out and 25 feet back. No acceleration or deceleration distance is needed because of the distance. Timing begins with the command "Go!" and ends when the starting line is crossed on the way back. The time is recorded on the scoring form. An assistive device may be used, and the type of device should be documented. Typically, demonstration is not needed on this task because walking is a familiar task.

Instructions to Patient: "I'd like you to walk out and back as quickly but as safely as you can. You will turn around at the end of the walkway and return to this spot. I will be timing you. Ready? Go!"

Clinical Relevance

- Completing the 50 ft (15.24 m) distance in 15 s is equal to a 1.0-m/s pace. You can calculate the patient's gait speed by dividing the distance walked by the time.
- Gait speeds of more than 0.8 m/s are typically required for safe community ambulation.[23]

Once the seven tasks are performed, the seven-item version of the PPT is complete. If you do not intend to have the patient perform stair climbing, add up the scores for the seven items now. If you are performing the M-PPT, the stairs are included.

8. Climbing One Flight of Stairs[a]

Testing Procedure: Explain to patient that they have the option of climbing up to four flights of stairs. Ask patient if they feel comfortable and are willing to perform these tasks. Ask patient to tell you of any symptom such as chest pain or shortness of breath, which should terminate the task. Vital signs should be monitored as indicated. Indications to monitor vital signs include evidence of more than ordinary effort expended in any previous task such as complaints of fatigue and the need to rest between tasks.

Ask patient to climb one flight of stairs that has 9 to 12 steps. Timing starts with the command "Go!" and ends when patient's first foot reaches the top step. Patient may use a handrail and/or assistive device, and this should be noted on the scoring form as well as the time taken to climb one flight of stairs.

Instructions to Patient: "This task involves climbing a flight of stairs as quickly but as safely as you can (Fig. 8.17). You may use the handrail if you need to. For this task, you are only required to go up to the landing. Stair climbing may require more than usual effort, so please let me know if you experience any tightness or pain in your chest or if you are short of breath and need to stop. OK? Go!"

FIGURE 8.17

If patient is willing, he or she may continue the stairs to achieve up to four flights. This effort is not timed.

9. Climbing Four Flights of Stairs

Testing Procedure: Patient is asked to climb up to four flights of stairs. Scoring is based on how many flights, up and down, patient completes. Patient descends the first flight of stairs, counted as one, and ascends the same flight up to four repetitions. This stair climbing and descent continue until the patient feels tired and wishes to stop, or until four flights, four ups and four downs total, have been completed.

Record the number of flights (maximum of four) climbed (up and down is one flight). A handrail and/or an assistive device may be used.

Instructions to Patient: "Now, the next task is to climb, up and down, as many times as you are comfortable, up to four times. You can determine how many flights you feel comfortable doing. Are you willing to try? How many flights do you think you can do? Ready? Go!"

Clinical Relevance

- Typically, a demonstration is not needed, and only one trial is given.
- Prior to beginning the stair tasks, it is helpful to ask the patient how many flights he or she thinks can be completed to give some idea of the anticipated level of performance.
- Patients should be gently encouraged, but not coerced or forced, to do more than they feel they can safely and comfortably do.
- Taking vital signs pre– and post–stair climbing or asking the patient to identify the level of exertion via the Borg Scale of Exertion may provide additional information to help inform the clinician's clinical decision-making.

The stair tasks complete the nine-item PPT. See Fig. 8.18 for the PPT scoring form. To complete the M-PPT, ask the patient to perform the next two tasks.

---

[a] The stair-climbing tasks (climbing one flight of stairs and climbing four flights of stairs) may be performed together, but they are scored separately. Generally, only one trial is given.

Physical Performance Test Scoring Sheet

			Time	Scoring	Score
				Physical Performance Test	
1	Writing task: (Write the sentence "Whales live in a blue ocean.")	Sec*		≤10 sec = 4 10.5–15 sec = 3 15.5–20 sec = 2 >20 sec = 1 unable = 0	
2	Eating task (simulated eating)	Sec		≤10 sec = 4 10.5–15 sec = 3 15.5–20 sec = 2 >20 sec = 1 unable = 0	
3	Lift a book and put it on a shelf Book: approximately 5.5 lbs Bed height: 23 in Shelf height: 46 in	Sec		≤2 sec = 4 2.5–4 sec = 3 4.5–6 sec = 2 >6 sec = 1 unable = 0	

4	Put on and remove a garment
	  1. Standing
	  2. Use of bathrobe, button-down shirt, or hospital gown
		Sec		≤10 sec = 4
				10.5–15 sec = 3
				15.5–20 sec = 2
				>20 sec = 1
				unable = 0	

5	Pick up a coin from the floor	Sec		≤2 sec = 4 2.5–4 sec = 3 4.5–6 sec = 2 >6 sec = 1 unable = 0	
6	Turn 360°		Discontinuous steps = 0 Continuous steps = 2 Unsteady (grabs, staggers) = 0 Steady = 2		
7	50-foot walk test (15.24 meters) <15 sec = 3.33 feet/sec or 1.0 m/sec	Sec		≤15 sec = 4 15.5–20 sec = 3 20.5–25 sec = 2 >25 sec = 1 unable = 0	
8	Climb one flight of stairs	Sec		≤5 sec = 4 5.5–10 sec = 3 10.5–15 sec = 2 >15 sec = 1 unable = 0	
9	Climb four flights of stairs		Number of flights of stairs up and down (maximum of 4)		
	TOTAL SCORE (maxium 36 for nine-item; 28 for seven-item)				
	*For time measurements, round to nearest 0.5 seconds			Total score	

Data from: Reuben DB, Siu AL. An objective measure of physical function of elderly outpatients (the Physical Performance Test). *Journal of the American Geriatric Society* 1990; 38(10): 1105-1112.

FIGURE 8.18 Physical Performance Test (PPT) Scoring Form.

Modified Physical Performance Test

The modified PPT does not include the PPT tasks 1 (writing) and 2 (simulating eating). Instead, the following balance test is done first, followed by the chair stand test. Then tasks 3 to 9 from the PPT are performed.

1. Testing Procedures for Standing Static Balance Tasks

These balance tasks examine the patient's ability to stand in three positions: side-by-side, semi-tandem, and full tandem. The three positions should be tested in order because they increase in difficulty. Duration of the three balance positions is timed. If patient cannot perform one position, then the next position is not performed but, rather, is scored as "unable." These positions are designed to maximally challenge balance, so clinician should be alert for balance difficulties and maintain patient's safety at all times.

Each balance position is timed for a maximum of 10 seconds. Semiscoring tandem and tandem positions are tested with each foot forward. No out-toeing is permitted. Foot positioning should be strictly observed. If patient cannot attain the proper position, the score is zero for that stance task. Only one trial is allowed for each position.

Each position is demonstrated before testing. If desired, ask patient to practice the position. Patient may be assisted to assume the positions, but when timing starts, no support is given. Once patient appears to be steady, clinician begins timing, relinquishing support if it was initially needed to assume the correct position. Timing is continued until the patient moves a foot, uses a hand for support, or 10 seconds have elapsed. Record any time less than 10 seconds to the nearest hundredth of a second on the test form.

a. Feet Together Stance

Testing Procedure: The first balance task is feet together stance. In this position, patient is asked to stand for 10 seconds with the feet together in a side-by-side stance position (Fig. 8.19).

Instructions to Patient: "These three balancing tasks require you to stand in three different positions for up to 10 seconds. You can use me to get into the position, but then, you have to stand by yourself. I will be timing you when you are ready."

"First, I want you to place your feet completely together, like this. Then hold the position as long as you can. Ready? Begin."

If patient was able to hold the position for 10 seconds, proceed to the next balance position. If position was held for less than 10 seconds, record the seconds and proceed to chair stand test.

b. Semi-tandem Stance

Testing Procedure: The second balance task is semi-tandem stance position. Demonstrate the position. Patient stands with heel of one foot placed to the side of and touching the big toe of the other foot. Either foot can be placed in the forward position. The position should be timed (Fig. 8.20). (Note: This task should be performed only in patients who were able to perform the previous feet together stance task for 10 seconds.) Score the worst performance.

Instructions to Patient: "Move one foot in front of the other so that the heel of the front foot is against the side of the big toe of the other foot, like this. Make sure you do not turn your foot out. You can choose whichever foot you like. Begin!"

If able to complete 10 seconds, proceed to the third balance test. If unable to hold the semi-tandem position for 10 seconds, record the time held and proceed to the chair stand test.

FIGURE 8.19   FIGURE 8.20

c. Full Tandem Stance

Testing Procedure: The third and final position is tandem stance position. Demonstrate the position. Ask patient to place heel of one foot directly in front of the toes of the other foot. Either foot can be placed in the forward position (Fig. 8.21). (Note: This task should be performed only in patients who were able to perform the semi-tandem stance for 10 seconds.)

Instructions to Patient: "Place the heel of one foot directly in front of the toes of the other foot, like this. Either foot can be placed in the forward position. Are you ready? Begin."

Clinical Relevance

- Allowing patient to choose which foot to place forward in the semi-tandem or full tandem stance may indicate which foot the patient feels is stronger. Only one foot-forward position is tested.
- The original instructions, stated here, were for research purposes. In the clinical situation, patients may not be able to assume the ideal position because of severe valgus, for example. Therefore, some latitude may be required.

2. Chair Stand (Five Repetition)

Testing Procedure: The chair stand task is a test of leg strength and mobility. Patient is asked to stand from the chair with the arms folded across the chest while the clinician observes. If patient is able to rise from the chair once, they are then asked to stand up and sit down five times as quickly as possible. Timing begins as soon as the command to stand is given and continues until patient is fully upright at the end of the fifth stand.

Position of Patient: Seated, with arms crossed over the chest. Feet are planted on the floor in a comfortable position (Fig. 8.22).

Instructions to Patient: "Fold your arms across your chest and sit so that your feet are on the floor. Then, stand up, keeping your arms folded across your chest." (After it is observed that patient can safely stand independently without use of arms, proceed to the timed five-repetition part of the chair stand task.) "Now stand up straight, as quickly as you can, five times, without stopping in between. Keep your arms folded across your chest. I'll be timing you with a stopwatch."

Clinical Relevance

- Place the chair against a wall to avoid any movement.
- Observe the quality of the movement such as the position of the hips, reflected in valgus.
- Refer to the chair stand test on page 340.

FIGURE 8.21

FIGURE 8.22

Scoring

Each task's performance is recorded on the PPT scoring form (see Fig. 8.18) or M-PPT scoring form (Fig. 8.23) using a scale of 0 to 4. Total possible scores for the seven-item version of the PPT is 28, whereas the nine-item version PPT is 36. The M-PPT total possible score is 36. Reuben and Siu established percentile reference scores for the PPT based on the performance of a 79-year-old male who is independent in all ADLs.[42]

25th percentile ... 21 (9 items), 15 (7 items)
75th percentile ... 29 (9 items), 22 (7 items)
90th percentile ... 31 (9 items), 24 (7 items)

See Table 8.7 for mean scores for men and women aged 60 to 101 for the PPT.[48] Reuben determined that the following scores indicated a degree of frailty.[42]

32 to 36 = not frail
25 to 32 = mild frailty
17 to 24 = moderate frailty
<17 = unlikely to be able to function in the community.

The minimal important difference in older adults is 2.4 points.[39]

Clinical Relevance

- Timing a patient during task performance should be done with the utmost awareness of the influence of timing. Many patients may move faster than is safe because of a competitive nature. In some cases, it may not be best practice to tell the patient the task is timed, especially in cases where balance is significantly impaired.
- It is recommended to use the lowest score because of the need to accurately record the patient's performance in the clinical setting. Although performance may improve with repeated trials, the most genuine real-life performance may be the lowest timed or poorest performance.

Table 8.7 SEVEN-ITEM PHYSICAL PERFORMANCE TEST SCORES[a]

Age	Male	Female
60–69	26	26.4 (0.9)
70–79	24.6 (1.7)	25.1 (0.9)
80–89	20.4 (4.8)	19.5 (3.8)
90–101	16.5 (6.4)	16.2 (6.0)

[a]Subjects were able to use an assistive device.

Data from Lusardi, M. M., Pellecchia, G. L., & Schulman M. (2003). Functional performance in community living older adults. *Journal of Geriatric Physical Therapy*, 26:14–22

Modified Physical Performance Test

1.	Standing Static Balance	Feet Together: ____sec	Semi-tandem: ____sec	Tandem: ____sec	Score
		❑ 10 sec	❑ 10 sec	❑ 10 sec	❑ 4
		❑ 10 sec	❑ 10 sec	❑ 3–9.9 sec	❑ 3
		❑ 10 sec	❑ 10 sec	❑ 0–2.9 sec	❑ 2
		❑ 10 sec	❑ 0–9 sec	Unable	❑ 1
		❑ 0–9 sec	Unable	Unable	❑ 0

			Time	Scoring values	Score
2.	Chair stand (5 × without arms)			≤11 sec = 4 11.1–14 sec = 3 14.1–17 sec = 2 >17 sec = 1 unable = 0	
3.	Lift a book and put it on a shelf			≤2 sec = 4 2.1–4 sec = 3 4.1–6 sec = 2 >6 sec = 1 unable = 0	
4.	Put on and remove a garment			≤10 sec = 4 10.1–15 sec = 3 15.1–20 sec = 2 >20 sec = 1 unable = 0	
5.	Pick up a coin from the floor			≤2 sec = 4 2.1–4 sec = 3 4.1–6 sec = 2 >6 sec = 1 unable = 0	
6.	Turn 360°		Discontinuous steps = 0 Continuous steps = 2		
			Unsteady (grabs, staggers) = 0 Steady = 2		
7.	50-foot walk			≤15 sec = 4 15.1–20 sec = 3 20.1–25 sec = 2 >25 sec = 1 unable = 0	
8.	Climb one flight of stairs			≤5 sec = 4 5.1–10 sec = 3 10.1–15 sec = 2 >15 sec = 1 unable = 0	
9.	Climb four flights of stairs		Number of flights of stairs up and down (maximum 4)		
TOTAL SCORE				9-item score	/36

FIGURE 8.23 Scoring Form for Modified Physical Performance Test (M-PPT).

Purpose: The timed up-and-go test (TUG) is a test of general mobility that involves standing from a standard-height chair, walking, turning, and sitting down.[49] The test can be performed with an assistive device.[50] Typically, the use of an assistive device indicates slower performance.

The TUG takes only seconds to perform and can be used in all healthcare settings because of the minimal equipment and space required. The test can be used to identify impairments related to mobility.

Essential Muscle Movements for Task Performance: Hip extension, hip abduction from a flexed position, hip external rotation, knee extension, ankle plantar flexion, ankle dorsiflexion and inversion,[3] and trunk extension and flexion. Hip flexion also contributes to walking velocity.[27] The reader is referred to the gait section of this chapter for a more specific list of muscles that are imperative for smooth and normal gait.

Reliability: r = 0.91 (interrater reliability) and 0.96 (intraobserver reliability).[51] In individuals with Alzheimer disease, ICC = 0.97.[52]

Validity: Construct validity is for independence in mobility (the time taken is strongly correlated to the level of functional mobility). Similar to gait speed, it can predict global health and new ADL difficulty. Those who required more than 20 seconds to perform the TUG had a 50% chance of having difficulty performing household chores.[53] It has limited ability to predict falls in community-dwelling older adults and should not be used in isolation to identify individuals at risk for falls.[54]

Equipment: Standard 17-in.-high chair with arms, stopwatch, and 3 m measured on the floor.

Testing Procedure: A chair with arms is placed against a wall to prevent the chair from moving. Measure a distance of 3 m from the front legs of the chair. A line or other object should indicate the 3-m mark (Fig. 8.24). Demonstrate the task for the patient, using an assistive device if the patient will be using one. Ask the patient to walk at a usual and comfortable speed of 3 m to a specified mark on the floor, turn around, and walk back to the chair, sitting all the way back in the chair. Timing starts on "Go!" rather than when the patient starts to rise. Be clear so that the patient knows you are about to start the test. Stop timing when the patient is fully seated with their back against the chair. A practice trial is given before the two test trials are performed. Stand to the side of patient. Clinician may choose to walk with patient if safety is a concern (Fig. 8.25).

Position of Patient: Seated in a chair with arms, feet on the floor, and back against the back of the chair.

Instructions to Patient: "On 'Go!' I want you to stand up and walk as quickly but as safely as you can to the mark on the floor, turn, and return to the chair, sitting down with your back against the back of the chair. I'll be timing you, OK? Go!"

FIGURE 8.24

FIGURE 8.25

Scoring

Fastest trial time taken to perform the TUG is the score. Ten seconds or faster indicates the patient is freely mobile. Thirty seconds or slower indicates the patient is dependent in mobility.[55]

A score greater than 9 seconds is predictive of developing disability within 2 years.[56]

MDCs for the TUG range between 1.0 and 2.1 seconds.[13,57,58]

Reference Scores

A total of 92% of community-dwelling older adults had TUG times of less than 12 seconds, whereas only 9% of institutionalized patients performed the TUG in that time. Community-dwelling women between 65 and 85 years of age should be able to perform the TUG in 12 seconds or less.[59]

TUG times are worse than average if they exceed 9.0 seconds for 60- to 69-year-olds, 10.2 seconds for 70- to 79-year-olds, and 12.7 seconds for 80- to 89-year-olds.[60] Table 8.8 lists reference values for the TUG test. Kenny et al.[61] provide reference values for the TUG based upon sex, height, and age for community-dwelling adults 50 years and older (n = 5,791) in Ireland.

Clinical Relevance

- Make sure the patient can hear you and waits for your "Go!"
- If using an object to mark the farthest point of the 3-m distance, make sure it is moved forward of the 3-m mark to avoid lengthening the course as the patient walks around the object (see Fig. 8.25).
- Always retest using the same assistive device as used in the original test.
- Avoid overcoaching. Valuable information that will inform clinical decision-making can be obtained from observing how the patient chooses to perform the test.
- Using the general procedure for the TUG, a timed performance can be obtained from any surface, such as a couch or car seat, to assist in clinical decision-making and objective documentation.
- Scoring may be either the fastest, the slowest, or an average of the trials. Each repeat test should reflect the same choice.

Table 8.8 **REFERENCE SCORES FOR THE TIMED UP AND GO TEST**

Age Group (Years)	Time in Seconds (95% Confidence Interval)
60–69	8.1 (7.1–9.0)
70–79	9.2 (8.2–10.2)
80–89	11.3 (10.0–12.7)

Data from Bohannon, R. W. Reference values for the timed up and go test: a descriptive meta-analysis. *Journal of Geriatric Physical Therapy*, 2006;29(2):64–68.

Purpose: The stair climb test assesses the ability to climb a flight of stairs. Qualitative and quantitative assessment can be made to determine the amount of assistance a patient needs, identify impairments that may contribute to stair climbing, and indicate how quickly and/or safely the patient can accomplish the task. The stair climb test is also used as a functional test of power.[62,63]

Essential Muscle Movements for Task Performance: Ascent: hip extension, knee flexion and extension, ankle plantar flexion, ankle dorsiflexion, spine extension, and core stability. Descent: eccentric knee extension, hip flexion, and core muscles. For a test that requires stability and balance, however, any lower extremity muscle or group will be used at some point during the task.

Reliability: ICC = 0.99[64]

Validity: Moderate validity as a functional measure with correlations to other functional measures such as TUG, gait speed, and STS movement.[65] Also correlates with balance tests and lower extremity strength and power.

Equipment: Any flight of stairs with a railing can be used. The pediatric version (timed up and down stairs) requires 11 stairs to compare the score with reference values.

Testing Procedure: Timing starts when patient's first foot is lifted from the floor and is stopped when both feet are on the top stair. Because descent is typically more difficult, clinician should time ascent and descent separately. Clinician should document use of handrails, assistive devices, gait belts, and number of stairs.

Position of Clinician: Safety of the patient should be the clinician's primary concern. Therefore, clinician may need to closely guard patient, ascending and descending the stairs with the patient (Fig. 8.26). If the clinician is confident of the safety of the patient, the clinician can choose to remain at the bottom of the flight of stairs during the test.

Instructions to Patient: "I want to see how safely and how quickly you can climb this flight of stairs. Do you feel safe to climb these stairs? You may hold onto the railing if you want to. Please stop at the top of the stairs before coming down so I can time how long it takes you to descend. Ready? Go!"

FIGURE 8.26

Scoring

Scoring the time it takes the patient to ascend and descend stairs must include the number of stairs. Time is calculated by dividing the number of stairs in the flight by the time taken to go up and down.

In nondisabled adult individuals, 0.5 seconds per stair (up and down) is typical (Table 8.9).[65] Stair ascent and descent (combined) decreases with age from 2.5 stairs per second in 20- to 39-year-olds to 1.2 stairs per second in 90+-year-olds.[66] In children ages 8 to 14, 8.1 seconds for 14 steps (0.58 seconds per step) was determined to be normal for combined ascent and descent (Table 8.10).[67]

Table 8.9 GROUP DATA FOR STAIR CLIMB TIME FROM SYSTEMATIC REVIEW

Age	Ascent	Descent
18–49	0.48 ± 0.14	0.50 ± 0.14
50–65	0.46 ± 0.17	0.54 ± 0.29
>65	0.65 ± 0.41	1.4 ± 0.55
>65 with decreased mobility	0.95 ± 0.44	1.11 ± 0.47
Neurological	1.01 ± 0.57	0.9 ± 0.47
Medical	0.6 ± 0.15	0.81 ± 0.15
Musculoskeletal	0.82 ± 0.33	0.96 ± 0.41

Data from Nightengale, E. J., Pourkazemi, F., & Hiller, C. E. (2014). Systemic review of timed stair tests. *Journal of Rehabilitation Research and Development*, 51(3):335–350.

Clinical Relevance

- Carefully observe patient's use of the handrail. Patient may use handrail for balance or may use handrail for weight-bearing to offload a painful joint or compensate for weakness. Watch for the patient pulling on the handrail. This observation can inform clinical decision-making.
- Note position of the feet during stair descent, which may indicate compensation for muscle weakness or pain.
- Stair climbing without a handrail typically increases ground reaction forces by seven times the body weight.[68,69]
- If a patient with eyeglasses has difficulty descending stairs, don't encourage him or her to move faster. Glasses sometimes cause the patient to see a step where there is none, and increased speed may result in a fall.
- It typically takes longer to ascend than descend stairs in the healthy population. Stair ascent and descent time increase with age, with stair descent time increasing to a greater extent.[65]
- Single-leg squats can identify independent stair negotiation ability in older adults.[70]
- Standardization recommendations include a flight of at least 10 stairs timing ascent and descent times separately and asking patient to perform as quickly as possible with handrail to be used for balance only.[65]

Table 8.10 TIME OF COMBINED ASCENT AND DESCENT ON FLIGHT OF 11 STAIRS (SECONDS/STAIR)

	3–9 YEARS		10–19 YEARS		20–59 YEARS		60+ YEARS	
	M	F	M	F	M	F	M	F
95th percentile	2.32	2.31	0.73	0.84	0.78	0.97	1.5	2.0

F, Female; M, male.

Data from McKay, M. J., Baldwin, J. N., Ferreira, P., et al. (2017). Normative reference values for strength and flexibility of 1,000 children and adults. *Neurology.* 88(1):36–43.

Purpose: Floor rise ability is necessary for a patient's safety and confidence and is used for a variety of functional and recreational activities, including housework, bathing, gardening, and some exercises like yoga.[71] Anyone who falls should be able to rescue themselves from the floor (unless they have become seriously injured or have a severe neuromuscular disease). The floor rise test assesses the patient's ability to rise from the floor, thereby identifying impairments and functional ability and informing clinical decision-making.

Essential Muscle Movements for Task Performance: Knee extension, ankle plantar flexion, hip extension, core stability, and trunk rotation. If arms are needed to assist, scapular adduction and downward rotation, scapular depression and adduction, elbow extension, and shoulder horizontal adduction.

Reliability: Excellent reliability (ICC = 0.94 in community-dwelling older adults[71] and ICC = 0.99[72] in community-dwelling older women). The MDC ranged from 2.4 to 2.8 s.[72]

Validity: An inability to rise from the floor is associated with older age, increased mortality, and lower functional abilities and risk for serious injury.[73] Inability to rise after a fall is also predictive of future falls.[74] Floor rise performance is significantly associated with age and gait velocity.[71]

Equipment: Stopwatch, chair with arms, and an unobstructed floor surface that allows the patient to lie flat.

Testing Procedure: Clinician should demonstrate the lowering of the body to the floor, lying supine, and rising again. During the test, patient should lie supine so that 75% of the body is in contact with the floor. Patient may choose to place the head and trunk flat on the floor, bending the knees or lying flat with only the head and shoulders raised (Fig. 8.27). Either position is acceptable. A chair should be nearby to be used by the patient if needed. Timing begins on "Go!" and ends when the patient is fully standing again and steady. Document the type of assistance needed to rise, as appropriate.

Instructions to Patient: "I want you to get onto the floor, without assistance if possible, lying flat so that most of your body is flat on the floor, then get up again. You may get up in any way you choose, and if you need to, you may use this chair. I can help you if you can't get up by yourself. I will demonstrate. I will be timing you and will stop timing when you are fully standing and steady. Are you ready? Good. Go!"

Scoring

The score is the time it takes to complete the floor transfer. The clinician may score only the time it takes to rise from the floor, rather than the combined floor descent and rise. The mean time to stand from a supine position was 2.08 seconds in children.[75] In adults, the average time was 2.6 seconds for young healthy adults (mean age, 23 years), 5.5 seconds for healthy older adults living independently (mean age, 73 years), and 17.1 seconds for congregate housing older adults (mean age, 81 years).[76] In the authors' experience, a patient taking more than 10 seconds for this test will often need assistance with the transfer.

FIGURE 8.27

Clinical Relevance

- When an individual has difficulty getting up from the floor, it often involves an inability to shift weight at the hips and roll onto the side as in side sitting to the knees.
- Clinician should note the "cause" of any difficulty in rising, such as pain, weakness, or an inability to motor plan. These causes may form the basis of a treatment plan.
- Because there are several ways to rise from the floor, the method used by the patient should be noted in the documentation. The position requiring the most strength is rising without assistance (Fig. 8.28), using one knee to rise requires less strength (Fig. 8.29), and using assistance such as a chair requires the least amount of strength (Fig. 8.30).

Floor rise (timed supine to stand) is a common test used to assess mobility in patients with muscular dystrophy. A Gower sign (using hands to push on and "climb up" legs to raise the body from a squatting position) is commonly observed in these patients due to the proximal weakness they have at the trunk, pelvis, and hips.[77]

FIGURE 8.29

FIGURE 8.28

FIGURE 8.30

Human gait is a remarkable feat. Each step is a complex integration of muscular and neural events, all of which have to occur in proper sequence and magnitude to prevent loss of balance and maintain a smooth and integrated forward progression with the least expenditure of energy.[78] Loss of muscle strength has a devastating effect on gait, particularly velocity, safety, and energy cost.[79] The reader is referred to an entire issue of the journal *Physical Therapy* devoted to this and related topics.[80]

This chapter segment is focused only on five events in the gait cycle that occur smoothly and successfully if the muscles involved are sufficiently strong. Weakness in the gluteus medius, tibialis anterior (TA), quadriceps, gluteus maximus, or gastroc soleus will significantly decrease gait velocity and interrupt the integration of gait events and the limb segments involved.

Because locomotion is so important to humans, rehabilitation is often focused on its restoration. The key to successful rehabilitation, however, is the identification of the muscles or muscle groups that are weak. What follows are some common deviations in the gait cycle that are directly linked to specific muscle weakness. These deviations are easily observed, and once observed, the clinician can perform specific muscle testing for confirmation.

Gluteus Medius Weakness

During the loading phase of the gait cycle, as the stance limb is accepting the entire weight of the body (single limb support), the gluteus medius contracts vigorously to keep the pelvis from dropping to the opposite side. With mild weakness of the gluteus medius, the clinician will often observe a positive Trendelenburg sign (excessive drop of the opposite pelvis during single-limb stance).[81] When electromyographic output during gait is measured and compared to the electromyographic output generated during a maximal isometric contraction, the demand on the gluteus medius appears to be approximately 25% of its maximum force capacity. Thus, in general, strength must be at least Grade 3 to prevent the pelvis from dropping.[82] If pelvic drop is observed, strength must be restored because gait velocity slows and the energy required to walk increases in the presence of gluteus medius weakness.[79]

Inman calculated the demand on the gluteus medius during single limb stance (most of the gait cycle) as 2.5 times the weight of the head, arms, and trunk.[83] Thus, for a 150-lb. individual, the gluteus medius must generate approximately 100 lb. of torque with each step. If the clinician is strength testing with a handheld dynamometer, a minimum of 100 lb. should be the expected value in a 150-lb. person.

Tibialis Anterior Weakness

Immediately following heel strike, the TA decelerates the foot to the floor.[79,82] This eccentric contraction is a rapid event that places high demand on the muscle, estimated at between 45% and 75% of its maximum strength.[82,84] A demand this high requires a manual muscle grade of at least 4. Weakness of the TA immediately eliminates the foot-lowering portion of the normal gait cycle. With moderate weakness (approximately Grade 3), the clinician will observe a foot flat gait.[82] Stride length is shortened to permit the foot flat landing. A shorter stride results in slower gait velocity. Thus, if the clinician observes a patient who fails to execute heel strike and approaches each step with a foot flat approach, muscle test the TA to confirm its strength loss. If there is severe weakness, clinician will observe (and hear) a foot slap gait.

Quadriceps Weakness

Another key event in the stance phase of gait is shock absorption at the knee shortly after heel strike.[82] During this instant in the gait cycle, the knee (in a normal person) rapidly goes from full extension to 15° of flexion, and the quadriceps absorb a high amount of force, estimated to be 75% of maximum.[82] With shock absorption, the quadriceps permit a smooth transition to mid-stance. If the quadriceps are weak, the entire shock absorption process disappears, which is another observable event. Instead of a brisk knee flexion following heel strike, the patient with weak quadriceps will shorten the stride and approach the entire first half of the stance phase with a nearly extended knee. No shock absorption takes place. Strength estimates vary, but the quadriceps must be at least a Grade 3 to absorb the shock of knee flexion immediately after heel strike.[82] If the clinician observes a failure of knee flexion during the initial phase of stance, quadriceps strength should be evaluated.

Gluteus Maximus Weakness

At heel contact when the stance phase is initiated, the gluteus maximus is already activated to extend the hip and prevent forward "jackknifing," or uncontrolled trunk flexion, over the femur.[81] If gluteus maximus muscle weakness is present, patient will exhibit a forward trunk lean of "jackknifing." This deviation of a forward trunk lean may occur during the entire stance phase or occur suddenly, a "pitching forward," suggesting a sudden failure of the muscles to hold the trunk upright. Gluteus maximus strength should be sufficient to hold and support the weight of the head, arms, and trunk, or about 60% of body mass.[82] If suspected gluteus maximus weakness exists, as evidenced by a forward trunk lean during stance, with subsequent slowing of gait, further muscle testing is indicated for confirmation. Strong activation of the gluteus maximus during mid-stance when the foot is firmly planted also assists indirectly with knee extension.[81]

Gastrocnemius-Soleus Weakness

The major burst of activity during gait from the gastrocnemius-soleus muscles occurs near heel off and decreases rapidly to near zero at toe off. During this period of the gait cycle, the muscles concentrically contract to create an ankle plantar flexion torque that participates in the forward propulsion of the body.[81] The soleus is one of the most important muscles of the leg because it works not just to control the foot and ankle complex but has a critical role in stabilizing the knee.[85] Equally important is the role of the soleus to prevent forward translation of the tibia toward the end of the stance phase. If the soleus is functioning adequately, the ankle is stable, and heel rise occurs.[82] The demand on the gastrocnemius and soleus is extremely high, measured at 75% of maximum for the gastrocnemius and at more than 80% for the soleus. When gastrocnemius-soleus muscle strength is at least Grade 4, the ankle will lock, and heel rise will occur, which is another key event in the gait cycle that markedly influences velocity.[86] If heel rise is noticeably diminished or nonexistent, further muscle testing is indicated.

Each of the five gait events described has been identified as one of the "critical determinants of gait."[85,86] Without these five critical determinants, gait velocity is markedly diminished, and as noted, if gait speed slows enough, community ambulation is no longer feasible and/or independence may be lost. Indeed, loss of gait function is a major reason for nursing home placement in a person's later years.[87]

Hicks and colleagues reported that a collective strength of 24% of normal is required to walk.[88] If strength is below 24% of normal, profound changes in gait speed have already occurred, and a person with this much weakness is on the threshold of frailty and loss of independence and in need of an assistive device.[89] Clinicians can recognize subtle but highly observable gait deviations long before strength losses become catastrophic. Muscle testing techniques as presented in this book permit identification of strength losses in the early phase of loss, when rehabilitation is more feasible and successful.

1. Jette AM. Toward a common language for function, disability and health. *Phys Ther*. 2006;86:726–734.

2. Eriksrud O, Bohannon RW. Relationship of knee extension force to independence in sit-to-stand performance in patients receiving acute rehabilitation. *Phys Ther*. 2003;83(6):544–551.

3. Gross MM, Stevenson PJ, Charette SL, et al. Effect of muscle strength and movement speed on the biomechanics of rising from a chair in healthy elderly and young women. *Gait Posture*. 1998;8(3):175–185.

4. Özüdoğru A, Canlı M, Ceylan İ, Kuzu Ş, Alkan H, Karaçay BÇ. Five times sit-to-stand test in people with non-specific chronic low back pain-a cross-sectional test-retest reliability study. *Ir J Med Sci*. 2022. https://doi.org/10.1007/s11845-022-03223-3. Epub ahead of print. PMID: 36376556.

5. Wang Z, Yan J, Meng S, et al. Reliability and validity of sit-to-stand test protocols in patients with coronary artery disease. *Front Cardiovasc Med*. 2022;9:841453. https://doi.org/10.3389/fcvm.2022.841453. PMID: 36093135. PMCID: PMC9452740.

6. Bohannon RW. Sit to stand test for measuring performance of lower extremity muscles. *Percept Mot Skills*. 1995;80:163–166.

7. Csuka M, McCarty DJ. A simple method for measurement of lower extremity muscle strength. *Am J Med*. 1985;78:77–81.

8. Jones CJ, Rikli RE, Beam WC. A 30-s chair stand test as a measure of lower body strength in community-residing older adults. *Res Q Exerc Sport*. 1999;70(2):113–119.

9. Lein DH, Alotaibi M, Almutairi M, Singh H. Normative reference values and validity for the 30-second chair-stand test in healthy young adults. *Int J Sports Phys Ther*. 2022;17(5):907–914. PMID: 35949374. PMCID: PMC9340829.

10. Goldberg A, Chavis M, Watkins J, et al. The five-times-sit-to-stand test: validity, reliability and detectable change in older females. *Aging Clin Exp Res*. 2012;24(4):339–344.

11. Deshpande N, Metter EJ, Guralnik J, et al. Predicting 3-year incident mobility disability in middle-aged and older adults using physical performance tests. *Arch Phys Med Rehabil*. 2013;94(5):994–997.

12. Zhang Q, Li YX, Li XL, et al. A comparative study of the five repetition sit-to-stand test and the 30-second sit-to-stand test to assess exercise tolerance in COPD patients. *Int J Chron Obstruct Pulmon Dis*. 2018;13:2833–2839. https://doi.org/10.2147/COPD.S173509. PMID: 30237707. PMCID: PMC6136403.

13. Alfonso-Rosa RM, Del Pozo-Cruz B, Del Pozo-Cruz J, Sañudo B, Rogers ME. Test-retest reliability and minimal detectable change scores for fitness assessment in older adults with type 2 diabetes. *Rehabil Nurs*. 2014;39(5):260–268. https://doi.org/10.1002/rnj.111. PMID: 23780835. Epub 2013 Jun 18.

14. Pua Y-H, Tay L, Clark RA, et al. Reference ranges for gait speed and sit-to-stand performance in a cohort of mobility-intact community-dwelling older adults from Singapore. *JAMDA*. 2022;23:1579–1584.

15. Guralnik Jack M, Fried Linda P, Simonsick Eleanor M, et al., eds. *The Women's Health and Aging Study: Health and Social Characteristics of Older Women with Disability*. Darby PA: Diane Pub Co; 1995:44.

16. Brown M. Quick tests to aid in the diagnosis of physical frailty. *GeriNotes*. 1998;15(4):15.

17. Makizako H, Shimada H, Doi T, et al. Predictive cutoff values of the five times sit-to-stand test and the timed "up & go" test for disability incidence in older people dwelling in the community. *Phys Ther*. 2017;97:417–424.

18. Klukowska AM, Staartjes VE, Vandertop WP, Schröder ML. Five-repetition sit-to-stand test performance in healthy individuals: reference values and predictors from 2 prospective cohorts. *Neurospine*. 2021;18(4):760–769. https://doi.org/10.14245/ns.2142750.375. PMID: 35000330. Epub 2021 Dec 31. PMCID: PMC8752709.

19. Makizako H, Kiyama R, Nakai Y, et al. Reference values of chair stand test and associations of chair stand performance with cognitive function in older adults. *AHR*. 2022;2(3):10090. https://www.sciencedirect.com/science/article/pii/S2667032122000361#:~:text=Reference%20values%20of%20chair%20stand%20performance%20by%20age%20and%20gender,are%20described%20in%20Table%202.

20. Gao S-Y, Xia Y, Wu Q-J, Chang Q, Zhao Y-H. Reference values for five-repetition chair stand test among middle-aged and elderly community-dwelling Chinese adults. *Front Med*. 2021;8,659107. https://doi.org/10.3389/fmed.2021.659107.

21. Kuo YL. The influence of chair seat height on the performance of community-dwelling older adults' 30-second chair stand test. *Aging Clin Exp Res*. 2013;25(3):305–309.

22. Eriksrud O, Bohannon RW. Relationship of knee extension force to independence in sit-to-stand performance in patients receiving acute rehabilitation. *Phys Ther*. 2003;83(6):544–551. PMID: 12775200.

23. Fritz S, Lusardi M. White paper: "Walking speed: the sixth vital sign". *J Geriatr Phys Ther*. 2009;32(2):2–5.

24. Dommershuijsen LJ, Ragunathan J, Ruiter R, et al. Gait speed reference values in community-dwelling older adults – cross sectional analysis from the Rotterdam study. *Exp Gerontol*. 2022;158:111646. https://www.sciencedirect.com/science/article/pii/S0531556521004289.

25. Neptune RR, Sasaki K, Kautz SA. The effect of walking speed on muscle function and mechanical energetics. *Gait Posture*. 2008;28:135–143.

26. John CT, Seth A, Schwartz MH, et al. Contributions of muscles to mediolateral ground reaction force over a range of walking speeds. *J Biomech*. 2012;45(14):2438–2443.

27. Chang RW, Dunlop D, Gibbs J, et al. The determinants of walking velocity in the elderly. An evaluation using regression trees. *Arthritis Rheum*. 1995;38(3):343–350.

28. Kim HJ, Park I, Lee HJ, et al. The reliability and validity of gait speed with different walking pace and distances against general health, physical function, and chronic disease in aged adults. *J Exerc Nutrition Biochem*. 2016;20(3):46–50.

29. Cabanas-Valdés R, García-Rueda L, Salgueiro C, Pérez-Bellmunt A, Rodríguez-Sanz J, López-de-Celis C. Assessment of the 4-meter walk test test-retest reliability and concurrent validity and its correlation with the five sit-to-stand test in chronic ambulatory stroke survivors. *Gait Posture*. 2023;101:8–13. https://doi.org/10.1016/j.gaitpost.2023.01.014. PMID: 36696822. Epub ahead of print.

30. Abellan van Kan G, Rolland Y, Andrieu S, et al. Gait speed at usual pace as a predictor of adverse outcomes in community-dwelling older people: an International Academy on Nutrition and Aging (IANA) task force. *J Nutr Health Aging*. 2009;13(10):881–889.

REFERENCES

31. Artaud F, Singh-Manoux A, Dugravot A, et al. Decline in fast gait speed as a predictor of disability in older adults. *J Am Geriatr Soc.* 2015;63(6):1129–1136.

32. Blain H, Carriere I, Sourial N, et al. Balance and walking speed predict subsequent 8-year mortality independently of current and intermediate events in well-functioning women aged 75 years and older. *J Nutr Health Aging.* 2010;14(7):595–600.

33. Ostir GV, Berges IM, Ottenbacher KJ, et al. Gait speed and dismobility in older adults. *Arch Phys Med Rehabil.* 2015;96(9):1641–1645.

34. Ng SS, Au KK, Chan EL, et al. Effect of acceleration and deceleration distance on the walking speed of people with chronic stroke. *J Rehabil Med.* 2016;48(8):666–670.

35. Ng SS, Ng PC, Lee CY, et al. Assessing the walking speed of older adults: the influence of walkway length. *Am J Phys Med Rehabil.* 2013;92(9):776–780.

36. Andrews AW, Chinworth SA, Bourassa M, et al. Update on distance and velocity requirements for community ambulation. *J Geriatr Phys Ther.* 2010;33(3):128–134.

37. Beauchamp MK, Hao Q, Kuspinar A, et al. Reliability and minimal detectable change values for performance-based measures of physical functioning in the Canadian longitudinal study on aging. *J Gerontol A Biol Sci Med Sci.* 2021;76(11):2030–2038. https://doi.org/10.1093/gerona/glab175. PMID: 34170316. PMCID: PMC8514069.

38. McFadyen BJ, Winter DA. An integrated biomechanical analysis of normal stair ascent and descent. *J Biomech.* 1988;21(9):733–744.

39. King MB, Judge JO, et al. Reliability and responsiveness of two physical performance measures examined in the context of a functional training intervention. *Phys Ther.* 2000;80(1):8–16.

40. Binder EF, Schechtman KB, Ehsani AA, et al. Effects of exercise training on frailty in community-dwelling older adults: results of a randomized, controlled trial. *J Am Geriatr Soc.* 2002;50(12):1921–1928. https://doi.org/10.1046/j.1532-5415.2002.50601.x. PMID: 12473001.

41. Beissner KL, Collins JE, Holmes H. Muscle force and range of motion as predictors of function in older adults. *Phys Ther.* 2000;80:556–563.

42. Reuben DB, Siu A. An objective measure of physical function of elderly outpatients: the physical performance test. *J Am Geriatr Soc.* 1990;38(10):1105–1112.

43. Reuben DB, Siu A, Kimpau S. The predictive validity of self-report and performance-based measures of function and health. *J Gerontol.* 1992;47:M106–M110.

44. Delbaere K, Van den Noortgate N, et al. The physical performance test as a predictor of frequent fallers: a prospective community-based cohort study. *Clin Rehabil.* 2006;20(1):83–90.

45. VanSwearingen JM, Paschal KA, Bonino P, et al. Assessing recurrent fall risk of community-dwelling, frail older veterans using specific tests of mobility and the physical performance test of function. *J Gerontol A Biol Sci Med Sci.* 1998;53A:M457–M464.

46. Briggs RA, Houck JR, Drummond MJ, Fritz JM, LaStayo PC, Marcus RL. Asymmetries identified in sit-to-stand task explain physical function after hip fracture. *J Geriatr Phys Ther.* 2018;41(4):210–217. https://doi.org/10.1519/JPT.0000000000000122. PMID: 28252470.

47. Brown M, Sinacore DR, Binder EF, et al. Physical and performance measures for the identification of mild to moderate frailty. *J Gerontol A Biol Sci Med Sci.* 2000;55A(6):M350–M355.

48. Lusardi MM, Pellecchia GL, et al. Functional performance in community living older adults. *J Geriatr Phys Ther.* 2003;26:14–22.

49. Herman T, Giladi N, Hausdorff JM. Properties of the 'timed up and go' test: more than meets the eye. *Gerontology.* 2010;57(3):203–210.

50. Mathias S, Nayak US, Isaacs B. Balance in elderly patients: the "get-up and go" test. *Arch Phys Med Rehabil.* 1986;67(6):387–389.

51. Bischoff HA, Stähelin HB, Monsch AU, et al. Identifying a cut-off point for normal mobility: a comparison of the timed 'up and go' test in community-dwelling and institutionalised elderly women. *Age Ageing.* 2003;32(3):315–320. https://doi.org/10.1093/ageing/32.3.315. PMID: 12720619.

52. Ries JD, Echternach JL, Nof L, et al. Test-retest reliability and minimal detectable change scores for the timed "up & go" test, the six-minute walk test, and gait speed in people with Alzheimer disease. *Phys Ther.* 2009;89(6):569–579.

53. Donoghue OA, Savva GM, Cronin H, et al. Using timed up and go and usual gait speed to predict incident disability in daily activities among community-dwelling adults aged 65 and older. *Arch Phys Med Rehabil.* 2014;95(10):1954–1961.

54. Barry E, Galvin R, Keogh C, et al. Is the timed up and go test a useful predictor of risk of falls in community dwelling older adults: a systematic review and meta-analysis. *BMC Geriatr.* 2014;14:14.

55. Steffen T, Seney M. Test-retest reliability and minimal detectable change on balance and ambulation tests, the 36-item short-form health survey, and the unified Parkinson disease rating scale in people with parkinsonism. *Phys Ther.* 2008;88(6):733–746.

56. Makizako H, Shimada H, Doi T, et al. Predictive cutoff values of the five times sit-to-stand test and the timed "up & go" test for disability incidence in older people dwelling in the community. *Phys Ther.* 2017;97:417–424.

57. Yuksel E, Unver B, Kalkan S, Karatosun V. Reliability and minimal detectable change of the 2-minute walk test and timed up and go test in patients with total hip arthroplasty. *Hip Int.* 2021;31(1):43–49. https://doi.org/10.1177/1120700019888614. PMID: 31928090. Epub 2020 Jan 13.

58. Donoghue OA, Savva GM, Börsch-Supan A, Kenny RA. Reliability, measurement error and minimum detectable change in mobility measures: a cohort study of community-dwelling adults aged 50 years and over in Ireland. *BMJ Open.* 2019;9(11):e030475. https://doi.org/10.1136/bmjopen-2019-030475. PMID: 31719075. PMCID: PMC6858113.

59. Bischoff HA, Stahelin HB, Monsch AU, et al. Identifying a cut-off point for normal mobility: a comparison of the timed "up and go" test in community-dwelling and institutionalised elderly women. *Age Ageing.* 2003;32(3):315–320.

60. Bohannon RW. Reference values for the timed up and go test: a descriptive meta-analysis. *J Geriatr Phys Ther.* 2006;29(2):64–68.

61. Kenny RA, Coen RF, Frewen J, Donoghue OA, Cronin H, Savva GM. Normative values of cognitive and physical function in older adults: findings from the Irish Longitudinal Study on Ageing. *J Am Geriatr Soc.* 2013;61(suppl 2):S279–S290. https://doi.org/10.1111/jgs.12195. PMID: 23662720.

62. Zech A, Steib S, Sportwiss D, et al. Functional muscle power testing in young, middle-aged, and community-dwelling

nonfrail and prefrail older adults. *Arch Phys Med Rehabil.* 2011;92(6):967–971.

63. Roig M, Eng JJ, MacIntyre DL, et al. Associations of the stair climb power test with muscle strength and functional performance in people with chronic obstructive pulmonary disease: a cross-sectional study. *Phys Ther.* 2010;90(12):1774–1782.

64. LeBrasseur NK, Bhasin S, Miciek R, et al. Tests of muscle strength and physical function: reliability and discrimination of performance in younger and older men and older men with mobility limitations. *J Am Geriatr Soc.* 2008;56:2118–2123.

65. Nightingale EJ. Systemic review of timed stair tests. *JRRD (J Rehabil Res Dev).* 2014;51(3):335–350.

66. Butler AA, Menant JC, Tiedemann AC, et al. Age and gender differences in seven tests of functional mobility. *J NeuroEng Rehabil.* 2009;6:31.

67. Zaino CA, Marchese VG, Westcott SL. Timed up and down stairs test: preliminary reliability and validity of a new measure of functional mobility. *Pediatr Phys Ther.* 2004;16(2):90–98.

68. Teh KC, Aziz AR. Heart rate, oxygen uptake, and energy cost of ascending and descending the stairs. *Med Sci Sports Exerc.* 2002;34:695–699.

69. Stolk J, Verdonschot N, Huiskes R. Stair climbing is more detrimental to the cement in hip replacement than walking. *Clin Orthop Relat Res.* 2002;405:294–305. Nightengale, 2014.

70. Hockings RL, Schmidt DD, Cheung CW. Single-leg squats identify independent stair negotiation ability in older adults referred for a physiotherapy mobility assessment at a rural hospital. *J Am Geriatr Soc.* 2013;61(7):1146–1151.

71. Klima DW, Anderson C, Samrah D, Patel D, Chui K, Newton R. Standing from the floor in community-dwelling older adults. *J Aging Phys Act.* 2016;24(2):207–213. https://doi.org/10.1123/japa.2015-0081. PMID: 26291641. Epub 2015 Aug 20.

72. Moffett MA, Avers D, Bohannon RW, Shaw KL, Merlo AR. Performance and clinimetric properties of the timed up from the floor completed by apparently healthy community-dwelling older women. *J Geriatr Phys Ther.* 2021;44(3):159–164.

73. Bergland A, Laake K. Concurrent and predictive validity of "getting up from lying on the floor". *Aging Clin Exp Res.* 2005;17(3):181–185.

74. Close JC, Hooper R, Glucksman E, Jackson SH, Swift CG. Predictors of falls in a high risk population: results from the prevention of falls in the elderly trial (PROFET). *Emerg Med J.* 2003;20(5):421–425. https://doi.org/10.1136/emj.20.5.421. PMID: 12954679. PMCID: PMC1726177.

75. Ng J, Conaway MR, Rigby AS, Priestman A, Baxter PS. Methods of standing from supine and percentiles for time to stand and to run 10 meters in young children. *J Pediatr.* 2013;162(3):552–556. https://doi.org/10.1016/j.jpeds.2012.08.030. PMID: 23058291. Epub 2012 Oct 9.

76. Ulbrich J, Raheja A, Alexander NB. Body positions used by healthy and frail older adults to rise from the floor. *J Am Geriatr Soc.* 2000;48(12):1626–1632. https://doi.org/10.1111/j.1532-5415.2000.tb03874.x. PMID: 11129753.

77. Shrestha S, Munakomi S, Gower S. [Updated 2022 Feb 17]. In: *StatPearls [Internet].* Treasure Island (FL): StatPearls Publishing; 2022.

78. Kuo AD, Donelan JM. Dynamic principles of gait and their clinical implications. *Phys Ther.* 2010;90:157–176.

79. Waters RL. The energy expenditure of normal and pathological gait. *Gait Posture.* 1999;9:207–231.

80. Perry J. Special issue: stepping forward with gait rehabilitation. *Phys Ther.* 2010;90(2):142–305.

81. Neumann DA. *Kinesiology of the Musculoskeletal System: Foundations for Rehabilitation.* St. Louis: Elsevier; 2017. ISBN: 978-0-323-28753-1.

82. Perry J, Burnfield JM. *Gait Analysis: Normal and Pathological Function.* 2nd ed. Thorofare NJ: Slack Inc; 2010:3–260.

83. Inman V. Functional aspects of the abductor muscles of the hip. *J Bone Joint Surg.* 1947;29:607–619.

84. Dubo HIC, Peat M, Winter DA, et al. Electromyographic temporal analysis of gait: normal human locomotion. *Arch Phys Med Rehabil.* 1976;57:415–420.

85. Kerrigan DC, Della Croce U, Marciello M, et al. A refined view of the determinants of gait: significance of heel rise. *Arch Phys Med Rehabil.* 2000;81:1077–1080.

86. Saunders JB, Inman VT, Eberhardt HD. The major determinants in normal and pathological gait. *J Bone Joint Surg.* 1953;35A:543–548.

87. Studenski S, Perera S, Patel K, et al. Gait speed and survival in older adults. *JAMA.* 2011;305:70–78.

88. Hicks GE, Shardell M, Alley DE, et al. Absolute strength and loss of strength as predictors of mobility decline in older adults: the InCHIANTI study. *J Gerontol A Biol Sci Med Sci.* 2012;67(1):66–73.

89. Bassey EJ, Fiatarone MA, O'Neill EF, et al. Leg extension power and functional performance in very old men and women. *Clin Sci.* 1992;52:321–327.

CHAPTER **9**

Handheld Muscle Dynamometry

Handheld Muscle
Dynamometry

   Introduction

   Instrumentation

Summary

Shoulder Flexion

Shoulder Extension

Shoulder Abduction

Shoulder External
Rotation

Shoulder Internal
Rotation

Elbow Flexion

Elbow Extension

Wrist Extension

Hip Flexion

Hip Extension

   Hip Extension Tests
   Modified for Hip
   Flexion Tightness

Hip Abduction

Hip External Rotation

Hip Internal Rotation

Knee Flexion

Knee Extension

Foot Dorsiflexion and
Inversion

INTRODUCTION

Handheld dynamometry (HHD) is a manual muscle testing (MMT) procedure by which a dynamometer is held in the hand of an examiner to quantitatively measure the strength or force of specific muscle actions of the limbs or trunk. Essentially, it is an extension of the human hand. HHD should not be confused with grip strength dynamometry (see page 227) in which an instrument held in the patient's hand is used to measure that patient's hand-grip strength. HHD measures force on a continuous scale in Newtons (N), pounds (lb), or kilograms (kg) from 3.6 N up to 1320 N (0.2 to 300 lb), depending on the device.

Research published over the past 100 years describes the use of at least a dozen different handheld dynamometers.[1] Although researchers have commonly used handheld dynamometers, they are less commonly used in the clinic, perhaps because the HHD technique is not routinely taught in entry-level programs. However, HHD has been used in a variety of settings that reflect the scope of clinical practice such as acute care,[2] inpatient rehabilitation,[3,4] home care,[5] and outpatient clinics.[6]

Handheld dynamometers are accurate, easy to use, portable, and afford an objectivity that is lacking in MMT. The continuous scale used in HHD allows the identification of subtle differences in side-to-side comparisons and can avoid the ceiling effect of MMT. HHD is also more responsive, making it possible to discern changes in strength within Grades 4 and 5. However, many of the issues and limitations of MMT discussed in Chapters 1 and 2 are relevant to the application of HHD. The reader is referred to these chapters to review the limitations of MMT and to extend the recommendations for enhancing the reliability of MMT to HHD, recognizing that the same procedures apply to HHD. The reader is reminded that HHD values are influenced by the tester's strength, position, ability to stabilize the body segment, and technique used, similar to MMT. Absolute values of force are subject to the limitations cited earlier and should be interpreted with much caution. For example, scores for large muscle forces (over 250 N) may not be accurate due to stabilization and tester strength issues.[7] The inability of some handheld dynamometers to record the high forces generated by strong muscles (e.g., quadriceps and plantar flexors), lack of clear meaning of the scores, and lack of standardization of positions are additional limitations of HHD.

INSTRUMENTATION

Many HHD devices exist and are used in the clinic and research studies. Some have pads for specific body parts. Unfortunately, different devices have characteristics unique to the device that prevent comparisons of reference scores. These characteristics include device design (attachments, handles), units of measurement, and upper force limit. The clinician should be aware of these issues and rely on one handheld dynamometer in a clinic to compare intraindividual and interindividual values.

Clinimetric Properties

The clinimetric properties of force measures obtained by HHD have been researched extensively over the past few decades. Research on HHD reveals conflicting results for both test-retest and intertester reliability, in part because of the methodological quality of studies and lack of standardization of method (e.g., lack of stabilization, patient position, rate of force applied, use of make or break tests).[8,9] Reliability tends to be lower when stronger actions, such as knee extension or plantar flexion, stronger patients, or weaker testers are involved.[10-12] Only reference scores from HHD used in the traditional test positions of this text are included.

Reliability

A systematic review of the intraexaminer reliability of HHD measurements obtained from the upper extremity demonstrated acceptable intrarater and interrater reliability (intercorrelation coefficient ([ICC] > 0.90) for shoulder internal and external rotation and elbow flexion and extension[8,13] but not for the lower extremity (e.g. hip adduction and extension, knee flexion and extension, and ankle dorsiflexion).[14] The insufficient reliability for the lower extremity may be due to a lack of standardization of positions in the studies included in this systematic review and insufficient stabilization (e.g. hip abduction, hip flexion, and ankle plantar flexion).[14] Abdominal flexor strength was found to be reliable when tested in a 25° inclined position.[15]

Strength measurements are internally consistent when performed by a tester with adequate strength,[13] perhaps making HHD on lower extremities feasible for nonathletes and older people.[16,17] but not to compare results with reference scores.[16,18] Intersession reliability is better than intrasession reliability.

Validity

The validity of HHD is supported by considerable research. Specifically, correlations between measurements obtained by HHD and measurements obtained by isokinetic dynamometry (concurrent validity) support the criterion validity of HHD.[9,15,19-20] Convergent validity is supported by correlations between lower limb strength measured by HHD and performance of activities such as dressing, toileting, and transferring[21]; bed mobility[1,22]; sit to stand[3,23]; level ground ambulation[24-25]; and stair negotiation.[26] Known group validity is upheld by differences in the dynamometrically measured strength of adults with and without pathologies and problems as diverse as renal failure,[24] stroke,[27] osteoporosis,[28] diabetes,[29] osteoarthritis,[30] dementia,[21] and fear of falling.[30-31]

Responsiveness

Responsiveness is described through reporting of minimal detectable change (MDC) and is variable and affected by HHD methods. Responsiveness in HHD is not well researched except in the upper limb. Various authors have suggested that strength differences between affected and nonaffected limbs should not exceed 10% to 15%, especially if returning to sport.[14] One study found a 22-N MDC in shoulder internal rotation and an 8-N MDC in external rotation.[32] Another recent systematic review and metanalysis demonstrated an MDC of under 15% for the strength measurement of shoulder internal and external rotation using HHD in a sitting position.[13] When measuring modified hip extension, the MDC of 14.8 Nm using HHD compared with 25.6 Nm using isokinetic dynamometry[20] (Fig. 6.28).

Reference Scores

Reference scores have been published for dynamometrically obtained measures of upper and lower limb strength.[7,33-38] These scores are limited by the positions and type of dynamometer used and the use of both make and break tests. Nevertheless, they provide some indication of what might be expected from healthy adults.

General Procedures

The tests described in this chapter use the same MMT positions described elsewhere in this book, and thus, the same testing procedures are followed. First, the position of the patient is described. Then the patient is asked to perform the test action against gravity to assess the quality and quantity of the action and to determine if application of resistance is appropriate (e.g., in the presence of pain or inflammation). Although HHD may be used on a muscle action that does not produce the full range, it is important to discern what impairments prevent the full range, such as weakness, joint restrictions, or pain. If weakness is below a Grade 3 (i.e., the patient cannot tolerate any resistance other than gravity), HHD may not be practical. Next, appropriate stabilization is applied; a critical element in HHD testing. The assistance of another person may be needed if the clinician suspects the patient's muscle action could overcome the clinician's strength or if adequate stabilization can only be achieved with extra help. Once adequate stabilization is achieved, place the HHD on the body segment and ask the patient to push or pull against the HHD with maximum effort. This effort should occur within 2 to 5 seconds, adhering to the procedures outlined on page 2. The use of a break test elicits a slightly stronger and eccentric contraction[38] than a make test, and thus it is used in this text, similar to the recommended procedure for MMT. However, there may be times when a make test is more appropriate (e.g., in the presence of joint instability, patient's ability to cooperate, or pain). To enhance reliability, an enthusiastic command such as "push, push, push" is provided. At the completion of the effort, the peak force score is read from the dynamometer. Although a single effort may suffice for the experienced clinician,[39] a second or third trial should be conducted for the inexperienced clinician and patient. If multiple efforts are attained, the tester can choose whether to average the results or use the highest or lowest result. Allow a rest of at least 30 seconds between efforts. Scoring is recorded in Newtons, rather than as muscle grades.

Testing Specific Actions

Various methods of testing for different actions of the limbs and trunk using HHD have been described in the literature. Procedures vary, revealing a lack of standardization. Therefore, we have chosen the standard muscle-testing positions described in this book, which are known to be valid testing positions. Consistent positions may encourage adoption and broader use, especially as validity studies on these positions are published. The clinician should review the helpful hints for each muscle action described in previous chapters.

Reference Scores

The lack of standardization of HHD makes the interpretation of scores difficult. Further, studies interchange the terms normative scores with reference scores. Because normative values imply scores from a very large cohort, and many scores come from small studies and are therefore not "normative," the term *reference scores* is used. Reference scores are defined as scores obtained from individuals presenting conditions that are similar to the tested subject.[40]

In this chapter, we have used reference data from studies using positions similar to the standard MMT positions. These positions often require some dynamic stabilization that may influence the amount of muscle force generated. Differences in results when compared with reference scores may reflect different positions or stabilization. For reference scores of the upper limb, the dominant side was used. The reader should be aware that in normal adults without pain or muscle disease, the stronger side generally does not exceed the weaker one by more than 22%.[7] Results from break tests are included whenever available. Because of the variability of reference scores across studies, we have opted to use mean scores and standard deviations using decade data. If more precise scores are desired, the reader is encouraged to read the referenced study. The mean scores should give the reader an idea of approximate scores for specific muscle actions.

Scores are recorded in Newtons. When reference scores were recorded in kilograms, they are converted to Newtons by multiplying kilograms by 9.8. However, recording scores in Newton-meters (taking into consideration the length of the lever arm and the weight of limb, however impractical) would be most accurate to establish reference scores.[40] Therefore, results derived from standard test positions may be underestimated.[40] The reader is also cautioned about placing undue emphasis on absolute scores or scores exceeding 250 N, because 250 N most likely exceeds the force necessary for the performance of most functional tasks[7] and may have reduced reliability compared to lower scores. Additionally, most clinicians will be unable to effectively stabilize or resist muscle forces exceeding 250 N. Examples of this phenomenon are the forces exerted by knee extensors and plantar flexors.

HHD has the potential of making MMT more objective through the use of continuous scaling. However, many issues exist that limit the usefulness of reference scores for HHD. It is hoped that issues of standardized positions and stabilization, type of instrument, type of measurement, type of verbal stimulation, and type of resistance will become more consistent to enable the clinician to interpret a patient's scores against meaningful reference data. As standardization of HHD procedures are published and accepted, those changes will be reflected in this text.

SHOULDER FLEXION

(Anterior deltoid, Supraspinatus, Clavicular portion of pectoralis major, and Coracobrachialis)

Position of Patient: Short sitting with arm at side, elbow slightly flexed, forearm pronated.

Instructions to Clinician: Stand at the test side. Ask patient to raise arm forward to shoulder height (see Fig. 5.51 on page 127). If application of resistance is appropriate, proceed to test. Position patient's arm in 90° of flexion with forearm in neutral rotation and arm in the sagittal plane. Ask patient to hold the position. Place hand with the dynamometer over the distal humerus just above the elbow. The other hand stabilizes shoulder (Fig. 9.1). Resistance is given in a downward direction.

Test: Patient holds shoulder in 90° of flexion without rotation or horizontal movement (see Fig. 9.1 and Fig. 5.51 on page 127). The scapula should be allowed to abduct and upwardly rotate.

Instructions to Patient: "Hold your arm. Don't let me push it down. Hold … hold … hold."

Reference Scores

Reference scores with standard deviations below are for a break test in sitting position[36]:
Mean for 20- to 59-year-old men = 203.4 (43.1)
Mean for 20- to 59-year-old women = 102.6 (35.6)

FIGURE 9.1

(Posterior deltoid, Latissimus dorsi, Teres major, Long head of triceps)

Position of Patient: Prone with arms at sides and shoulder internally rotated (palm up). Head turned toward side being tested (see Fig. 5.57 on page 131).

Instructions to Clinician: Stand at test side. Ask patient to lift arm as high as possible. If application of resistance is appropriate, proceed to test. Position arm in full extension. Ask patient to hold the position. Place hand with the dynamometer over the posterior arm just above the elbow. Stabilization is provided by the prone position. Resistance is applied in a downward direction (Fig. 9.2).

Test: Patient holds arm off the table, with the elbow straight (see Fig. 5.59 on page 131).

Instructions to Patient: "Hold your arm. Don't let me push it down. Hold … hold … hold."

Reference Scores

Reference scores with standard deviations below are for a break test in the sitting position[36]:
Mean for 20- to 59-year-old men = 162.9 (41.7)
Mean for 20- to 59-year-old women = 80.9 (31.3)

FIGURE 9.2

SHOULDER ABDUCTION

(Middle deltoid and Supraspinatus)

Position of Patient: Short sitting with arm at side and elbow slightly flexed.

Instructions to Clinician: Stand behind patient. Ask patient to lift the arm out to the side at shoulder level with the forearm in neutral, thumb pointed up. If application of resistance is appropriate, proceed to test. Position patient's arm in 90° of abduction in the frontal plane. Ask patient to hold the position. Place the hand with the dynamometer over the arm, just above the elbow. Resistance is given in a downward direction. Stabilize at the top of the shoulder, if needed (Fig. 9.3).

Test: Patient abducts arm to 90°, arm in neutral rotation and elbow straight (see Fig. 5.66 on page 135).

Instructions to Patient: "Hold your arm. Keep your elbow straight. Don't let me push it down. Hold ... hold ... hold."

Reference Scores

Reference scores with standard deviations below are for a break test in sitting position[36]:
Mean for 20- to 59-year-old men = 167.0 (47.2)
Mean for 20- to 59-year-old women = 84.4 (31.8)

FIGURE 9.3

Position of Patient: Short sitting, with elbow flexed to 90° and forearm in neutral.

Instructions to Clinician: Stand in front of or sit beside patient. Ask patient to move the forearm away from the trunk (see Fig. 5.87 on page 148). If application of resistance is appropriate, proceed to test. Position patient's arm in neutral shoulder rotation with elbow flexed to 90°. Ask patient to hold the position. Place hand with the dynamometer over the dorsal (extensor) surface of the forearm, just proximal to the wrist. The other hand stabilizes the medial aspect of the elbow. Resistance is given with a medially directed force on the outside of the forearm. Because this is not an antigravity position, maximal resistance should be used, if appropriate (Fig. 9.4).

Test: Patient holds shoulder and forearm in neutral position against a medially directed force.

Instructions to Patient: "Push your forearm against my hand. Hold it. Don't let me move it. Hold … hold … hold."

Reference Scores

Reference scores with standard deviations below are for a break test in sitting position[36]:
Mean for 20- to 59-year-old men = 107.4 (31.5)
Mean for 20- to 59-year-old women = 59.2 (22.9)
    Reference scores for a make test in sitting position[33]:
Mean for 20- to 59-year-old men = 134.7 (39.6)
Mean for 20- to 59-year-old women = 82.2 (20.9)
Mean for 60- to 80-year-old and older men = 96.7 (25.3)
Mean for 60- to 80-year-old and older women = 63.3 (19.2)

FIGURE 9.4

SHOULDER INTERNAL ROTATION

(Subscapularis)

Position of Patient: Short sitting with elbow flexed to 90° and forearm in neutral.

Instructions to Clinician: Stand in front of or sit beside patient and ask patient to move the forearm toward the trunk (see Fig. 5.95 on page 153). If application of resistance is appropriate, proceed to test. Position shoulder in neutral rotation with the elbow flexed to 90°. Ask patient to hold the position. Place hand with the dynamometer over the volar (flexor) surface of the forearm, just proximal to the wrist. The other hand stabilizes the lateral aspect of the elbow with one hand. Resistance is given in a lateral direction away from the trunk (Fig. 9.5). Because this is not an antigravity position, maximal resistance should be used if appropriate.

Test: Patient holds shoulder and forearm in neutral against a laterally directed force.

Instructions to Patient: "Pull your forearm in toward your stomach. Hold it. Don't let me move it. Hold … hold … hold."

Reference Scores

Reference scores with standard deviations below are for a break test in sitting position[36]:
Mean for 20- to 59-year-old men = 112.7 (44.0)
Mean for 20- to 59-year-old women = 52.4 (22.1)

FIGURE 9.5

Position of Patient: Short sitting with arms at sides. Elbow flexed with forearm supinated.

Instructions to Clinician: Stand in front of patient toward the test side. Ask patient to bend the elbow. If the application of resistance is appropriate, proceed to test. Position patient's elbow in midrange of elbow flexion with shoulder in the sagittal plane and forearm in supination (Fig. 9.6). Ask patient to hold the position. Place hand holding the dynamometer over the volar (flexor) surface of the forearm proximal to the wrist in the direction of elbow extension (Fig. 9.7). The other hand provides stabilization on the anterior surface of the shoulder. Resistance is given in a downward direction toward elbow extension.

Test: Patient holds elbow position.

Instructions to Patient: "Hold the position. Don't let me move it. Hold … hold … hold."

Reference Scores

Reference scores with standard deviations below are for a break test in sitting position[36]:
Mean for 20- to 59-year-old men = 287.5 (83.8)
Mean for 20- to 59-year-old women = 163.3 (49.6)
 Reference scores for a make test in supine position[33]:
Mean for 60- to 80-year-old and older men = 209.4 (48.4)
Mean for 60- to 80-year-old and older women = 129.7 (33.9)

FIGURE 9.6

FIGURE 9.7

ELBOW EXTENSION

(Triceps brachii)

Position of Patient: Prone on the table with patient's head facing toward test side. Patient starts the test with shoulder in 90° of abduction and elbow flexed to 90° and in neutral rotation with thumb pointed down. Forearm hangs over the side of the table (see Fig. 5.113 on page 164).

Instructions to Clinician: Stand to side of patient. Ask patient to straighten elbow. If the application of resistance is appropriate, proceed to test. Position the elbow in 160° (not full extension to avoid hyperextension or "locking"). Ask patient to hold the position. Place the hand with the dynamometer on the distal surface of the extended forearm just proximal to the wrist. Provide support of the arm just above the elbow with one hand. No stabilization is needed in this position. Resistance is applied in a downward direction (Fig. 9.8).

Test: Patient holds the position of elbow extension.

Instructions to Patient: "Hold it. Don't let me bend your elbow. Hold … hold … hold."

Reference Scores

Reference scores with standard deviations below are for a break test in sitting position[36]:

Mean for 20- to 59-year-old men = 184.2 (46.7)

Mean for 20- to 59-year-old women = 120.0 (34.3)

Reference scores below are for a make test in supine position.[33]

Mean for 60- to 80-year-old and older men = 162.1 (36.8)

Mean for 60- to 80-year-old and older women = 102.8 (25.3)

FIGURE 9.8

(Extensor carpi radialis longus, Extensor carpi radialis brevis, and Extensor carpi ulnaris)

Position of Patient: Short sitting with elbow flexed and forearm supported on a table. Forearm is fully pronated.

Instructions to Clinician: Sit or stand at a diagonal in front of patient. Ask patient to lift the hand. If resistance is appropriate, proceed to test. Position wrist in full extension with forearm fully pronated. (Fig. 9.9). Ask patient to hold the position. Place hand holding the dynamometer over the dorsal (extensor) surface of the hand. Stabilization is provided by the resting position of the forearm on the table. Resistance is given in a distal and downward direction (Fig. 9.10).

Test: For the combined test of the three wrist extensor muscles, patient holds wrist in full wrist extension. Do not permit extension of the fingers.

Instructions to Patient: "Hold your wrist. Don't let me push it down. Hold … hold … hold."

Reference Scores

Reference scores with standard deviations below are for a break test in sitting position[36]:
Mean for 20- to 59-year-old men = 186.1 (48.8)
Mean for 20- to 59-year-old women = 107.9 (41.2)

FIGURE 9.9

FIGURE 9.10

HIP FLEXION

(Psoas major and Iliacus)

Position of Patient: Short sitting with thighs fully supported on the table and legs hanging over the edge. Patient may use the arms to provide trunk stability by grasping the table edge or with hands on the table at each side.

Instructions to Clinician: Stand next to the limb being tested. Ask patient to lift the thigh off the table (see Fig. 6.5 on page 238). If the application of resistance is appropriate, proceed to test. Position the hip in maximum hip flexion. Ask patient to hold the position. Place hand holding the dynamometer over the distal thigh just proximal to the knee joint. Stabilization is provided by patient's arms. Resistance is given in a downward direction (Fig. 9.11).

Test: Patient holds hip at end range, clearing the table and maintaining neutral rotation.

Instructions to Patient: "Sit tall and hold your thigh up. Don't let me push it down. Hold … hold … hold."

Reference Scores

Reference scores with standard deviations below are for a make test in supine position[33]:
Mean for 20- to 59-year-old men = 247.0 (17.0)
Mean for 20- to 59-year-old women = 80.0 (22.0)
   Reference scores below are for a break test in supine position[33]:
Mean for 60- to 69-year-old men = 247.0 (17.0)
Mean for 60- to 69-year-old women = 167.0 (20.0)

FIGURE 9.11

Test is for the aggregate of all hip extensor muscles.

Position of Patient: Prone. Arms may be at the side of body or abducted to hold the sides of the table. (Note: If there is a hip flexion contracture, immediately go to the test described for hip extension modified for hip flexion tightness; see Fig. 6.28).

Instructions to Clinician: Stand at the level of the pelvis on side of limb to be tested. (Note: Fig. 9.12 shows the clinician on the opposite side to avoid obscuring activity.) Ask patient to lift leg off the table as high as possible while keeping knee straight. Pelvis should remain stabilized against the table. Stabilization can be applied over the gluteus maximus to keep the pelvis from rising if needed. If application of resistance is appropriate, proceed to test. Position leg in full extension with no pelvic rotation. Ask patient to hold position. Place hand holding the dynamometer on posterior thigh just above the knee. Resistance is applied in a downward direction (Fig. 9.12).

Test: Patient holds thigh off table in the maximum available range.

Instructions to Patient: "Lift your leg off the table as high as you can. Don't bend your knee. Hold it. Don't let me push it down. Hold … hold … hold."

Reference Scores

Not available.

HIP EXTENSION TEST MODIFIED FOR HIP FLEXION TIGHTNESS

Position of Patient: Patient stands with hips flexed and leans over table so that the anterior superior iliac spine (ASIS) is "hooked" on the end of table. Arms are used to "hug" the table for support. Knee of the non–test limb should be flexed to allow test limb to rest on the floor at the start of the test.

Instructions to Clinician: Stand at the side of the limb to be tested. (Note: Fig. 9.13 shows the clinician on the opposite side to avoid obscuring the test position.) Ask patient to lift leg toward the ceiling. If application of resistance is appropriate, proceed to test. Place hand holding the dynamometer over posterior thigh just above knee. Opposite hand stabilizes pelvis laterally to maintain hip and pelvis position. Resistance is applied downward, toward the floor (Fig. 9.13),

Test: Patient holds hip in full extension.

Instructions to Patient: "Lift your leg off the floor as high as you can. Keep your knee straight. Don't let me push it down. Hold … hold … hold."

Reference Scores

Not available

FIGURE 9.12

FIGURE 9.13

HIP ABDUCTION

(Gluteus medius and Gluteus minimus)

Position of Patient: Side lying with test leg uppermost. Patient's hip is slightly extended beyond the midline and pelvis rotated slightly forward (see Fig. 6.48 on page 262). Lowermost leg is flexed for stability.

Instructions to Clinician: Stand behind patient. Ask patient to lift leg as high as possible with verbal cues as needed to prevent leg from rotating and hip from flexing. The raised ankle should be in line with the pelvis. Stabilization on the hip may be needed. If application of resistance is appropriate, proceed to test. Position leg into approximately 30° abduction with the ankle in line with the iliac crest. Place HHD just proximal to knee. Resistance is applied in a downward direction (Fig. 9.14).

Test: Patient holds the abducted hip at about range of motion without flexing the hip or rotating it in either direction.

Instructions to Patient: "Hold your leg. Don't let me push it down. Hold … hold … hold."

Reference Scores

Side-lying hip abduction using a strap to fix the hand-held dynamometer to the distal thigh (not shown) has a high reliability (ICC = 0.95)[26] and may improve scores and reliability. Widler[41] found a 30% higher force value in the side-lying position, using a fixed dynamometer compared to supine using a fixed dynamometer. However, reference scores do not exist for the side-lying position in large sample sizes.

Reference scores with standard deviations below are for a make test in the supine position[33]:
Mean for 20- to 59-year-old men = 170.7 (43.9)
Mean for 20- to 59-year-old women = 113.1 (32.4)
Mean for 60-year-old and older men = 124.8 (32.8)
Mean for 60-year-old and older women = 83.8 (23.5)

FIGURE 9.14

(Gluteus maximus [posterior])

Position of Patient: Short sitting with thighs fully supported on the table and legs hanging over the edge. (Trunk may be supported by placing hands flat or fisted at patient's side on the table.)

Instructions to Clinician: Sit on a low stool or kneel beside limb to be tested. Ask patient to turn leg in toward other leg without moving thigh (see Fig. 6.39 on page 256).

If application of resistance is appropriate, proceed to test. Position leg into neutral rotation. Place hand with dynamometer on medial aspect of ankle just above malleolus. Extra padding may be needed under dynamometer for patient's comfort (not shown). The other hand, which will offer counterpressure, is contoured over the lateral aspect of the distal thigh just above knee. Resistance is applied as a laterally directed force at the ankle. Stabilization is provided in a medially directed force at the knee counteracting the resistance provided at the ankle. The two forces are applied in counterdirections for this rotary motion (Fig. 9.15).

Test: Patient attempts to externally rotate hip against maximum resistance.

Instructions to Patient: "Hold your leg. Don't let me turn your leg out. Hold … hold … hold."

Reference Scores

Reference scores with standard deviations below are for a make test in sitting position[33]:

Mean for 20- to 59-year-old men = 169.4 (45.8)
Mean for 20- to 59-year-old women = 100.7 (29.1)
Mean for 60- to 80-year-old and older men = 125.5 (33.9)
Mean for 60- to 80-year-old and older women = 76.3 (23.7)

FIGURE 9.15

HIP INTERNAL ROTATION

(Glutei minimus and Gluteus medius; Tensor fasciae latae)

Position of Patient: Short sitting with thighs fully supported on the table and legs hanging over the edge. (Trunk may be supported by placing hands flat or fisted at patient's sides on the table.)

Instructions to Clinician: Sit or kneel in front of patient. Ask patient to move lower leg out, away from other leg without letting thigh move (see Fig. 6.44 on page 259). If application of resistance is appropriate, proceed to test. Position leg in mid-position between internal and external rotation. Place hand with dynamometer on lateral surface of ankle just above malleolus. The other hand, which offers counterpressure, is contoured over the medial surface of the distal thigh just above the knee. Resistance is given in a medially directed force at the knee as a counterforce (Fig. 9.16).

Test: Patient holds the midrange of hip rotation against resistance.

Reference Scores

Reference scores with standard deviations described later are for a make test in sitting position[33]:

Mean for 20- to 59-year-old men = 217.0 (62.4)

Mean for 20- to 59-year-old women = 136.1 (44.0)

Mean for 60- to 80-year-old and older men = 169.7 (55.0)

Mean for 60- to 80-year-old and older women = 108.4 (33.8)

FIGURE 9.16

(All Hamstring muscles)

Position of Patient: Prone with legs straight and toes hanging over the edge of the table. A towel roll placed just above the knee may make this position more comfortable.

Instructions to Clinician: Stand next to limb to be tested. Ask patient to flex knee as far as possible (see Fig. 6.79 on page 276). If application of resistance is appropriate, proceed to test. Position knee in about 45° of knee flexion (midrange). Ask patient to hold the position. Place hand holding the dynamometer on posterior surface of leg just above ankle. Extra padding under the handheld dynamometer may be needed. The other hand provides stabilization over hamstring tendons on posterior thigh (optional). Firm pressure with this hand may offset any cramping of the hamstring muscles. Resistance is applied downward in direction of knee extension (Fig. 9.17).

Test: Patient holds knee in 45° of knee flexion.

Instructions to Patient: "Hold your leg. Don't let me straighten your knee. Hold … hold … hold."

Reference Scores

Reference scores not available.

FIGURE 9.17

KNEE EXTENSION

(Quadriceps femoris)

Patient Position: Short sitting. Place either a wedge or a hand under patient's distal thigh to cushion the thigh from the surface. Patient's hands rest on the table on either side of the body for stability or may grasp the table edge. Patient should be allowed to lean backward slightly to relieve hamstring muscle tension. Do not allow patient to hyperextend the knee.

Instructions to Clinician: Stand at the side of the limb to be tested. Ask patient to straighten knee. If application of resistance is appropriate, proceed to test. Position knee in approximately 45° of knee flexion (midrange and avoiding the ability of patient to "lock" the knee). Ask patient to hold position. Place hand holding dynamometer over anterior surface of distal leg just above ankle. Padding under the handheld dynamometer may be necessary for patient comfort. Resistance is applied in a downward direction toward the floor with both hands if necessary (Fig. 9.18).

Very often, the patient's strength can overpower the clinician's strength during this muscle action. To prevent patient's pelvis from rising (a common occurrence in a maximum-effort test), a belt or strap may be used to secure the patient to the testing surface.

Test: Patient holds knee in 45° (midrange) of knee flexion.

Instructions to Patient: "Hold your leg. Don't let me bend it. Hold … hold … hold."

Reference Scores

Reference scores with standard deviations below are for a make test in sitting position[37]:

Mean for 20- to 59-year-old men = 551.2 (86.1) (20 subjects surpassed 650 N)

Mean for 20- to 59-year-old women = 398.7 (94.48) (1 subject surpassed 650 N)

Mean for 60- to 79-year-old men = 386.9 (94.2)

Mean for 60- to 79-year-old women = 241.9 (81.6)

FIGURE 9.18

Position of Patient: Supine with the foot at the end of the table.[a]

Instructions to Clinician: Stand at the foot of the table with patient's heel resting on the table. Ask patient to bring foot up and in, toward the body. If application of resistance is appropriate, proceed to test. Position foot in maximum dorsiflexion. Ask patient to hold the position. Place hand holding dynamometer over dorsum of foot just proximal to toes. Stabilization of the body to keep it from sliding may be needed. Resistance is given by pulling down and out (Fig. 9.19). You may need to use both hands to appropriately resist this potentially strong muscle action.

Test: Patient holds position of full ankle dorsiflexion and inversion, keeping toes relaxed.

Instructions to Patient: "Bring your foot up and in. Hold it. Don't let me pull it down. Hold … hold … hold."

Reference Scores

Reference scores with standard deviations below are for a make test in long sitting[33]:
Mean for 20- to 59-year-old men = 224.6 (48.2)
Mean for 20- to 59-year-old women = 166.5 (41.6)
Mean for 60- to 80-year-old and older men = 173.3 (44.0)
Mean for 60- to 80-year-old and older women = 131.5 (38.9)
    Reference scores with standard deviations below are for a break test in supine[35]:
Mean for 20- to 59-year-old men = 279.3 (23.0)
Mean for 20- to 59-year-old women = 240.3 (26.0)
Mean for 60- to 69-year-old men = 266.0 (30.0)
Mean for 60- to 69-year-old women = 216.0 (31.0)

FIGURE 9.19

---

[a]We recommend the supine position, rather than an antigravity position, because of the mechanical advantage afforded the clinician in providing adequate resistance to this very strong muscle.

REFERENCES

1. Bohannon RW. Hand-held dynamometry: adoption 1900-2005. *Percept Mot Skills.* 2006;103:3–4.
2. Vanpee G, Hermans G, Segers J, Gosselink R. Assessment of limb muscle strength in critically ill patients: a systematic review. *Crit Care Med.* 2014;42(3):701–711. https://doi.org/10.1097/CCM.0000000000000030. PMID: 24201180.
3. Eriksrud O, Bohannon RW. Relationship of knee extension force to independence in sit-to-stand performance in patients receiving acute rehabilitation. *Phys Ther.* 2003;83:544–551.
4. Buckinx F, Croisier JL, Reginster JY, et al. Reliability of muscle strength measures obtained with a hand-held dynamometer in an elderly population. *Clin Physiol Funct Imaging.* 2017;37(3):332–340.
5. Bohannon RW. Hand-held dynamometer measurements obtained in a home environment are reliable but not correlated strongly with function. *Int J Rehabil Res.* 1996;19:345–347.
6. Visser J, Mans E, de Visser M, et al. Comparison of maximal voluntary isometric contraction and hand-held dynamometry in measuring muscle strength of patients with progressive lower motor neuron syndrome. *Neuromuscul Disord.* 2003;13:744–750.
7. van der Ploeg RJO, Dosterhuis H, Reuvekamp J. Measuring muscle strength. *J Neurol.* 1984;231:200–203.
8. Schrama PP, Stenneberg MS, Lucas C, et al. Intraexaminer reliability of hand-held dynamometry in the upper extremity: a systematic review. *Arch Phys Med Rehabil.* 2014;95(12):2444–2469.
9. Stark T, Walker B, Phillips JK, et al. Hand-held dynamometry correlation with the gold standard isokinetic dynamometry: a systematic review. *PMR.* 2011;3(5):472–479.
10. Stone CA, Nolan B, Lawlor PG, et al. Hand-held dynamometry: tester strength is paramount, even in frail populations. *J Rehabil Med.* 2011;43(9):808–811.
11. Wikholm JB, Bohannon RW. Hand-held dynamometer measurements: tester strength makes a difference. *J Orthop Sports Phys Ther.* 1991;13:191–198.
12. Wadsworth CT, Nielsen DH, Corcoran DS, et al. Interrater reliability of hand-held dynamometry: effects of rater gender, body weight, and grip strength. *J Orthop Sports Phys Ther.* 1992;16:74–81.
13. Chamorro C, Arancibia M, Trigo B, Arias-Poblete L, Jerez-Mayorga D. Absolute reliability and concurrent validity of hand-held dynamometry in shoulder rotator strength assessment: systematic review and meta-analysis. *Int J Environ Res Public Health.* 2021;18(17):9293. https://doi.org/10.3390/ijerph18179293. PMID: 34501883; PMCID: PMC8430567.
14. Chamorro C, Armijo-Olivo S, De la Fuente C, Fuentes J, Javier Chirosa L. Absolute reliability and concurrent validity of hand held dynamometry and isokinetic dynamometry in the hip, knee and ankle joint: systematic review and meta-analysis. *Open Med.* 2017;12:359–375. https://doi.org/10.1515/med-2017-0052. PMID: 29071305; PMCID: PMC5651404.
15. Tarca BD, Wycherley TP, Meade A, et al. Validity and reliability of hand-held dynamometry for abdominal flexion muscular assessment. *J Sport Rehabil.* 2020;30(2):343–346. https://journals.humankinetics.com/view/journals/jsr/30/2/article-p343.xml?content=pdf.
16. Arnold CM, Warkentin KD, Chilibeck PD, Magnus CR. The reliability and validity of handheld dynamometry for the measurement of lower-extremity muscle strength in older adults. *J Strength Cond Res.* 2010;24(3):815–824. https://doi.org/10.1519/JSC.0b013e3181aa36b8. PMID: 19661831.
17. Wang CY, Olson SL, Protas EJ. Test-retest strength reliability: hand-held dynamometry in community-dwelling elderly fallers. *Arch Phys Med Rehabil.* 2002;83(6):811–815. https://doi.org/10.1053/apmr.2002.32743. PMID: 12048660.
18. Grootswagers P, Vaes AMM, Hangelbroek R, Tieland M, van Loon LJC, de Groot LCPGM. Relative validity and reliability of isometric lower extremity strength assessment in older adults by using a handheld dynamometer. *Sports Health.* 2022;14(6):899–905. https://doi.org/10.1177/19417381211063847. Epub 2022 Feb 4. PMID: 35120409; PMCID: PMC9631031.
19. Holt KL, Raper DP, Boettcher CE, et al. Hand-held dynamometry strength measures for internal and external rotation demonstrate superior reliability, lower minimal detectable change and higher correlation to isokinetic dynamometry than externally-fixed dynamometry of the shoulder. *Phys Ther Sport.* 2016;21:75–81.
20. Keep H, Luu L, Berson A, Garland SJ. Validity of the handheld dynamometer compared with an isokinetic dynamometer in measuring peak hip extension strength. *Physiother Can.* 2016;68(1):15–22. https://doi.org/10.3138/ptc.2014-62. PMID: 27504043; PMCID: PMC4961312.
21. Suzuki M, Kirimoto H, Inamura A, et al. The relationship between knee extension strength and lower extremity functions in nursing home residents with dementia. *Disabil Rehabil.* 2012;34(3):202–209.
22. Bohannon RW. Rolling to the nonplegic side: influence of teaching and limb strength in hemiplegic stroke patients. 3:215–218.
23. Schurr K, Sherrington C, Wallbank G, et al. The minimum sit-to-stand height test: reliability, responsiveness and relationship to leg muscle strength. *Clin Rehabil.* 2012;26(7):656–663.
24. Bohannon RW, Smith J, Hull D, et al. Deficits in lower extremity muscle and gait performance among renal transplant candidates. *Arch Phys Med Rehabil.* 1995;76:547–551.
25. Moore AM, Krauss EM, Parikh RP, et al. Fermoral nerve transfers for restoring tibial nerve function:an anatomical study and clinical correlation: a report of 2 cases. *J Neurosurg.* 2017;129(4):1024–1033. https://thejns.org/view/journals/j-neurosurg/129/4/article-p1024.xml.
26. Alnahdi AH, Zeni JA, Snyder-Mackler L. Hip abductor strength reliability and association with physical function after unilateral total knee arthroplasty: a cross-sectional study. *Phys Ther.* 2014;94(8):1154–1162.
27. Andrews AW, Bohannon RW. Short-term recovery of limb muscle strength after acute stroke. *Arch Phys Med Rehabil.* 2003;84:125–130.
28. McGrath RP, Kraemer WJ, Vincent BM, et al. Muscle strength is protective against osteoporosis in an ethnically diverse sample of adults. *J Strength Cond Res.* 2017;31(9):2586–2589.
29. McGrath R, Vincent BM, Al Snih S, et al. The association between muscle weakness and incident diabetes in older Mexican Americans. *J Am Med Dir Assoc.* 2017;18(5):452.e7–452.e12.
30. Pua YH, Wrigley TV, Cowan SM, et al. Intrarater test-retest reliability of hip range of motion and hip muscle strength measurements in persons with hip osteoarthritis. *Arch Phys Med Rehabil.* 2008;89(6):1146–1154.

31. Oliveira CC, McGinley J, Lee AL, et al. Fear of falling in people with chronic obstructive pulmonary disease. *Respir Med*. 2015;109:483–489.

32. Cools AM, De Wilde L, Van Tongel A, et al. Measuring shoulder external and internal rotation strength and range of motion: comprehensive intra-rater and inter-rater reliability study of several testing protocols. *J Shoulder Elbow Surg*. 2014;23(10):1454–1461.

33. McKay MJ, Baldwin JN, Ferreira P, et al. Normative reference values for strength and flexibility of 1,000 children and adults. *Neurology*. 2017;88(1):36–43.

34. Andrews AW, Thomas MW, Bohannon RW. Normative values for isometric muscle force measurements obtained with hand-held dynamometers. *Phys Ther*. 1996;76:248–259.

35. Phillips BA, Lo SK, Mastaglia FL. Muscle force measured using "break" testing with a hand-held myometer in normal subjects aged 20 to 69 years. *Arch Phys Med Rehabil*. 2000;81:653–661.

36. Van Harlinger W, Blalock L, Merritt JL. Upper limb strength: study providing normative data for a clinical handheld dynamometer. *PMR*. 2015;7(2):135–140.

37. Bohannon RW. Reference values for extremity muscle strength obtained by hand-held dynamometry from adults aged 20 to 79 years. *Arch Phys Med Rehabil*. 1997;78(1):26–32.

38. van der Ploeg RJ, Oosterhuis HJ. The "make/break test" as a diagnostic tool in functional weakness. *J Neurol Neurosurg Psychiatry*. 1991;54(3):248–251.

39. Bohannon RW, Chu J, Portz M. Measurement of hip extension strength with a portable device: description, reliability and validity of a procedure. *Isokinet Exerc Sci*. 2015;23:271–274.

40. Morin M, Duchesne E, Bernier J, et al. What is known about muscle strength reference values for adults measured by hand-held dynamometery: a scoping review. *Arch Rehabil Res Clin Transl*. 2022;4:100172. www.ncbi.nlm.nih.gov/pmc/articles/PMC8904874/.

41. Widler KS, Glatthorn JF, Bizzini M, et al. Assessment of hip abductor muscle strength. A validity and reliability study. *J Bone Joint Surg Am*. 2009;91(11):2666–2672.

CHAPTER 10

Case Studies

Introduction

Case 1: Shoulder Pain

Case 2: Compromised Gait and Function Secondary to Muscle Weakness

Case 3: Fatigue Secondary to Muscle Weakness

Case 4: Muscle Weakness Following Nerve Injury

Case 5: Muscle Weakness Following Hip Surgery

Case 6: Muscle Weakness Following Childbirth

INTRODUCTION

This chapter serves as a brief summary of the muscle testing performance concepts presented throughout this book. Concepts are amplified using a series of case studies that illustrate the need for various forms of muscle testing. Each case features a real patient with a need for specific data to verify clinical findings and understand functional deficits. An overview of the problem-solving approach used by the clinician is presented for each to aid in the development of the student clinician's clinical decision-making skills.

The variety of tests available to clinicians is illustrated in these case studies. The diagnoses presented are common, and each case is intended to highlight the rationale for specific muscle test selection.

 Case 1: Shoulder Pain

The patient was a 56-year-old male investment banker who developed right shoulder pain after a weekend of working with his arms extended over his head while painting the ceilings in his home. Initial observation reveals forward shoulders and abducted scapulae.

Questions to Consider:

1. What other information might you want to have to develop a preliminary clinical impression?
2. What muscles do you want to test?
3. What information will muscle testing give you to aid in developing your clinical impression?

Summary

Because of his forward shoulder posture, weakness of scapular stabilizers was suspected. Testing of scapular upward rotators revealed Grade 3 strength. Muscle testing of glenohumeral muscles revealed Grade 3 of right external rotators (teres minor and infraspinatus) and Grade 4 strength of shoulder abductor (middle deltoid), with pain that limited full effort. Shoulder internal rotation, flexion, and extension strength were all Grade 5 and nonpainful and considered noncontributing. Given his response of pain to shoulder abduction and weakness of scapular upward rotators, faulty scapular-thoracic and glenohumeral mechanics were suspected as contributing to pain at the shoulder.

Attention to scapular function was part of the evaluation because glenohumeral joint movement is only possible if the scapula also moves simultaneously. Focusing on the glenohumeral joint would not resolve this patient's problem because of weakness of scapulohumeral muscles, specifically the serratus anterior and lower trapezius. Strengthening of scapular stabilizers repositions the scapula. When the scapula is repositioned through strength and muscle reeducation, the humerus will be reseated properly in the glenoid fossa, thus opening the subacromial space and allowing more freedom for the supraspinatus to slide beneath the acromion process. This is likely to improve joint mechanics, relieve pain, and possibly prevent a recurrence.

This case example reflects a typical patient who is referred to an outpatient clinic. The original symptom was pain, but the patient's discomfort was the consequence of mechanical dysfunction related to muscle weakness. Knowledge of anatomy, kinesiology, and manual muscle testing enabled the clinician to isolate the root causes of the patient's painful condition.

Case 2: Compromised Gait and Function Secondary to Muscle Weakness

The patient is a 68-year-old retired man. Two weeks ago, he went to the movies with his wife and, after 2 hours of sitting, found he could not get up from the chair without a great amount of effort. This embarrassing incident prompted him to seek help, and he referred himself to an older-adult wellness clinic.

Evaluation revealed a pleasant-appearing gentleman with flexed hips (~20°) and knees (~15°) when standing upright. With clinician cueing, his lower extremity positioning could be corrected to a more erect posture, but only momentarily. He is of average height (68 inches) but is overweight, stating that he weighs approximately 240 lb. (body mass index = 36, which is obese).

Questions to Consider:

1. What other information might you want to know?
2. What do you want to examine and why?
3. What are effects of a sedentary lifestyle on mobility (e.g., walking, rising from the floor, stair climbing, rising from a chair)?
4. What functional tests might be valuable?
5. What muscle tests might be valuable and why?

Summary

Observation revealed clear difficulty rising from the standard 17-inch chair in the waiting room, as evidenced by using his arms and rocking back and forth several times before he could stand up with notable effort. A physical activity history showed low activity, sitting being the predominant activity, and difficulty walking three blocks. Clinical impression was sarcopenia secondary to physical inactivity and age. Functional testing was conducted first to focus on the muscle strength exam. Gait evaluation revealed the following: slow usual gait speed (2 mph or 0.9 m/s), forward trunk lean during the entire gait cycle, pelvic drop bilaterally during the stance phase (exhibited by a "waddling" gait), failure to flex the knee at loading, and an absence of heel rise at the end of the stance phase as exhibited by a flat foot and shortened stride. These observations suggested possible weakness of the following muscle groups: core, hip extensors, hip abductors, knee extensors, and plantar flexors. Thus, additional muscle testing was done.

Because this man was large, it became immediately apparent to the clinician that manual muscle testing was not feasible given the clinician's size in relation to the patient's size. Therefore, alternative testing using the leg press and the one-repetition maximum (1-RM) method was chosen. The patient was also tested using the standard 25× heel rise test for plantar flexors (described on page 286).

Total Lower Extremity Strength Testing

Leg press provides a composite value for total lower extremity extension (ankle plantar flexion, knee extension, and hip extension). Leg press is ideal because reference scores are available for men and women of all ages (see Table 7.4, page 318). Initial resistance was based on the reference scores for a 68-year-old man that were 1.4 times his body weight.

However, because of this patient's difficulty in rising from a chair, a functional task that requires a minimum of 50% of the body's weight (120 pounds), RM testing was started at 120 pounds (50% of body weight). However, he could not move the weight stack, aiding the clinician as to why the patient had difficulty rising from a chair unassisted. Further adjustments downward over two trials achieved a 3-RM at 90 pounds (~40% body weight).

Hip Extension

Prone hip extension test was performed bilaterally, and the patient was able to lift one thigh from the table but not complete full range. He was unable to lift the other leg from the table (Grade 2 bilaterally). To establish the appropriate amount of resistance for effective strengthening, RM testing was chosen next. Cuff weights were attached to his ankle (one side at a time) to provide resistance. In a standing position, the patient was able to extend his hip with 7 lb. for six repetitions on the right side, at which point he could not perform a seventh repetition, and 5 lb. for six repetitions on the left (unable to lift a seventh repetition) while using arm support for balance and stability.

Knee Extension

An RM using the leg extension machine (open-chain approach) was used to isolate the knee extensors. The patient was seated on the leg extension machine, and initially, 50 lbs. was selected from the weight stack to test one leg at a time. Fifty pounds was chosen because it is slightly less than half of the bilateral leg press 1-RM. The patient was not able to complete the full range, so weight was decreased by 10 pounds. He was then able to complete full range with utmost effort (7/10 on modified Borg Scale of Perceived Exertion). To confirm the RM, the patient was asked to perform as many repetitions as possible. He was unable to do another repetition with full range; therefore, his 1-RM for the first leg was 40 pounds. The test was then repeated on the other side and achieved a 4-RM at 30 pounds. (Note: Open-chain movements generally produce less force than what is achieved on the leg press because of isolation of the knee extensors.)

Hip Abduction

Manual muscle testing in a side-lying position revealed an inability to lift either leg against gravity (Grade 2) that was confirmed with the ability to abduct each leg in supine through full range. To provide an RM to inform the exercise prescription, an elastic loop of medium resistance was placed around both ankles. The patient stood holding onto the back of a chair for balance and stability. He was asked to abduct his right leg strongly toward a position of 5 o'clock as if he was in the center of the clock. The goal was midrange (Fig. 10.1). The patient was able to achieve the target position six times before starting to lean on his arms, indicating muscle fatigue and a 6-RM. The same procedure was repeated for the left leg with similar results. Because the gluteus medius must stabilize

Continued

Case 2: Compromised Gait and Function Secondary to Muscle Weakness—cont'd

FIGURE 10.1

the upper half of the body, a tremendous amount of strength is required, which the patient did not have, indicating why he has difficulty with the sit-to-stand task. An optimal starting point for exercise would be using the same resistance band with a goal of progressing to 10 to 12 repetitions before proceeding to the next level of resistance.

Plantar Flexion

The patient's plantar flexors were tested using a standing plantar flexion test because of its ease and functionality. Given a lack of heel rise during gait, it was expected the patient would be in the lower part of the range of normal. Testing of each leg revealed an ability to accomplish five repetitions on the right and four on the left, which corresponds to a Grade 4. The traditional plantar flexion test (see page 286) requires 25 repetitions of at least 2-inch clearance.[1] Norms for a male of 60+ years require completing from 4 to 27 heel raises of at least 2-inch clearance.[2]

Core Testing

Core testing was conducted using a modified plank test, as the patient was unable to assume a full plank secondary to inflexible feet. Core testing was conducted because of the patient's flexed posture and fatigue when walking three blocks. The RM was 4 seconds. A "normal" plank is 60 seconds in a full plank (legs extended and weight on toes). His result is consistent with individuals who exhibit a forward-leaning posture such as when using a walker, indicating back extensor fatigue and weakness.

In summary, this patient's knee extension strength was Grade 4 with a 4-RM of 30 pounds and 40 pounds, hip extensors were Grade 2 with 6 and 5 pounds at 6-RM, hip abductors were Grade 2 with RM of 6 reps with moderate resistance, and plantar flexors were Grade 4 with a 4- and 5-RM. Modified plank for core strength equaled 4 seconds. These grades indicate muscle weakness of a magnitude that compromises physical activity, alters normal gait pattern, and explains his inability to rise from a chair without using the arms. The specific tests provided objective numbers that could be used in context with body weight demands of daily activities and help establish the appropriate amount of resistance for an effective exercise program. It should be noted that this individual walked into the clinic unassisted and yet demonstrated profound muscle weakness when isolated testing was performed. This scenario is quite common.

Case 3: Fatigue Secondary to Muscle Weakness

The patient was a health care professions student participating in the muscle testing laboratory. During testing, it was noticed that he could not walk on his toes symmetrically, and on questioning, he admitted that he had calf muscle fatigue after walking across campus, which seemed to affect his ability to walk quickly. On further questioning, he reported a history of multiple left ankle sprains, the most recent being 6 months earlier while playing volleyball. Initially, he treated the sprain with ice and compression and had limited his weight bearing until the swelling decreased. He never sought the consultation of a clinician after any of his sprains. It took several months for the ankle stiffness to resolve, and he reported there was some swelling after activities such as walking across campus. He was playing volleyball once again but did not feel he had regained his ability to jump, cut side to side, or go for a ball with confidence.

Questions to Consider:

1. What other information might you want to have to develop a preliminary clinical impression?
2. What muscles do you want to test?
3. What information will muscle testing give you to aid in developing your clinical impression?

There was no ankle pain at examination, but there was limited range of motion at end range of dorsiflexion, eversion, and inversion. Strength was evaluated using manual muscle testing. Manual muscle testing was chosen for the following reasons: the clinician can compare strength values side to side, forces produced by the evertors and invertors are small enough to resist manually, and body weight resistance is used to challenge plantar flexors.

Standing plantar flexion test revealed his ability to rise 25 times on the unaffected ankle, clearing at least 2 inches with each repetition (Grade 5). On the sprained side, he completed three repetitions with difficulty before muscle fatigue occurred, as evidenced by the inability to lift his heel the required 2 inches (Grade 4).

Inversion and eversion were then tested using manual resistance.

The unaffected side was tested first and was evaluated as Grade 5 in both movements secondary to a negative break test against maximum resistance. Strength on the affected side was Grade 5 for inversion but Grade 3 for eversion. It took minimal resistance before the fibularis longus and brevis (i.e., peroneal muscles) failed to hold against resistance. There was no pain with muscle resistance.

This case reflects a common finding: residual muscle strength deficits following what appears to be a simple injury. His involved plantar flexors were Grade 4, and his evertors were Grade 3. Given his commonplace injury, he expected a complete return of strength and range and did not seek the services of a clinician. He could have gone through life unable to fully participate in sports at his level of inherent skill and strength. It was the serendipity of being a student in a clinical program that resulted in evaluation and subsequent treatment. How many other men and women are "getting by" with diminished strength following a simple injury?

Case 4: Muscle Weakness Following Nerve Injury

The patient is a 34-year-old male who was referred to the clinic because of weakness in his forearm, wrist, and hand. History taking revealed the patient was caught in an earthquake 7 months prior and suffered a crush injury of the arm when a portion of a wall collapsed on it. He had open reduction and internal fixation surgery to repair the crush damage to the radius and ulna, and his arm and forearm were in a cast for 3 months (due to a lack of orthopedic follow-up). After cast removal, he was placed in a wrist immobilizer that permitted some movement at the elbow, wrist, and fingers. The patient wore the wrist immobilizer for approximately 4 more months again because of the inconsistency of medical personnel providing follow-up care. He had his first therapy visit 2 months after removal of the wrist immobilizer (7 months postinjury). At that time, his fractures were healed, and he was cleared for all resistance activities for the upper extremity, including wrist and hand.

The patient complained of an inability to hold onto objects, including a water glass. A wrist drop deformity was noted with the patient's wrist in flexion. The patient's fingers were swollen and stiff, but movement was observable toward finger closure and spreading the fingers a small distance (abduction). Thumb movement was minimal in all directions. Gross sensory testing revealed diminished sensation along the forearm over the muscle bellies of the wrist extensors and over the dorsum of the thumb. Sensation was also diminished on the thumb pad and over the skin of the thumb web.

The initial findings were severe muscle weakness following almost 1 year of reduced mobility; generalized hand/finger stiffness; reduced range of motion throughout the forearm, wrist, and hand; and diminished sensation at multiple sites. The clinician suspected a radial nerve injury and chose to do a manual muscle test to rule out or confirm nerve injury.

Establishing a strength and muscle involvement baseline was needed in this case. Muscle tests performed:

Elbow flexion and extension: To confirm that nerve damage is below the elbow.

Elbow flexion: Grade 5

Elbow extension: Grade 5

Radial nerve: Wrist extension (extensor carpi radialis longus and brevis, extensor carpi ulnaris), metatarsophalangeal (MP) extension (extensor digitorum communis), thumb MP and interphalangeal (IP) extension (extensor pollicis brevis and longus), thumb abduction (abductor pollicis longus), and index small finger extension (extensor indicis and extensor digiti minimi).

Results

Wrist extension: Grade 2

Finger extension: Grade 2

Thumb MP: Grade 2

Thumb IP extension: Grade 2

Index finger extension: Grade 1

Small finger extension: Grade 1

Median nerve: pronation (pronator teres and quadratus), wrist flexion (flexor carpi radialis), MP flexion and IP extension of index/middle fingers (lateral two lumbrical muscles), proximal interphalangeal (PIP) flexion (flexor digitorum superficialis), distal interphalangeal (DIP) flexion of index and middle fingers (flexor digitorum profundus), thumb MP and IP flexion (flexor pollicis brevis and longus), thumb abduction (abductor brevis), and thumb opposition (opponens pollicis)

Results

Wrist flexion: Grade 3

PIP flexion: Grade 2

DIP flexion of index and middle fingers: Grade 2

MP flexion: Grade 2

Thumb opposition: Grade 2

Thumb PIP flexion: Grade 2

Thumb abduction: Grade 2

Thumb IP flexion: Grade 2

Ulnar nerve: wrist flexion (flexor carpi ulnaris), finger abduction (dorsal interossei) and adduction (palmar interossei), thumb adduction (adductor pollicis), MP flexion and IP extension (interossei and medial 2 lumbrical muscles), small finger flexion (flexor digiti minimi), small finger abduction (abductor digiti minimi), and opposition of small finger (opponens digiti minimi)

Results

Finger abduction and adduction: Grade 3

Thumb adduction: Grade 3

Grip strength was measured with a handheld dynamometer and revealed 40 lb. on uninvolved extremity and 4 lb. on involved extremity, barely enough to hold a glass of water.

Based upon patient's symptoms and objective muscle and sensory testing, the clinician confirmed suspicions of a radial nerve injury below the elbow. In addition, weakness and muscle atrophy along the median and ulnar nerve distribution were noted likely from prolonged immobilization, lack of availability of care, and decreased use of the extremity. With therapy and a solid home exercise program, the patient began to report signs of recovery. The therapist expected improvement in strength along the median and ulnar-supplied musculature within 3 months of beginning therapy and was hopeful for recovery from radial nerve injury with functional use of the hand within 1 to 2 years postinjury.

Manual muscle testing was ideal in this instance because there were small muscles involved where the therapist could apply appropriate resistance and easily position the limbs and segments. In addition, specific knowledge was needed to define muscle loss. Grip strength testing could not have provided the important insights gained through individualized muscle testing necessary to diagnose the nerve injury.

Case 5: Muscle Weakness Following Hip Surgery

The patient is a 78-year-old woman weighing 170 lb. (BMI = 26.6) who broke her right hip after a fall from her bicycle. She had an open reduction internal fixation of the hip 7 months ago and had physical and occupational therapy for 5 weeks immediately following the surgery in a long-term care setting.

A posterior approach that bisects the gluteus maximus and medius was performed for the fracture repair, affecting strength. Following surgery, she was non–weight bearing for nearly 3 months and used a walker to ambulate. At month 4, she was permitted toe-touch ambulation and, over the next few months, progressed to walking with a single-point cane. Currently, the patient is reluctant to return to road cycling for fear of falling, so she elected to regain her fitness level by training on a stationary cycle. Immediately after beginning her stationary cycling, she found her right leg (affected side) would not perform as well as her left. Gait observation indicated a shorter stride length on the right and a gluteus medius limp (positive Trendelenburg sign) that was masked by the cane. As soon as the patient placed the cane on her arm and attempted to walk unaided, her gluteus medius limp became evident, and the short stride on the right became even shorter. Her complaint was "lack of push power" on the right and that her leg "wore out" in seconds rather than minutes. Her goal was to cycle vigorously for 30 minutes daily and take a brisk walk every other day.

Questions to Consider:

1. What does a gluteus medius limp indicate? How would you confirm your suspicion?
2. What muscles are most important to walking? The least?[3]
3. What muscles would you test in order of importance? Describe your technique for each group.

Summary

Given the age and sex of the patient and the likely muscles involved, a manual muscle test was selected for use. In addition, a single-limb leg press was used bilaterally to provide side-to-side comparisons. Two functional tests were utilized, the 30-second chair rise test and the timed stair climb for

one flight and the total number of consecutive flights. Manual muscle testing for the gluteus medius was performed side lying. The patient was unable to lift her involved side against gravity (Grade 2). Her uninvolved side was Grade 4. Manual muscle testing of the hip adductors, extensors, and internal and external rotators was performed, beginning with active range against resistance and then applying resistance, if successful, or changing the position to a Grade 2 if unsuccessful. Also tested were muscles above and below the affected site, knee flexors and extensors, and core (abdominals, back extensors) because it is rare that weakness is present at one segment only. A standing heel rise test was performed bilaterally. The modified plank position was used for core muscles, as the patient could not attain a full plank or perform a lateral plank.

Results

Core: Grade 3 via the plank test
Hip extensors: Grade 4 left, Grade 2 right
Hip abductors: Grade 4 left, Grade 2 right
Hip adductors: Grade 4 left, Grade 3 right
Internal rotation: Grade 4 left, Grade 4 right
External rotation: Grade 4 left, Grade 3 right
Knee flexion: Grade 4 left, Grade 4 right
Plantar flexion: 4 on the left; 0 on the right.
Unilateral leg press: 140 pounds left, 45 pounds right
Chair rises: Without using chair arms, the patient was able to do one chair rise, and this one repetition required multiple attempts.
Stair climb: The patient ascended one flight of nine stairs up and down in 39 seconds.

This case illustrates the fairly classic scenario of the effects of prolonged immobilization and being discharged long before rehabilitation is complete. Fortunately, the patient had a long exercise history, with her current state of weakness and reduced function unacceptable to her. Thus, she was a prime candidate for a home program of strengthening and endurance work and a continuing community exercise program.

Case 6: Muscle Weakness Following Childbirth

The patient gave birth to her second child 2 years ago. Post-partum exercises were never initiated, and she had no history of engaging in any routine physical activity other than childcare. Now she is having difficulty with urine leakage when laughing, coughing, and lifting her toddler. The stress incontinence prompted her to seek help.

Muscles of the pelvic floor and abdomen elongate enormously to accommodate pregnancy and childbirth. In many women, the stretched musculature fails to return to its pre-partum strength and length. This pelvic floor/abdominal weakness scenario is especially likely in women who have had multiple births, particularly if they did not perform postpartum exercises.

For this woman, manual muscle testing of the abdominals and pelvic floor was chosen because these muscles are often found to be weak following childbirth. Muscle testing revealed the following.
Abdominal curl: seven repetitions with difficulty
Prone plank: 3 seconds
Pelvic floor (manual test): Grade 3

In summary, childbirth weakened the pelvic floor and abdominal musculature. Even though this weakness is present in nearly all women after delivery, too few are counseled to perform pelvic floor exercises or strengthen abdominals. If the condition persists, urinary incontinence is likely. Standard muscle testing techniques were used to identify weakness.

REFERENCES

1. Lunsford BR, Perry J. The standing heel-rise test for ankle plantar flexion: criterion for normal. *Phys Ther*. 1995;75:694–698.
2. Jan MH, Chai HM, Lin YF, et al. Effects of age and sex on the results of an ankle plantar-flexor manual muscle test. *Phys Ther*. 2005;85:1078–1084.
3. van der Krogt MM, Delp SL, Schwartz MH. How robust is human gait to muscle weakness?. *Gait Posture*. 2012 May;36(1):113–119. https://doi.org/10.1016/j.gaitpost.2012.01.017. PubMed PMID: 22386624. Epub 2012 Mar 3. PMID: . PMCID: PMC4890623.

Page numbers followed by "*f*" indicate figures, "*t*" indicate tables, and "*b*" indicate boxes.

A

Abdominals, strength exercises for, 69*b*
Abductor digiti minimi
  finger abduction and, 205
  finger MCP extension and, 200*t*–201*t*
Abductor pollicis brevis
  metacarpals, stabilization of, 220, 220*f*
  opposition (thumb to little finger) and, 225*t*
  palpation of, 220, 220*f*
  substitution in, 220*b*
  thumb abduction and, 218–220, 218*t*
Abductor pollicis longus
  substitution in, 219*b*
  tendon, palpation of, 219, 219*f*
  thumb abduction and, 218–220, 218*t*, 219*b*
Acromioclavicular joint, 98, 98*f*
Active resistance test, 3
Activities of daily living (ADLs), 18, 338
Acute care facilities, manual muscle testing (usage), 17
Acute rehabilitation facilities, manual muscle testing (usage), 17
Adductor magnus, 268–272, 268*f*
Adductor pollicis
  palpation of, 223, 223*f*
  thumb adduction and, 221–223, 221*t*
Adjoining fingers, middle phalanx (grasping) of, 206, 206*f*
ADLs. *See* Activities of daily living
Alternate rhomboid test, 118
American College of Sports Medicine (ACSM), 315
  for partial curl up, 74, 74*t*
Ankle plantar flexion, 283–289, 283*f*, 283*b*, 284*t*
Anterior deltoid, shoulder flexion and, 125
Anterior superior iliac spine, 242
Arms
  abduction of
    cross section of, 172*f*
    elbow extension (accomplishment) in, 166*b*
    external rotation and, 171*b*
  adduction of, 117, 117*f*
  hand resistance in, 101, 101*f*
  maintenance, 103, 103*f*
  support of, 113, 113*f*
    in flexion/abduction range, 144, 144*f*
    in shoulder abduction, 150, 150*f*
    in shoulder position, 117, 117*f*, 160
  weight, support of, 110, 110*f*
ASIS. *See* Anterior superior iliac spine
Available range of motion, 6
Axilla (inferior margin), teres minor (palpation) on, 149, 149*f*

B

Belly press test, 156*b*
Biceps
  antecubital space, tendon (palpation) in, 160, 160*f*
  elbow flexion and, 157
  shoulder abduction and, 134*t*
  shoulder flexion and, 126*t*
  suggested exercise for, 161*b*

Biceps brachii
  elbow flexion and, 158*t*
  forearm supination and, 158, 158*f*, 168–172, 169*t*
  substitution in, 137*b*
Biceps femoris, 276
Body-weight testing
  pull-ups (chin-ups) test, 333, 333*t*
  push-ups test, 334, 334*t*–335*t*
Book, lifting, 348, 348*f*
  in modified physical performance test, 346
Brachialis
  elbow flexion and, 157, 158*t*
    forearm, in pronation, 159, 159*f*
  suggested exercise for, 161*b*
Brachioradialis
  elbow flexion and, 157, 158*t*
  forearm and
    lateral surface, palpation of, 160, 160*f*
    in mid position, 159, 159*f*
  suggested exercise for, 161*b*
Break test, 2
  alternatives of, 2
Bulbocavernosus, in pelvic floor, 90*t*

C

Capital extension
  grade 2, grade 1, and grade 0, 35
  grade 3, 34–35, 34*f*
  grade 5 and grade 4, 34–35, 42*f*
  muscles in, 33*t*
  posterior, 27*f*
  range of motion, 27*b*
Capital extensors
  palpation of, 30
  weakness, 27*f*
Capital flexion (chin tuck), 26
  anterior view of, 36*f*
  clinical relevance, 39*b*
  deep muscles of, palpation of, 39*b*
  forward head posture in, 39*b*
  grade 2, grade 1, and grade 0, 39, 39*f*
  grade 3, 38
  grade 5 and grade 4, 38, 38*f*
  muscles in, 36*t*
  patient, starting position of, 37–39, 37*f*
  range of motion, 36*b*
Carpometacarpal (CMC) joint, angle of, 212
Case studies, 393–400
  in knee extension, 395*b*–396*b*
  in muscle weakness
    compromised gait and function secondary to, 395*b*–396*b*
    fatigue secondary to, 397*b*
    following childbirth, 399*b*
    following hip surgery, 399*b*
    following nerve injury, 398*b*
    in plantar flexion, 395*b*–396*b*
    in shoulder pain, 394*b*
Ceiling effect, manual muscle testing, 21
Cervical flexion
  anterior, 40*f*
  grade 2, grade 1, and grade 0, 43, 43*f*
  grade 3, 42, 42*f*
  grade 5 and grade 4, 42–43, 42*f*
  muscles of, 41*t*
  range of motion, 40*b*
  substitution, 43*b*

Cervical rotation
  grade 2, grade 1, and grade 0, 45–46
  grade 5, grade 4, and grade 3, 45–46
  muscles in, 45*b*
Chair stand, 340–341, 342*b*
  arms extended in, 342*b*
  feet position in, 340, 340*f*
  five-repetition, 354, 354*f*, 354*b*
  in moderately disabled women, 343
  modified physical performance test and, 358*t*
  normal range of, 341*t*
  quality of movement in, 340, 340*f*
  sit-to-stand move in, 342*b*
  testing of gluteus medius in, 342*b*
  30-second version, 341
  timed five-repetition version, 340
  trunk, excessive bending forward of, weak quadriceps and, 342*b*
Chest, cross sections of arm muscles in, 123*f*
Childbirth, muscle weakness following, case study in, 399*b*
Chin tuck. *See* Capital flexion
Clavicle (medial half), pectoralis major (palpation) on, 144, 144*f*
Clavicular head
  cervical flexion, 41*t*
  grades 5/4, shoulder horizontal adduction and
    patient instructions in, 143
    patient position in, 142–144
    test of, 143
    therapist instruction in, 143, 143*f*
Clavicular part
  shoulder horizontal adduction and, 142*t*
  shoulder internal rotation and, 152*t*
Closed chain, 316*b*
Cocontraction, 70
Coin, picking up of, 349, 349*f*, 349*b*
  in modified physical performance test, 346
Community mobility requirements, manual muscle testing, 18*b*
Compromised gait, secondary to muscle weakness, case study in, 395*b*–396*b*
Contractile activity, detection ability of, 15
Contracture, impact, 6
Coracobrachialis, shoulder flexion and, 125, 126*t*
Core muscles, 70, 70*f*–72*f*
  tests for, 70–76, 71*t*
    alternate form of prone plank testing, 73, 73*b*
    front abdominal power test, 75, 75*f*
    isometric trunk flexor endurance test, 75, 75*f*
    prone plank test (prone bridge test), 72, 72*f*, 72*t*
    side bridge endurance test, 73, 73*f*, 73*b*
    timed partial curl up test, 74, 74*f*
    unilateral supine bridge test, 76, 76*f*
Core strength, 70–76
Core strengthening, strength exercises for, 76*b*
Core testing, 70–76, 395*b*–396*b*
Cuff muscles, shoulder abduction and, 134*t*
Cyriax method of testing contractile lesions, 334–335

D

Deep back muscles, in trunk rotation, 65t
Deep cervical flexors, 37. *See also* Capital flexion (chin tuck)
Delirium, presence of, 15
Deltoid
   palpation of, 136, 136f
   superior/anterior surfaces, palpation of, 128, 128f
   supraspinatus, work (combination) and, 137b
   testing, 124
Deltoid (anterior)
   shoulder flexion and, 126t
   shoulder horizontal adduction and, 142t
   suggested exercise for, 128b
Deltoid (middle)
   shoulder abduction and, 134t
   shoulder horizontal adduction and, 138t
   suggested exercise for, 132b, 137b
Deltoid (posterior)
   shoulder extension and, 130t
   shoulder external rotation and, 147t
   shoulder horizontal abduction and, 138t
   suggested exercise for, 132b
Diagnostic validity, manual muscle testing, 21
Diaphragm, 77f, 79
   maximal expiratory pressure, 79–80
   maximum inspiratory pressure, 79–80
   in quiet inspiration, 77f, 79, 81
Digastric muscle, in capital flexion, 36t
Direct force measurements, 5
Distal interphalangeal (DIP) finger flexion, muscles and, 190t
Distal interphalangeal (DIP) tests, 194
   for flexor digitorum profundus, 194
   grade 2, grade 1, and grade 0 of, 194
   grade 5, grade 4, and grade 3 of, 194, 194f
   substitutions in, 194b
Distal phalanx, of thumb, 216, 216f
Dorsal interossei
   finger abduction and, 204
   finger MCP extension and, 198t, 200t–201t
   palpation of, 205, 205f
Duchenne muscular dystrophy, intrarater reliability of, 20

E

Eating task, physical performance test and, 346
Elastic band testing, 324, 324t, 326b
Elbow extension, 162–165, 166b, 380, 380f
   cross section level of, 162f
   grade 2, grade 1, and grade 0 of, 165
   grade 5, grade 4, and grade 3 of, 164–165, 164f
   illustration of, 162f
   limb, parallel position of, 165, 165f
   muscles and, 163t
   posterior view of, 162f
   prone position test for, 166b
   range of motion of, 163b
   substitutions in, 166b
      via external rotation, 166b
      via horizontal adduction, 166b
   triceps brachii and, 162
   triceps tendon, tension in, 165, 165f
Elbow flexion, 115–116, 115f, 157–161, 161b, 379, 379f
   anterior view of, 157f
   biceps and, 157
   brachialis and, 157
   brachioradialis and, 157
   cross section level of, 157f

Elbow flexion *(Continued)*
   forearm supination in, 158, 158f
   grade 1 and grade 0 of, 161
   grade 2 of, 160
   grade 5, grade 4, and grade 3 of, 158–161
   illustrations of, 157f
   manual resistance, absence of, 139f
   muscle and, 158f
   range of motion of, 158b
   scapular adduction in, 109–110, 109f
   sitting position, alternate, 160, 160f
Elbows
   counterforce at, 155, 155f
   cupping of, 159, 159f
   distal humerus, resistance of, 112–113, 112f
   extension of, 101, 101f
   flexors, position of, 160
   hand resistance in, 135, 135f
      posterior arm contour in, 139, 139f
   outside, stabilization of, 153, 153f
   resistance of, 115–116, 115f
      downward, 143, 143f
      outward, 143, 143f
   stabilization, hand resistance of, 148, 148f
   straightness of, 131, 131f
   support of, 102, 102f
Endurance, 70–76, 89
Equipment-based strength testing
   elastic band testing, 324, 324t, 326b
   free weights testing, 321–322, 322f
   interpretation of, 317
   isokinetic testing, 323
   latissimus dorsi pull-down test, 320, 320f
   leg press test, 318–319, 318f
   sitting unilateral knee extension test, 317–326, 317f
Erector spinae, in core, 71t
Exercises, of muscle test, 10
Extensor carpi radialis brevis, wrist extension and, 182, 183t, 186
Extensor carpi radialis longus
   elbow flexion and, 158t
   wrist extension and, 182, 183t, 186
Extensor carpi ulnaris, wrist extension and, 182, 183t, 186
Extensor digiti minimi
   finger MCP extension and, 195–197, 196t, 200t–201t
   test of, 197
   wrist extension and, 183t
Extensor digitorum
   finger MCP extension and, 195–197, 196t, 200t–201t
   test of, 197
   wrist extension and, 183t
Extensor indicis
   finger MCP extension and, 195–197, 196t
   test of, 197
   wrist extension and, 183t
Extensor pollicis brevis
   first metacarpal base, abductor pollicis longus tendon (palpation) of, 219, 219f
   thumb abduction and, 218t
   thumb MCP and IP extension and, 214–217, 215t
Extensor pollicis longus
   tendon, palpation of, 217, 217f
   thumb MCP and IP extension and, 214–217, 215t

F

Fast, 89
Fatigue, secondary to muscle weakness, case study in, 397b
FHP. *See* Forward head posture
Fibularis longus and brevis, 296–299
   isolation of, 299

Fifth metacarpal (radial side), opponens digiti minimi (palpation) on, 227, 227f
Finger abduction, 204–205
   dorsal interossei and, 204
      dorsal view of, 204f
      grade 2, grade 1, and grade 0 of, 205
      grade 5 and grade 4 of, 204–205, 204f
      illustration of, 204f
      range of motion of, 204b
   palmar interossei and, 206, 207b
      adjoining fingers, middle phalanx (grasping) of, 206, 206f
      grade 2, grade 1, and grade 0 of, 207
      grade 5 and grade 4 of, 206–207
      illustration of, 206f
      palmar view of, 206f
      range of motion of, 206b
      resistance of, 206, 206f
      substitution in, 207b
   thumb muscles and, 208
Finger MCP extension, 195–197
   extensor digitorum, extensor indicis, and extensor digiti minimi, 195–197, 197b
      cross section level of, 195f
      dorsal views of, 195f
      illustration of, 195f
      long finger, dorsal interossei (test) of, 205, 205f
      muscles and, 196t
      range of motion of, 196b
      grade 2, grade 1, and grade 0 of, 197
      grade 5, grade 4, and grade 3 of, 197
   interossei and lumbricals, 198, 203b
      grade 2, grade 1, and grade 0 of, 203
      grade 5, grade 4, and grade 3 of, 202, 202f
      illustration of, 199f
      muscles and, 200t–201t
      palmar view of, 199f
      range of motion of, 199b
      substitution of, 203b
   IP joints, in flexion, 197, 197f
   substitution in, 197b
Finger PIP and DIP flexion, 189–191
   cross section level of, 189f
   flexor digitorum profundus and, 189–191, 190t
   flexor digitorum superficialis and, 189–191, 190t
   grade 5, grade 4, and grade 3 of, 191, 191f
   illustration of, 189f
   palmar view of, 189f
First metacarpal, opponens pollicis (palpation) of, 227, 227f
Five-repetition chair stand, 354, 354f, 354b
Flexor carpi radialis
   elbow flexion and, 158t
   forearm pronation and, 174t
   tendons, palpation of, 181, 181f
   test of
      grade 3 of, 180, 180f
      grade 5 and 4 of, 179, 179f
      wrist flexion and, 177–181, 179f
Flexor carpi ulnaris
   elbow flexion and, 158t
   tendons, palpation of, 181, 181f
   test of
      grade 3 of, 180, 180f
      grade 5 and 4 of, 179, 179f
      wrist flexion and, 177–181, 179f
Flexor digiti minimi brevis, finger MCP extension and, 200t–201t
Flexor digitorum profundus
   DIP tests for, 194
   finger MCP extension and, 200t–201t
   finger PIP and DIP flexion and, 189–191, 190t
   wrist flexion and, 179f

Flexor digitorum superficialis
finger MCP extension and, 200*t*–201*t*
finger PIP and DIP flexion and, 189–191, 190*t*
muscle and, 190*t*
palpation of, 193, 193*f*
range of motion of, 190*b*
wrist flexion and, 179*f*
Flexor pollicis brevis
opposition (thumb to little finger) and, 225*t*
thumb MP/IP flexion and, 210, 211*t*
Flexor pollicis longus
tendon location/palpation of, 212, 212*f*
thumb MP/IP flexion and, 210, 211*t*
wrist flexion and, 179*f*
Floor rise, 361, 362*b*
assistance in, 362*b*
head and shoulders raised, 361, 361*f*
strength in, requirement for, 362*b*
Foot dorsiflexion and inversion, 290–292, 290*f*, 291*t*, 291*b*, 389, 389*f*
clinical relevance, 292*b*
grades, 291–292, 291*f*–292*f*
substitution, 292*b*
Foot eversion with plantar flexion, 296–299, 296*f*, 297*t*, 297*b*
clinical relevance, 299*b*
grade 1 and grade 0, 299
grade 5, grade 4, grade 3, and grade 2, 298–299, 298*f*
strength exercises for, 299*b*
Foot inversion, 294*t*, 389, 389*f*
clinical relevance, 295*b*
grade 1 and grade 0, 295, 295*f*
grade 5, grade 4, grade 3, and grade 2, 294–295, 294*f*
substitution, 295*b*
Forced expiration, 82, 82*f*, 82*b*
muscles of, 87*t*–88*t*
Forearm pronation, 173–176, 173*f*, 176*b*
cross section level of, 173*f*
grade 1 and grade 0 of, 176
grade 5, grade 4, and grade 3 of, 175
illustrations of, 173*f*
muscles and, 174*t*
palmar view of, 173*f*
pronator quadratus and, 173–176
pronator teres and, 173–176
palpation of, 176*b*
range of motion of, 174*b*
resistance, absence of, 175, 175*f*
shoulder rotation/abduction of, 176*b*
substitution in, 176*b*
volar (flexor) surface, hypothenar eminence (resistance application) over, 175, 175*f*
Forearms
cross section of, 172*f*
distal surface support of, 140, 140*f*
dorsal surface, hand (downward resistance) on, 164, 164*f*
hanging, 164, 164*f*
lateral surface, palpation of, 160
in mid position
brachioradialis, 159, 159*f*
elbow support, 180, 180*f*
movement of, 148*f*
friction elimination in, 149, 149*f*
positions, of elbow flexion, 159
in pronation, brachialis, 159, 159*f*
in supination, biceps brachii, 158, 158*t*
volar (flexor) of
hand resistance at, 153, 153*f*
wrist, hand resistance over, 158*f*, 159
Forearm supination, 168–172, 171*b*
anterior view of, 168*f*
biceps brachii and, 168
cross section level of, 168*f*

Forearm supination (*Continued*)
grade 1 and grade 0, 171–172
grade 5, grade 4, and grade 3, grade 2 of, 169–170
hands, grasping of, 169, 169*f*
illustration of, 168*f*
muscles and, 169*t*
partial range of motion of, 170, 170*f*
range of motion of, 169*b*
substitution in, 171, 171*f*
supinator and, 168, 169*t*
support, supinator palpation in, 171, 171*f*
wrist, in neutral position, 179, 179*f*
finger, test of, 191, 191*f*
Forward head posture (FHP), 37
Fourth dorsal interossei, finger test for, 205, 205*f*
Frailty, 18
Free weights testing, 321–322, 322*f*
Functional abilities, representation by, 338
Functional assessment tests, 338
Functional movement, muscles essential for, 339*t*
Functional performance
measurement of, 339
testing of, 337–368, 340*f*
Functional task performance, measurement of, 339
Functional testing, 17, 338

G

Gait, 363–364
compromised, secondary to muscle weakness, case study in, 395*b*–396*b*
critical determinants of, 364
Gait speed, 342–344, 344*b*
conversions for, 344*t*
mean usual gait speed, 345*t*
self-selected walking speed in, 343*f*
timing of, beginning of, 343, 343*f*
Garment, putting and taking off of, 348–349, 348*f*–349*f*
modified physical performance test and, 346
Gastrocnemius and soleus, 283–289
clinical relevance, 288*b*
combined test
grade 1 and grade 0, 287–289, 287*f*
grade 2, 287
grade 5, grade 4, and grade 3, 285–289, 285*f*, 286*f*, 286*t*
strength exercises, 288*b*
Gastrocnemius, weakness of, 364
Geniohyoid muscle, in capital flexion, 36*t*
Gluteus maximus
in core, 71*t*
hip extension, 244*f*
posterior, 256
strength exercises for, 253*b*
weakness of, 363
Gluteus medius, 258–260, 262
Trendelenburg sign in, 6
weakness of, 363–364
Gluteus minimus, 258–260, 262
Grade 0 muscle, 5
Grade 1 muscle, 5
Grade 2 muscle, 5
Grade 3 muscle, 5
Grade 4 muscle, 4–5
revisited, 6
Grade 5 muscle, 4
Gravity, elimination of, 149
Grip strength, 229–230, 229*b*–230*b*
patient instructions in, 227*f*, 229
patient position in, 227*f*, 229
scoring of, 229–230, 229*t*–230*t*
therapist instruction in, 227*f*, 229

H

Hallux and toe DIP and PIP flexion, 304–306, 304*f*, 305*t*, 305*b*, 307*f*, 308*b*, 309*f*
clinical relevance, 306*b*
grades 5 to 0, 306, 306*f*, 308–309, 308*f*
Hallux and toe MP and IP extension, supplemental video resources, 310*b*
Hallux metatarsophalangeal (MP) flexion, 300–303, 300*f*, 300*b*, 301*t*
clinical relevance, 302*b*
grades 5 to 0, 302
strength exercises for, 303*b*
Hamstring muscle, 274
in aggregate, 275, 275*f*
grading, 276
lateral hamstring test, 276
medial hamstring test, 275
strength exercises for, 277*b*
Hamstrings, in core, 71*t*
Handheld dynamometry (HHD), 369–392
clinimetric properties in, 370–371
elbow extension in, 380, 380*f*
elbow flexion in, 379, 379*f*
foot dorsiflexion and inversion in, 389, 389*f*
general procedures in, 371
hip abduction in, 384, 384*f*
hip extension in, 383, 383*f*
hip external rotation in, 385, 385*f*
hip flexion in, 382, 382*f*
hip internal rotation in, 386, 386*f*
knee extension in, 388, 388*f*
knee flexion in, 387, 387*f*
reference scores in, 371–372
shoulder abduction in, 376, 376*f*
shoulder extension in, 375, 375*f*
shoulder external rotation in, 377, 377*f*
shoulder flexion in, 374, 374*f*
shoulder internal rotation in, 378, 378*f*
testing specific actions in, 371
wrist extension in, 381, 381*f*
Handheld myometry. *See* Handheld dynamometry
Hands
elevation, wrist support and, 185, 185*f*
friction, elimination of, 149, 149*f*
muscles of, testing of, 188
extrinsic, 188
intrinsic, 198*t*
palm, resistance (application) over, 179, 179*f*
Head, position of, 107, 107*f*
Heel rise, failure of, 6
HHD. *See* Handheld dynamometry
Hip abduction, 261*t*, 268–272, 269*t*, 384, 384*f*
case study in, 395*b*–396*b*
from flexed position, 266–267, 266*t*
grade 5, grade 4, and grade 3, 267, 267*f*
and pelvic stabilization, 262
clinical relevance, 265*b*
grade 1 and grade 0, 264
grade 2, 263, 263*f*
grade 5, grade 4, and grade 3, 262–264, 262*f*
strength exercises, 265*b*
substitution, 264*b*
Hip adduction
clinical relevance, 272*b*
grade 1 and grade 0, 272
grade 2, 271, 271*f*
grade 5, grade 4, and grade 3, 270–272, 270*f*
substitution, 272*b*
Hip adductors
posterior, 273*f*
strength exercises for, 272*b*

Hip extension, 245*t*, 383, 383*f*
 case study in, 395*b*–396*b*
 gluteus maximus, 244*f*
 grade 1 and grade 0, 247, 247*f*
 grade 2, 247, 247*f*, 247*b*
 grade 5, grade 4, and grade 3, 246–247, 246*f*, 246*b*
 rotation, 254*f*, 255*t*, 255*b*
Hip extension rotation, 254*f*, 255*t*, 255*b*
 grade 1 and grade 0, 257, 257*f*, 257*b*
 grade 2 alternate test, 257
 grade 5, grade 4, grade 3, and grade 2, 256–257, 256*f*
Hip extension test
 to isolate gluteus maximus, 248–249
  grade 1 and grade 0, 249, 249*b*
  grade 2, 249, 249*f*
  grade 5, grade 4, and grade 3, 248, 248*f*
 modified for hip flexion tightness, 250–251
  grade 2, grade 1, and grade 0, 250–251, 250*f*
  grade 5, grade 4, and grade 3, 250
 supine hip extension test, 252–253
Hip external rotation, 385, 385*f*
Hip flexion, 236–239, 236*f*, 237*t*, 382, 382*f*
 abduction, and external rotation with knee flexion, 241–243, 241*f*, 242*t*
  distal leg, medial-anterior surface of, 242, 242*f*
  grade 1 and grade 0, 243, 243*f*, 243*b*
  grade 2, 243, 243*f*
  grade 5, grade 4, and grade 3, 242–243, 242*f*
  muscles, 242*f*
  sartorius, 241*f*, 242, 243*b*
  substitution, 247*b*
 anterior, 236*f*
 grade 1 and grade 0, 239
 grade 2, 239
 innervation, 236*f*
 range of motion, 237*b*
 substitutions, 240*b*
 tightness, hip extension tests modified for, 383, 383*f*
Hip internal rotation, 258*t*, 386, 386*f*
 alternate grade 2 for patient who cannot sit, 260
 grade 1 and grade 0, 260
 grade 5, grade 4, grade 3, and grade 2, 259–260, 259*f*
Hip surgery, muscle weakness following, case study in, 399*b*
Home health setting, manual muscle testing, 18
Hop and standing long jump tests, 332, 332*f*
Horizontal adduction, usage of, 166*b*
Humeral head, forearm pronation and, 174*t*
Hypothenar eminence
 resistance application with, 175, 175*f*
 usage of, 179, 179*f*
Hypothenar, finger MCP extension and, 198*t*

I

Iliococcygeus, in pelvic floor, 90*t*
Iliocostalis cervicis, in cervical extension, 33*t*
Iliocostalis lumborum, in pelvic elevation, 56*t*
Inferior oblique head, in cervical flexion, 41*t*
Infraspinatus
 shoulder abduction and, 134*t*
 shoulder external rotation and, 146, 147*t*
 shoulder horizontal abduction and, 138*t*
 suggested exercise for, 150*b*

Inspiratory training, strength exercise for, 81*b*
Intercostales externi, in quiet inspiration, 83*t*–84*t*
Intercostales interni
 in forced expiration, 87*t*–88*t*
 in quiet inspiration, 83*t*–84*t*
Intercostales intimi, in quiet inspiration, 83*t*–84*t*
International Classification of Functioning (ICF) disablement model, 338
Interphalangeal (IP) joints
 extension of, 203, 203*f*
 of hallux, 308*t*
 MCP joints, in flexion, 197, 197*f*
 position of, 212, 212*f*
Interspinales cervicis, in cervical extension, 33*t*
Intertransversarii cervicis, in cervical extension, 33*t*
Intrinsics-plus test, 201, 201*f*
Ischiococcygeus, in pelvic floor, 90*t*
Isokinetic dynamometry, 370
Isokinetic testing, 323

J

Jobe test, 134*t*
Joint range of motion (limitation), contracture/fixed joint limitation (impact), 6

K

Kegel exercise, 89*b*
Kendall examination, 16*b*
Key movements, 17
Kinetic chain, 316*t*
Knee extension, 278–281, 278*f*, 279*t*, 388, 388*f*
 case study in, 395*b*–396*b*
 clinical relevance, 282*b*
 grade 1 and grade 0, 281, 281*f*
 grade 2, 281
 grade 5, grade 4, and grade 3, 280–281, 280*f*
Knee flexion, 274*t*, 387, 387*f*
 clinical relevance, 277*b*
 grade 1 and grade 0, 277
 grade 2, 276–277, 276*f*
 grade 5, grade 4, and grade 3, 275
 substitutions, 277*b*

L

Lateral hamstring test, 276
Lateral head, elbow extension and, 163*t*
Latissimus dorsi
 alternate test for, 122–123
 in forced expiration, 87*t*–88*t*
 grade 5, grade 4, and grade 3, grade 2, and grade 1 of, 121–123, 121*f*
 illustrations of, 119*f*
 muscle and, 120*t*
 in pelvic elevation, 56*t*
 posterior view of, 119*f*
 scapular depression/adduction and, 112*t*, 119–123
 shoulder extension and, 130*t*
 shoulder internal rotation and, 152*t*
 suggested exercise for, 122*b*
Latissimus dorsi pull-down test, 320, 320*f*
Leg, cross sections of, 289*f*
Leg extension machine, in knee extension, 395*b*–396*b*
Leg press test, 318–319, 318*f*
Levator ani, in pelvic floor, 90*t*
Levatores costarum, in quiet inspiration, 83*t*–84*t*

Levator scapulae
 in cervical extension, 33*t*
 in cervical rotation, 45*b*
 scapular adduction (retraction) and, 109*t*
 scapular adduction/downward rotation and, 115*t*
 scapular elevation and, 106*t*
Limbs, parallel position of, 165
Locomotion, importance of, 363
Long finger dorsal interossei, test for, 205, 205*f*
Long head, elbow extension and, 163*t*
Longissimus cervicis, in cervical extension, 33*t*
Long-term care facilities, manual muscle testing, 18
Longus capitis
 in capital flexion, 36*t*
 in cervical rotation, 45*b*
Longus colli
 in cervical flexion, 41*t*
 inferior oblique, in cervical rotation, 45*b*
Lumbar multifidus (LM), 50
Lumbricals, finger MCP extension and, 198*t*, 200*t*–201*t*

M

Manual muscle examination, documentation of, 8*f*–10*f*
Manual muscle testing (MMT), 14
 accuracy of, 3
 acute care facilities, 17
 acute rehabilitation facilities, 17
 ceiling effect, 21
 community mobility requirements, 18*b*
 diagnostic criteria for frailty, 18*b*
 diagnostic validity, 21
 handheld dynamometers and, 370
 in hip abduction, 395*b*–396*b*
 history of, 14
 home health setting, 18
 limitations of, 20–21
 long-term care facilities, 18
 objectivity, 20
 outpatient clinics, 18–19
 patient, influence of, 15
 population variation, 20
 principles of, 2–10
 range of motion values, deviation of, 15
 relevance of, 14
 reliability of, 20
 results, fatigue of, 15
 sensitivity, 20–21
 strength testing technique of, 14
 tester strength, 21
 therapist shortcuts, avoidance of, 15
 validity of, 20
 wellness clinics, 19
Manual muscle testing alternatives, 313–336
 body-weight testing
  pull-ups (chin-ups) test, 333, 333*t*
  push-ups test, 334, 334*t*–335*t*
 considerations, 314
 Cyriax method of testing contractile lesions, 334–335
 equipment-based strength testing
  elastic band testing, 324, 324*t*, 326*b*
  free weights testing, 321–322, 322*f*
  interpretation of, 317
  isokinetic testing, 323
  latissimus dorsi pull-down test, 320, 320*f*
  leg press test, 318–319, 318*f*
  sitting unilateral knee extension test, 317–326, 317*f*
 multiple-repetition maximum test, 316, 316*t*–317*t*

Manual muscle testing alternatives *(Continued)*
   one-repetition maximum test, 315–316
   power testing, 326–332
     hop and standing long jump tests, 332, 332*f*
     Margaria-Kalamen stair sprint test, 327, 328*t*
     medicine ball throw test, 329, 329*f*
     shot put test, 329–330, 330*f*
     vertical jump test, 330, 330*f*, 331*t*
   tips for, 314*b*
Margaria-Kalamen stair sprint test, 327, 328*t*
Mat table, firmness of, 7
Maximal expiratory pressure (MEP), 79–80
Maximum inspiratory pressure (MIP), 79–80
Medial hamstring test, 275
Medial head, elbow extension and, 163*t*
Medicine ball throw test, 329, 329*f*
Metacarpals, stabilization of, 219, 219*f*
   in thumb adduction, 222, 222*f*
Metatarsophalangeal joints of toes, 308*t*
Middle deltoid, shoulder abduction and, 133–136
Middle finger, finger adduction toward, 207, 207*f*
MMT. *See* Manual muscle testing
Moderately disabled women, chair stand in, 343
Modified Oxford Scale, 88–89
Modified physical performance test, 346–355
   chair stand (five-repetition) and, 354, 354*f*, 354*b*
   full tandem stance in, 354*f*
   lifting book in, 346
   picking up a coin in, 346
   scoring of, 355*t*, 355*b*
     form for, 356*f*
   standing static balance task in, 353
     feet together stance in, 353, 353*f*
     full tandem stance in, 354, 354*b*
     semi-tandem stance in, 353, 353*f*
Multifidi
   in cervical extension, 33*t*
   in core, 71*t*
Multiple-repetition maximum test, 316, 316*t*–317*t*
Muscle mass, 16
Muscles
   belly, grasping (avoidance), 15
   contour and bulk, differences (sensitivity) in, 15
   essential for functional movements, 339*t*
   fibers, direction of, 15
   function of, 15
   location and anatomic features of, 15
   scapular adduction (retraction) and, 109*t*
Muscle strength scoring convention, 2
Muscle test, 2–7
   available range of motion of, 6
   contractile activity, detection ability of, 15
   contractions, types of, 11*b*
   criteria for assigning, 4–6
     grade 0 muscle, 5
     grade 1 muscle, 5
     grade 2 muscle, 5
     grade 3 muscle, 5
     grade 4 muscle, 4–5
     grade 4 muscle revisited, 6
     grade 5 muscle, 4
     plus (+) or minus (−) grades, 5
   exercises of, 10
   method, standardization of, 15
   numeric 0 to 5 system of, 2
   patient, position, importance of, 7
   positioning, usage (consistency) of, 15
   preparation for, 7
   prime movers of, 7–10

Muscle test *(Continued)*
   principles of, 2–10
   range of motion values, deviation of, 15
   results, fatigue of, 15
   surface friction, control, 7
   therapist shortcuts, avoidance of, 15
Muscle weakness, case study in
   compromised gait and function secondary to, 395*b*–396*b*
   fatigue secondary to, 397*b*
   following childbirth, 399*b*
   following hip surgery, 399*b*
   following nerve injury, 398*b*
Muscular endurance, 70
Mylohyoid muscle, in capital flexion, 36*t*

N
Nagi model of Disablement, 338
Neck
   flexion and extension of, 31*f*
   muscles of, testing, 26, 45*b*
Nerve injury, muscle weakness following, case study in, 398*b*
Nondominant arm, force (elicitation) of, 176*b*

O
Objectivity, manual muscle testing, 20
Oblique head, thumb adduction and, 221*t*
Obliquus capitis inferior, in cervical rotation, 45*b*
Obliquus externus abdominis
   in forced expiration, 87*t*–88*t*
   in trunk flexion, 60*t*
   in trunk rotation, 65*t*
Obliquus externus, in pelvic elevation, 56*t*
Obliquus internus abdominis
   in forced expiration, 87*t*–88*t*
   in pelvic elevation, 56*t*
   in trunk flexion, 60*t*
   in trunk rotation, 65*t*
Omohyoid muscle, in cervical flexion, 41*t*
One-repetition maximum test, 315–316, 316*t*
Open chain, 316*b*
Opponens digiti minimi
   finger MCP extension and, 200*t*–201*t*
   opposition (thumb to little finger) and, 225–227, 225*t*
   resistance for, 226, 226*f*
Opponens pollicis
   opposition (thumb to little finger) and, 225–227, 225*t*
   resistance, application of, 226, 226*f*
Opposition (thumb to little finger), 225–227, 228*b*
   fifth metacarpal (radial side), opponens digiti mini (palpation) on, 227, 227*f*
   first metacarpal, opponens pollicis (palpation) of, 227, 227*f*
   grade 5 to grade 0 of, 226–227, 226*f*
   illustration of, 225*f*
   muscles and, 225*t*
   opponens digiti minimi and, 225–227
   opponens pollicis and, 225–227
   palmar view of, 225*f*
   range of motion of, 225*b*
   substitutions in, 228*b*
Outpatient clinics, manual muscle testing, 18–19

P
Palmar interossei
   finger adduction and, 206–207, 207*f*
   finger MCP extension and, 198*t*, 200*t*–201*t*

Palmaris longus, thumb abduction and, 218*t*
Paradoxical breathing, 79
Pectoralis major
   clavicular fibers
     palpation of, 144, 144*f*
     shoulder flexion and, 126*t*
   in quiet inspiration, 83*t*–84*t*
   scapular depression/adduction and, 112*t*
   shoulder horizontal abduction and, 141–144, 144*b*
   shoulder internal rotation and, 152*t*
   suggested exercise for, 144*b*
Pectoralis minor
   scapular abduction and upward rotation and, 100*t*
   scapular depression/adduction and, 112*t*
Pelvic floor, 90
   anatomy of, 86–91, 86*f*
   muscles, 85*f*, 88–89, 88*f*, 90*t*
   risk management considerations, 90
Pelvic stabilization, and hip abduction, 262
Pelvis elevation, 55–58, 56*t*
   clinical relevance, 58*b*
   grade 1 and grade 0, 58
   grade 3 and grade 2, 57, 57*f*
   grade 5 and grade 4, 57–58, 57*f*
   muscles, 56*t*
   posterior, 55*f*
   range of motion, 55*b*
   substitution, 58*b*
Peroneus longus and brevis. *See* Fibularis longus and brevis
Physically active older adults, chair stand normative ranges for, 341, 341*t*
Physical performance test, 346–355
   climbing stairs in
     four flights of, 351, 351*b*
     one flight of, 351, 351*f*
   eating task in, 346, 347*f*
   lifting book in, 348, 348*f*
   modified, 346–355
     feet together stance in, 353, 353*f*
     scoring for, 355*t*, 356*f*
     semi-tandem stance in, 353, 353*f*
     standing static balance task in, 353
   picking up a coin from the floor in, 349, 349*f*, 349*b*
   putting on and taking off a garment, 348–349, 348*f*–349*f*
   scoring form for, 352*f*
   360° turn in, 350, 350*f*, 350*b*
   timed 50-foot walk in, 350, 350*b*
   writing a sentence in, 347, 347*f*
Plantar flexion
   ankle, 283–289, 283*f*, 283*b*, 284*t*
   case study in, 395*b*–396*b*
Plinth, firmness of, 7
Plus (+) or minus (−) grades, 5
Population variation, manual muscle testing, 20
Posterior deltoid
   fibers, palpation of, 140, 140*f*
   shoulder horizontal abduction and, 138*t*, 140*b*
   suggested exercise for, 140*b*
Postoperative patient, strength assessment in, 17
Power testing, 326–332
   hop and standing long jump tests, 332, 332*f*
   Margaria-Kalamen stair sprint test, 327, 328*t*
   medicine ball throw test, 329, 329*f*
   shot put test, 329–330, 330*f*
   vertical jump test, 330, 330*f*, 331*t*
Pronator quadratus, forearm pronation and, 173–176, 174*t*

Pronator teres
elbow flexion and, 158*t*
forearm pronation and, 173–176, 174*t*
palpation of, forearm pronation and, 176*b*
Proximal interphalangeal (PIP) finger flexion, muscles and, 190*t*
Proximal interphalangeal (PIP) tests, 192, 193*b*
for flexor digitorum superficialis, 192
palpation of, 193, 193*f*
grade 2, grade 1, and grade 0 of, 193
grade 5, grade 4, and grade 3 of, 192–193, 192*f*
range of motion, resistance (absence) of, 192–193, 192*f*
substitutions in, 193*b*
Proximal phalanx, base, dorsal interosseus (palpation) of, 205, 205*f*
Psoas major, in trunk flexion, 60*t*
Psoas minor, in trunk flexion, 60*t*
Pubococcygeus, in pelvic floor, 90*t*
Puborectalis, in pelvic floor, 90*t*
Pull-ups (chin-ups) test, 333, 333*t*
Push-ups test, 334, 334*t*–335*t*

Q

Quadratus lumborum, in pelvic elevation, 56*t*
Quadriceps, 278–281, 278*f*
strength exercises for, 282*b*
weakness of, 363
Quiet inspiration, 77–81, 77*f*
diaphragm, 77*f*, 79, 81
intercostals, 81
muscles of, 83*t*–84*t*
range of motion, 78*b*

R

Range of motion, availability of, 6
Rectus abdominis
in core, 71*t*
in forced expiration, 87*t*–88*t*
in trunk flexion, 60*t*
Rectus capitis anterior, in capital flexion, 36*t*
Rectus capitis lateralis, in capital flexion, 36*t*
Rectus capitis posterior major, in cervical rotation, 45*b*
Reliability
manual muscle testing, 20–21
of muscle testing, 26
Repetitions, 89
Resistance, 1-RM, 315
Rhomboid major
scapular adduction (retraction) and, 109*t*
scapular adduction/downward rotation and, 115*t*
scapular elevation and, 106*t*
shoulder horizontal abduction and, 138*t*
Rhomboid minor
scapular adduction (retraction) and, 109*t*
scapular adduction/downward rotation and, 115*t*
scapular elevation and, 106*t*
Rhomboids, suggested exercise for, 118*b*
Rhomboid test, alternate, 118
Rib cage, scapula, proximity of, 97
Rotator cuff, 145
Rotatores cervicis
in cervical extension, 33*t*
in cervical rotation, 45*b*

S

Scalenus anterior
in capital flexion, 36*t*
in cervical flexion, 41*t*
in quiet inspiration, 83*t*–84*t*

Scalenus medius
in cervical flexion, 41*t*
in cervical rotation, 45*b*
in quiet inspiration, 83*t*–84*t*
Scalenus posterior
in cervical flexion, 41*t*
in cervical rotation, 45*b*
in quiet inspiration, 83*t*–84*t*
Scapulae
axillary borders, fingers, extension of, 98
cardinal planes of, 96*f*
observation of, 97, 97*f*
position of, 97–99, 97*f*
abnormality, 99, 99*f*, 99*b*
range of motion of, 98
rest, position (abnormality), 99, 99*f*, 99*b*
symmetry of, 97–99, 97*f*
vertebral border motion of, 98, 98*f*
winging of, 97
Scapular abduction
direction of, 118, 118*f*
muscles and, 100*t*
range of motion of, 98
serratus anterior, 100
grading of, 101
trapezius, middle fibers and rhomboid major and minor, 108–110
upward rotation and, 100–103, 100*t*, 104*b*
grade 1 and grade 0 of, 103
grade 2 of, 102
grade 5, grade 4, and grade 3 of, 101–103
muscles and, 100*t*
range of motion of, 100*b*
Scapular adduction (retraction), 108–110, 110*b*
cross section level of, 108*f*
grade 2, grade 1, and grade 0 of, 110
grade 5, grade 4, and grade 3 of, 109, 109*f*–110*f*
illustrations of, 108*f*
muscles and, 109*t*
range of motion of, 109*b*
substitution in, 110*b*
Scapular adduction (retraction)/downward rotation, 114–118, 118*b*
alternate Rhomboid test, 118
cross section level of, 114*f*
grade 2, grade 1, and grade 0 of, 117
grade 5, grade 4, and grade 3 of, 115–118, 116*f*
illustration of, 114*f*
manual resistance, absence of, 116, 116*f*
maximal resistance in, 116, 116*f*
muscles and, 115*t*
posterior view of, 114*f*
range of motion of, 115*b*
rhomboids and, 114–118
Scapular depression/adduction, 111–113, 113*b*
cross section level of, 111*f*
grade 2, grade 1, and grade 0 of, 113
grade 5, grade 4, and grade 3 of, 112–113, 112*f*
illustration of, 111*f*
muscles and, 112*t*
range of motion of, 111*b*
trapezius, lower and middle fibers, 111–113
Scapular elevation, 105–107, 107*b*
cross section level of, 105*f*
grade 2, grade 1, and grade 0 of, 107
grade 5, grade 4, and grade 3 of, 106–107, 107*f*
illustration of, 105*f*
muscles in, 106*t*
posterior view of, 105*f*
range of motion of, 106*b*
trapezius, upper fibers and levator scapula, 106

Scapular vertebral border, 115*f*, 116
Scapulohumeral rhythm, 97
Screening tests, 7*b*
Second dorsal interossei, finger test for, 205, 205*f*
Selective tissue tension (STT) method, 335
Semispinalis capitis, in cervical rotation, 45*b*
Semispinalis cervicis
in cervical extension, 33*t*
in cervical rotation, 45*b*
Sensitivity, manual muscle testing, 20–21
Serratus anterior
alternate test for, 103, 103*f*
scapular abduction and, 100
origin/insertion of, 100*t*
suggested exercise for, 104*b*
weakness, sign of, 97
Shot put test, 329–330, 330*f*
Shoulder abduction, 133–136, 137*b*, 176*b*, 376, 376*f*
arm
by sliding, 136, 136*f*
support, 150, 150*f*
biceps brachii substitution and, 137*b*
cross section level of, 133*f*
grade 1 and grade 0 of, 136
grade 2 of, 136
grade 5, grade 4, and grade 3 of, 135–136
illustration of, 133*f*
lateral view of, 133*f*
manual resistance of, 135, 135*f*
middle deltoid and, 133–136
muscle and, 134*t*
range of motion of, 133*b*
supraspinatus and, 133–136
Shoulder abductors, testing, 326
Shoulder extension, 129–132, 375, 375*f*
cross section level of, 129*f*
grade 1 and grade 0 of, 132, 132*f*
grade 5, grade 4, and grade 3 of, 131–132, 131*f*
illustration of, 129*f*
lateral view of, 129*f*
latissimus dorsi and, 129
long head of triceps and, 129
muscles and, 130*t*
posterior deltoid and, 129
range of motion of, 130*b*
teres major and, 129
Shoulder external rotation, 146–150, 150*b*, 377, 377*f*
cross section level of, 146*f*
dorsal view of, 146*f*
grade 2, grade 1, and grade 0 of, 149
grade 5, grade 4, and grade 3 of, 148
alternate position for, 150
illustration of, 146*f*
infraspinatus and, 146
manual resistance, absence of, 148
muscles and, 147*t*
range of motion of, 147*b*
teres minor and, 146
Shoulder flexion, 125–128, 374, 374*f*
anterior deltoid and, 125
anterior view of, 125*f*
clavicular portion of pectoralis major and, 125
coracobrachialis and, 125
grade 2, grade 1, and grade 0 of, 128
grade 5, grade 4, and grade 3 of, 127–128, 127*f*
illustration of, 125*f*
muscles and, 126*t*
range of motion of, 126*b*
rotator cuff and, 125
substitutions in, 128*b*
supraspinatus and, 127
Shoulder girdle strength testing, 97–99, 99*b*

Shoulder horizontal abduction, 138–140
  pectoralis major and, 141–144, 144*b*
    cross section level of, 141*f*
    grade 2, grade 1, and grade 0 of, 144
    grade 5 and grade 4 of, 142–144
    illustrations of, 141*f*
    muscles and, 142*t*
    range of motion of, 142*b*
  posterior deltoid and, 138, 140*b*
    grade 2, grade 1, and grade 0 of, 140
    grade 5, grade 4, and grade 3 of, 139
    illustration of, 138*f*
    muscle and, 138*t*
    posterior view of, 138*f*
    range of motion of, 138*b*
    triceps brachii substitution in, 140*b*
Shoulder internal rotation, 151–156, 156*b*,
    378, 378*f*
  anterior view of, 151*f*
  belly press test for, 156*b*
  cross section level of, 151*f*
  grade 2, grade 1, and grade 0 of, 154,
    154*f*
  grade 5, grade 4, and grade 3 of, 153
    alternate test for, 155–156, 156*f*
  illustration of, 151*f*
  muscles and, 152*t*
  range of motion of, 152*b*
  subscapularis and, 151
Shoulder pain, case study in, 394*b*
Shoulders
  elevates (shrugs), 106, 106*f*
  girdle strength testing, 97–99
    preliminary examination of, 97–99
  gravity, elimination of (shoulder external
    rotation test), 149
  internal rotation of, 115–116, 115*f*
    arm extension/adduction, 117, 117*f*
    pronation, attempt, 176*b*
  joints, deltoid, superior/anterior surfaces
    (palpation) of, 128, 128*f*
  range of motion, improvement of, 98
  stabilization of, 127, 127*f*
    hand, usage of, 127, 127*f*
  superior aspect, stabilization of, 140, 140*f*
  supine position, rotation (testing) during,
    149
Sitting position, alternate, 160, 160*f*
Sitting unilateral knee extension test,
    317–326, 317*f*, 318*b*
Soleus
  heel rise, failure of, 6
  weakness of, 364
Special considerations, acute rehabilitation
    setting, 17
Sphincter urethrae, in pelvic floor, 90*t*
Spinal extensors' muscle, 50
Spinalis cervicis, in cervical extension, 33*t*
Splenius capitis, in cervical rotation, 45*b*
Splenius cervicis
  in cervical extension, 33*t*
  in cervical rotation, 45*b*
Stability, 70–76
Stair climb test, 359–360, 359*f*, 360*t*, 360*b*
  four flights of, 351, 351*b*
  in modified physical performance test, 346
  one flight of, 351, 351*f*
Standing static balance task, 353
  feet together stance, 353, 353*f*
  full tandem stance in, 354, 354*b*
  semi-tandem stance in, 353, 353*f*
Starting weight, in one-repetition maximum
    test, 315
Sternal head
  in cervical flexion, 41*t*
  grades 5/4, shoulder horizontal adduc-
    tion and
    patient instructions in, 143
    patient position in, 142–144

Sternal head *(Continued)*
    test of, 143
    therapist instruction in, 143, 143*f*
Sternal part, shoulder horizontal adduction
    and, 142*t*
Sternoclavicular joints, 98, 98*f*
Sternocleidomastoid muscle
  in cervical flexion, 41*t*
  in cervical rotation, 45*b*
  flexion to isolate
    grade 2, grade 1, and grade 0, 44, 44*f*
    grade 5, grade 4, and grade 3, 44, 44*f*
    range of motion, 44
Sternohyoid muscle, in cervical flexion, 41*t*
Sternothyroid muscle, in cervical flexion, 41*t*
Strength
  assessment, indications of, 14, 17
  clinimetric properties of, handheld dyna-
    mometry in, 370
  curvilinear relationship (conceptual
    design), 338*f*
  testing, total lower extremity, case study
    in, 395*b*–396*b*
Strength exercises
  for abdominals, 69*b*
  for core strengthening, 76*b*
  for foot eversion, 299*b*
  for gastrocnemius and soleus, 288*b*
  for hallux and toe MP flexion, 303*b*
  for hamstring muscle, 277*b*
  for hip abduction, 265*b*
  for hip adductors, 272*b*
  for hip internal rotation, 260*b*
  for iliopsoas, 240*b*
  for inspiratory training, 81*b*
  for quadriceps, 282*b*
  for tibialis anterior, 295*b*
Stylohyoid muscle, in capital flexion, 36*t*
Subscapularis
  shoulder abduction and, 134*t*
  shoulder internal rotation and, 151, 152*t*
  suggested exercise for, 156*b*
  tendon, palpation for, 154, 154*f*
Superior oblique head, in cervical flexion,
    41*t*
Supination, occurrence of, 149
Supinator
  forearm supination and, 168, 169*t*
  palpation, forearm support in, 171,
    171*f*
Supine hip extension test
  grade 5, grade 4, grade 3, and grade 2,
    252–253, 252*f*
Supine (grade 0) muscle, shoulder horizontal
    abduction (alternate test) for, 140
Supraspinatus
  peak activation of, 137*b*
  shoulder abduction and, 133–136, 134*t*
  shoulder external rotation and, 147*t*
  shoulder flexion and, 126*t*
  suggested exercise for, 128*b*, 137*b*
  testing, 134*b*

T

Tensor fasciae latae (TFL), 258–260,
    266–267
Teres major
  shoulder extension and, 130*t*
  shoulder internal rotation and, 152*t*
  suggested exercise for, 144*b*
Teres minor
  palpation of, 149, 149*f*
  shoulder abduction and, 134*t*
  shoulder external rotation and, 146,
    147*t*
  shoulder horizontal abduction and, 138*t*
  suggested exercise for, 150*b*
Tester strength, manual muscle testing, 21

Thenar eminence
  abductor pollicis brevis palpation in, 220,
    220*f*
  flexor pollicis longus tendon (palpation)
    in, 212, 212*f*
Thenar, finger MCP extension and, 198*t*
Thoracic wall (lateral aspects), latissimus
    dorsi (fiber palpation) on, 122, 122*f*
360° turn, 350, 350*f*, 350*b*
  in modified physical performance test, 346
Thumb abduction, 218–220
  abductor pollicis brevis and, 218–220
    grade 2, grade 1, and grade 0 of, 220
    grade 5, grade 4, and grade 3 of, 220
    substitution in, 220*b*
  abductor pollicis longus and, 218–220,
    219*b*
    grade 5 to grade 0 of, 219
    substitution in, 219*b*
  dorsal view of, 218*f*
  illustration of, 218*f*
  muscles and, 218*t*
  palmar view of, 218*f*
  range of motion of, 218*b*
Thumb adduction, 221–223, 224*b*
  adductor pollicis and, 221–223
    palpation of, 223, 223*f*
  grade 2 and grade 1 of, 223
  grade 5, grade 4, and grade 3 of, 222
  illustration of, 221*f*
  metacarpals, stabilization of, 222, 222*f*
  muscles and, 221*t*
  palmar view of, 221*f*
  range of motion of, 221*b*
  substitutions in, 224*b*
  wrist, stabilization of, 223, 223*f*
Thumb MCP and IP extension, 214–217,
    217*b*
  cross section level of, 214*f*
  dorsal views of, 214*f*
  extensor pollicis brevis and, 214–217
  extensor pollicis longus and, 214–217
  grade 2, grade 1, and grade 0 of, 217
  grade 5, grade 4, and grade 3 of, 216–217
  illustration of, 214*f*
  joint extension in, 217, 217*f*
  muscles and, 215*t*
  range of motion of, 215*b*
  substitution in, 217*b*
Thumb MCP and IP flexion, 210
  cross section level of, 210*f*
  distal phalanx, resistance of, 213, 213*f*
  flexor pollicis brevis and, 210
  flexor pollicis longus and, 210
  grade 5 to grade 0 of, 212
  illustration of, 210*f*
  muscles and, 211*t*
  palmar view of, 210*f*
  range of motion of, 211*b*
  substitution in, 212*b*–213*b*
Thumbs
  in adduction, 212
  distal joint extension of, 217, 217*f*
  distal phalanx of, 216, 216*f*
  medial rotation of, 226, 226*f*
  motions of, 209*f*
  muscles of, 208
Thyrohyoid muscle, in cervical flexion, 41*t*
Tibialis anterior, 290–292, 292*f*–293*f*,
    292*b*–293*b*, 295*b*
  weakness of, 363
Timed 50-foot walk, 350, 350*b*
Timed up and go (TUG), 357–358, 357*f*
  reference scores, 358, 358*t*, 358*b*
Toe DIP and PIP flexion, 304–306, 304*f*,
    305*t*, 305*b*, 307*f*, 308*b*, 309*f*
  clinical relevance, 306*b*
  grades 5 to 0, 306, 306*f*, 308–309,
    308*f*

Toe metatarsophalangeal (MP) flexion
  clinical relevance, 302b
  grades 5 to 0, 303
Toe MP and IP extension, supplemental
    video resources, 310b
Toes, metatarsophalangeal joints of, 308t
Total lower extremity strength testing, case
    study in, 395b–396b
Transverse head, thumb adduction and, 221t
Transversus abdominis (TA), 50
  in core, 71t
  in forced expiration, 87t–88t
Transversus perinei profundus, in pelvic
    floor, 90t
Transversus perinei superficialis, in pelvic
    floor, 90t
Transversus thoracis, in forced expiration,
    87t–88t
Trapezius
  in cervical extension, 33t
  on slack, 137b
Trapezius (lower)
  scapular abduction and upward rotation
      and, 100t
  scapular adduction (retraction) and, 109t
  scapular depression/adduction and, 112t
  suggested exercise for, 113b
Trapezius (middle)
  fibers, palpation of, 110, 110f
  scapular adduction (retraction) and, 109t
  scapular depression/adduction and, 112t
  shoulder horizontal abduction and, 138t
  suggested exercise for, 110b
Trapezius (upper)
  in cervical rotation, 45b
  scapular abduction and upward rotation
      and, 100t
  scapular adduction (retraction) and, 109t
  scapular elevation and, 106t
  suggested exercise for, 107b
Trendelenburg sign, positive value of, 6
Triceps brachii
  elbow extension and, 162, 163t
  long head
    shoulder extension and, 130t
    substitution by, 140b
  suggested exercise for, 167b
Triceps tendon, tension in, 165, 165f
Trunk extension
  lumbar spine, 51
  muscles, 49t–50t
  posterior, 48f
  range of motion, 48b
  thoracic spine, 52–54, 53f–54f, 54b
Trunk flexion, 59–64
  anterior, 59f
  assisted forward lean, 64, 64f
  clinical relevance, 64b
  cough, 64, 64f

Trunk flexion (Continued)
  grade 2, grade 1, and grade 0, 63–64, 63f
  grade 3, 62, 62f
  grade 4, 62, 62f
  grade 5, 61–64, 61f
  muscles, 60t
  range of motion, 59b
Trunk rotation
  anterior, 65f
  grade 1 and grade 0, 69, 69f
  grade 2, 68, 68f
  grade 3, 67, 67f
  grade 4, 67
  grade 5, 66–69, 66f
  muscles, 65t
  substitution, 66b
TUG. See Timed up and go

U

Ulnar head, forearm pronation and, 174t
Unilateral knee extension test, sitting,
    317–326, 317f, 318b
Unilateral supine bridge test (USBT), 76,
    76f
Upper extremity, muscles of, 95–234
Upper trapezius, scapular elevation and, 106t
Upward rotation and scapular abduction,
    100–103, 100t, 104b
  grade 1 and grade 0 of, 103
  grade 2 of, 102
  grade 5, grade 4, and grade 3 of, 101–103
  muscles and, 100t
  range of motion of, 100b

V

Validity, manual muscle testing, 20–21
Vertical intermediate head, in cervical flex-
    ion, 41t
Vertical jump test, 330, 330f, 331t
Volar (flexor) surface, hand resistance over,
    158f, 159

W

Walking
  speed, gender/age differentiation of, 343,
      343f
  task, in modified physical performance
      test, 346
  timed 50-foot, 350, 350b
Warm-up, 1-RM, 315
Wellness clinics, manual muscle testing, 19
Whole muscle, grades 5/4, shoulder hori-
    zontal adduction and
  patient position in, 142
  test of, 143

Wrist
  dorsal surface of
    resistance, application, 169, 169f
    tendon palpation, 186, 186f
  dorsum, tendon palpation on, 186, 186f
  flexor muscles, relaxation of, 160
  lateral palmar aspect, flexor carpi radialis
      (location) on, 179f, 181
  neutral position of, finger, test, 192–193,
      192f
  palmar surface, palpation of, 193, 193f
Wrist extension, 182–186, 187b, 381, 381f
  cross section level of, 182f
  dorsal surface, tendon palpation on, 186,
      186f
  dorsal views of, 182f
  dorsum, tendon palpation on, 186, 186f
  extensor carpi radialis brevis and, 182,
      183t
  extensor carpi radialis longus and, 182,
      183t
  extensor carpi ulnaris and, 182, 183t
  extensor digit minimi and, 183t
  extensor digitorum and, 183t
  extensor indicis, and, 183t
  grade 1 and grade 0 of, 186
  grade 2 of, 185
  grade 5, grade 4, and grade 3 of,
      183–186, 183f–184f
  illustration of, 182f
  muscles and, 183t
  range of motion of, 183b
  substitution in, 186b
  suggested exercise of, 187b
  wrist support, hand elevation and, 185,
      185f
Wrist flexion, 177–181, 181b
  cross section level of, 177f
  elbow support in, 180, 180f
  flexor carpi radialis and, 177–181
    tendons, palpation of, 181, 181f
  flexor carpi ulnaris and, 177–181
    tendons, palpation of, 181, 181f
  grade 1 and grade 0 of, 181
  grade 2 of, 180
  grade 3 of, 180
  grade 5 and grade 4 of, 179
  illustration of, 177f
  muscles and, 178t
  neutral position, forearm supination in,
      179, 179f
  palmar view of, 177f
  range of motion of, 178b
Writing task, physical performance test and,
    346